CANCER AND CHEMOTHERAPY

Volume III

CANCER AND CHEMOTHERAPY

CANCER AND CHEMOTHERAPY

Volume III

Antineoplastic Agents

Edited by

Stanley T. Crooke

Research and Development
Smith Kline & French Laboratories
Philadelphia, Pennsylvania
and
Department of Pharmacology
Baylor College of Medicine
Texas Medical Center
Houston, Texas

Archie W. Prestayko

Research and Development
Bristol Laboratories
Syracuse, New York
and
Department of Pharmacology
Baylor College of Medicine
Texas Medical Center
Houston, Texas

Editorial Assistant

Nancy Alder

1981

ACADEMIC PRESS
A Subsidiary of Harcourt Brace Jovanovich, Publishers
New York   London   Toronto   Sydney   San Francisco

ACADEMIC PRESS, INC.
111 Fifth Avenue, New York, New York 10003

United Kingdom Edition published by
ACADEMIC PRESS, INC. (LONDON) LTD.
24/28 Oval Road, London NW1 7DX

Library of Congress Cataloging in Publication Data
Main entry under title:

Cancer and chemotherapy.

   Includes bibliographies and index.
   CONTENTS: v. 1. Introduction to neoplasia and
antineoplastic chemotherapy--v. 2. Introduction
to clinical oncology--v. 3. Antineoplastic
agents.
   1. Cancer--Chemotherapy. 2. Antineoplastic
agents. I. Crooke, Stanley T. II. Prestayko,
Archie W. [DNLM: 1. Neoplasms--Drug therapy.
2. Antineoplastic agents. QZ267.C214]
RC667.C28   616.99'4061   79-8536
ISBN 0-12-197803-6 (v. 3)

PRINTED IN THE UNITED STATES OF AMERICA

81 82 83 84   9 8 7 6 5 4 3 2 1

CONTENTS

**PART II   MOLECULAR PHARMACOLOGY OF SELECTED
ANTINEOPLASTIC AGENTS**

PART III   CLINICAL PHARMACOLOGY OF SELECTED NEOPLASTIC AGENTS

LIST OF CONTRIBUTORS

Numbers in parentheses indicate the pages on which the authors' contributions begin.

Richard A. Bender (273), Department of Biochemistry, Scripps Clinic and Research Foundation, La Jolla, California 92037

J. R. Bertino (311, 359), American Cancer Society, Yale University School of Medicine, New Haven, Connecticut 06510

Bruce A. Chabner (3), Clinical Pharmacology Branch, Division of Cancer Treatment, National Cancer Institute, Bethesda, Maryland 20014

Michael Colvin (25, 287), Pharmacology Laboratory, Johns Hopkins Oncology Center, Baltimore, Maryland 21205

William A. Creasey (79), Department of Pharmacology, University of Pennsylvania School of Medicine, Philadelphia, Pennsylvania 19104

Stanley T. Crooke (49, 97, 111, 221, 343), Research and Development, Smith Kline & French Laboratories, Philadelphia, Pennsylvania 19101, and Department of Pharmacology, Baylor College of Medicine, Houston, Texas 77025

Virgil H. DuVernay (233), Department of Pharmacology, Baylor College of Medicine, Houston, Texas 77025

Manuel L. Gutierrez (155), Clinical Cancer Research, Bristol Laboratories, Syracuse, New York 13101

Elwood V. Jensen (187), The Ben May Laboratory for Cancer Research, The University of Chicago, Chicago, Illinois 60637

Archie W. Prestayko (133, 303, 351), Research and Development, Bristol Laboratories, Syracuse, New York 13201, and Department of Pharmacology, Baylor College of Medicine, Houston, Texas 77025

Steven D. Reich (61, 325, 377), Division of Clinical Pharmacology, University of Massachusetts Medical Center, Worcester, Massachusetts 01605

Philip S. Schein (37), Vincent T. Lombardi Cancer Research Center, Georgetown University School of Medicine, Washington, D.C. 20007

Daniel D. Von Hoff (207), Department of Medicine, Division of Oncology, University of Texas Health Science Center, San Antonio, Texas 78284

GENERAL PREFACE

With the rapid development of new chemotherapeutic approaches and new agents used in the treatment of patients with cancer, a basic textbook describing in some detail the drugs currently employed, current therapeutic approaches, and agents in development is essential. However, to understand fully cancer chemotherapeutic agents and their use, one must understand various aspects of anticancer drug development, the molecular and cellular biology of malignant disease, and the clinical characteristics of the most common neoplasms. Only with this information can a detailed discussion of anticancer drugs be presented.

It was with these thoughts in mind that "Cancer and Chemotherapy" was developed; the goal: to provide in a single text the information necessary for a detailed understanding of the major antineoplastic agents. Thus, Volume I is designed to provide the fundamental information concerning the molecular and cellular biology of cancer, carcinogenesis, and the basics of anticancer drug development. Volume II provides clinical information relative to the most common human malignancies and discusses the use of chemotherapeutics in the treatment of those diseases. In Volume III the antineoplastic agents are discussed. It contains reviews of all the major anticancer drugs and a review of agents in development. Furthermore, in two sections—the molecular pharmacology of selected antitumor drugs, and the clinical pharmacology of selected antitumor drugs—significantly more detailed discussions of certain drugs are provided. These drugs were selected because they have interesting characteristics and adequate data are available to allow a more detailed discussion. These two sections should be of particular value to individuals who have an interest in certain aspects of particular drugs.

Stanley T. Crooke
Archie W. Prestayko

PREFACE TO VOLUME III

In this volume, a discussion is presented in Part I of clinically useful anticancer drugs with respect to their mechanism of action, pharmacology, and pharmacokinetics, clinical utility, and associated toxicities. The various drug classes include alkylating agents (cyclophosphamide, nitrosoureas, mitomycin C, and others), plant alkaloids (vinca alkaloids, podophyllotoxin derivatives, maytansine), antibiotics (bleomycin, anthracyclines), platinum-containing complexes, antimetabolites and hormones. A brief description of investigational agents is provided. This section is concluded by a discussion of a new technique that is used to grow tumor cells in culture and to test the sensitivity of these cells to various anticancer drugs.

Part II presents a detailed discussion of the molecular pharmacology of several major drug classes.

Part III presents an in-depth discussion of the clinical pharmacology of several antitumor drugs. This section is limited to the drugs for which suitable assays have been developed and sufficient clinical data have been obtained.

Stanley T. Crooke
Archie W. Prestayko

Part I
General Reviews

1
NUCLEOSIDE ANALOGUES
Bruce A. Chabner

I. INTRODUCTION

The nucleoside analogues form a chemically large group and represent attempts to prepare new antineoplastics by rational synthesis. They can be divided into several structural groups, and a number of the agents are important drugs.

CANCER AND CHEMOTHERAPY, VOL. III

II. CYTOSINE ARABINOSIDE

Cytosine arabinoside (1-β-D-arabinofuranosylcytosine) (Fig. 1), also known as ara-C, was synthesized in 1959 and has since been recognized as the most active antimetabolite for remission induction in adult nonlymphocytic leukemia (Ellison, 1968). It is currently used with anthracyclines in the standard induction regimens for this disease, achieving 60–70% complete remissions in unselected cases (Kremer, 1975). It has also found limited usefulness in the treatment of meningeal leukemia or lymphoma for patients resistant to methotrexate or in patients experiencing methotrexate-related neurotoxicity (Band *et al.*, 1973).

A. Mode of Action

Cytosine arabinoside functions as an analogue of the naturally occurring nucleoside 2'-deoxycytidine (Fig. 1). The primary cytotoxic effect of cytosine arabinoside is believed to be inhibition of DNA polymerase by cytosine arabinoside triphosphate (ara-CTP), although the drug is also known to be incorporated into both RNA and DNA to a limited extent (Chu, 1971; Momparler, 1972; Rashbaum and Cozzarelli, 1976). Both semiconservative, or replicative, DNA synthesis, and unscheduled, or "repair," synthesis are inhibited, although the former appears to be more sensitive to inhibition; although maximum sensitivity of cells occurs during the S- or DNA-synthetic phase of the cell cycle, treatment of cells in other phases, such as G_2 or G_1, leads to chromatid deletions (Brewen and Christie, 1967; Hiss and Preston, 1978). Cells exposed to ul-

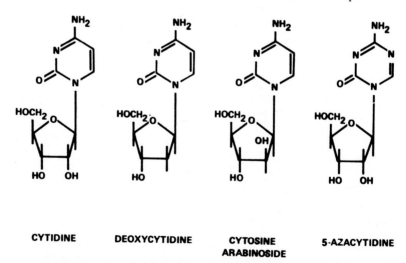

CYTIDINE   DEOXYCYTIDINE   CYTOSINE ARABINOSIDE   5-AZACYTIDINE

Fig. 1.   Structure of cytidine, deoxycytidine, and antitumor analogues.

traviolet irradiation are unable to repair single-strand breaks in DNA in the presence of ara-C (Hiss and Preston, 1978).

In order to achieve activation to ara-CTP, the nucleoside must enter the target cell, a process believed to occur by facilitated diffusion. Thereafter, a series of phosphorylation steps occurs (see Fig. 2), utilizing the same enzymes required by the physiologic nucleoside deoxycytidine in its activation to a triphosphate. The slight alteration in structure of the sugar moeity of ara-C renders it a somewhat less favorable substrate for deoxycytidine kinase, but a more active substrate for deoxycytidine monophosphate kinase (the second step in the pathway) (Hande and Chabner, 1978). The drug is also susceptible to degradation by cytidine deaminase, an enzyme found in liver, gastrointestinal tract, plasma, and some tumor cells and by deoxycytidine monophosphate deaminase, which is also found in leukemic cells as well as spleen and liver. The products of deamination of ara-C and cytosine arabinoside monophosphate (ara-CMP) are both inactive in terms of cytotoxicity. The nucleoside deaminase, found in high concentrations in human liver (Stoller *et al.*, 1978), is primarily responsible for ara-C elimination, but the possible role of these enzymes in resistance of tumors to ara-C requires further evaluation. Preliminary studies (Stoller *et al.*, 1975) indicate that the monophosphate deaminase is present in higher concentrations than the nucleoside deaminase in malignant cells.

Multiple mechanisms of drug resistance have been described in animal tumor systems, including deletion of the activating enzyme, deoxycytidine kinase (Draharosky and Kreis, 1970), and increased *de novo* synthesis of dCTP

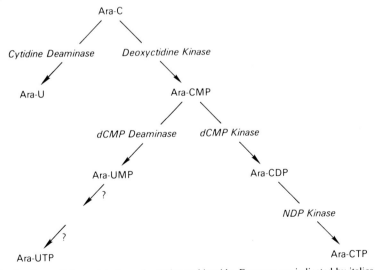

Fig. 2. Intracellular metabolism of cytosine arabinoside. Enzymes are indicated by italics. Tetrahydrouridine blocks cytidine deaminase, the first catabolic enzyme in the pathway.

(Momparler *et al.*, 1968); however, other potential mechanisms of drug resistance suggested by biochemical studies of enzyme activation (Stoller *et al.*, 1975) have not been investigated in detail. Chou *et al.* (1977) have shown that some human cells resistant to ara-C were still able to synthesize ara-CTP in high concentrations but appeared to be clinically resistant to its effects, implicating a possible change in affinity of DNA polymerase for the inhibitor.

The prediction of sensitivity or resistance for human leukemic cells, based on *in vitro* studies of enzyme concentrations or the ability of cells to activate ara-C to the nucleotide level, has been the subject of several clinical investigations that, thus far, have yielded conflicting results. Steuart and Burke (1971) were the first to suggest that pretreatment measurement of enzyme levels might be an accurate predictor of response; they found a direct relationship between high levels of cytidine deaminase and both *de novo* and acquired resistance to ara-C. In some patients, greater than 10-fold increases in the concentration of this enzyme were found in leukemic cells as the patients became clinically resistant to therapy. Tattersall *et al.* (1974), Smyth *et al.* (1976), and Chang *et al.* (1977) were unable to demonstrate a positive correlation between remission induction and cytidine deaminase activity. Tattersall found more convincing evidence for decreased activating enzyme activity (decreased deoxycytidine kinase) in resistant patients, a finding not confirmed by Chang *et al.* (1977). A somewhat different approach has been taken by Rustum *et al.* (1978), who have found a strong correlation between remission duration and the ability of leukemic cells to maintain peak concentration of ara-CTP after exposure to ara-C in culture. This observation, if true, points toward the importance of nucleotide degradative enzymes, such as alkalkine phosphatases, in determining the level of active metabolite in the target cell. The preceding investigations relating enzyme levels or drug activation to remission induction are complicated by two important factors that cloud their interpretation: (1) Most studies of leukemia induction therapy are yielding high response rates (at or above 70%); the few failures can be attributed to advanced age or infectious complications and not to primary drug resistance; and (2) in induction regimens, patients are treated with at least two agents. Thus a positive response does not necessarily connote sensitivity to both agents. The duration of complete response has been proposed as a more appropriate yardstick of drug sensitivity, but this figure is also likely to be a function of several factors: the fraction of cell kill during induction, the efficacy of maintenance therapy, and the kinetics of regrowth of the tumor cell population. Thus it may be difficult, if not impossible, to study prognostic factors for drug response, given the complicated nature of current therapeutic regimens.

B. Pharmacokinetics

Following intravenous bolus doses of 100 mg/m^2, peak plasma concentrations of 10^{-4} are achieved. Cytosine arabinoside is rapidly degraded by hepatic cytidine deaminase, leading to a primary elimination half-life of 30 min, although this half-life may be considerably prolonged in some individuals. The relationship between hepatic dysfunction and drug elimination has not been clarified, and guidelines are not available for dosage alteration in patients with liver failure. Approximately 80% of an administered intravenous dose of ara-C is recovered in the urine, 90% of this total being the inactive metabolite uracil arabinoside (Ho and Frei, 1971). More complete studies of ara-C pharmacokinetics have been hindered by the lack of availability of a suitable assay for routine plasma level determination.

Ara-C penetrates the blood–brain barrier with moderate efficiency producing cerebrospinal fluid concentrations approximately 40% of those in plasma in the few measurements reported. Direct intrathecal administration of the drug is effective in treating meningeal neoplasia; in the absence of deamination, spinal fluid half-life of ara-C (2 hr) is considerably longer than that in plasma (Ho and Frei, 1971).

C. Dose Schedule and Clinical Toxicity

Because of the rapid elimination of ara-C and the necessity to expose cells during their most active phase of DNA synthesis, most therapeutic regimens employ ara-C in continuous infusion or multiple intravenous doses per day. To simplify the clinical use of ara-C several alternative measures have been tested. Cyclocytidine, the 2'-2-OH ester of ara-C, is slowly hydrolyzed to produce the parent compound and thus produces sustained plasma concentrations of the active derivative. However, cyclocytidine has the uncomfortable side effects of causing parotid pain and postural hypotension in addition to the expected mucositis and myelosuppression produced by ara-C (Burgess et al., 1977). A second approach to the prolongation of ara-C plasma half-life has been the concomitant use of tetrahydrouridine, a potent inhibitor of cytidine deaminase (Kreis et al., 1977) (Fig. 2). Preliminary clinical trials of the ara-C-tetrahydrouridine combination indicate that greatly reduced doses of ara-C are required to produce limiting toxicity because of marked prolongation of the plasma half-life. Whether these advantages will be translated into improved clinical response has not been determined.

The primary toxicity of ara-C is exerted on the gastrointestinal epithelium and bone marrow. Mucositis and myelosuppression typically occur, reaching a maximum in the week following therapy, and recovery takes place within 2 weeks for patients with otherwise normal bone marrow. Mild and transient elevation of liver enzyme levels has been seen in 10–20% of patients but rarely leads to permanent hepatic damage and does not warrant discontinuation of treatment. Although infrequently used, intrathecal ara-C has been reported to cause acute arachnoiditis and chronic neurologic toxicity, including altered mental status and motor dysfunction similar to that caused by methotrexate (Band et al., 1973).

III. 5-AZACYTIDINE

A new cytidine analogue, 5-azacytidine, has shown promising activity against adult nonlymphocytic leukemia. This agent was synthesized in Czechoslovakia in 1964 and received extensive clinical testing in Europe prior to its introduction to the United States in 1970. For further clinical information the reader is referred to the extensive review of this agent by Von Hoff *et al.* (1976).

A. Mode of Action

The mode of action of this agent is unclear at present. Despite substitution of a nitrogen at the 5 position in the pyrimidine ring, 5-azacytidine functions as a cytidine analogue and requires activation to 5-azacytidine triphosphate, but the initial enzyme in this pathway, uridine-cytidine kinase, has poor affinity for this compound, with a K_m of 11 mM (Drake *et al.*, 1977). Small amounts of 5-azacytidine are incorporated into DNA, but its primary effects appear to be on RNA synthesis and function (Li *et al.*, 1970). 5-Azacytidine triphosphate is a weak inhibitor of RNA polymerase, but the monophosphate is incorporated into RNA, producing alterations in RNA processing, translation, and polyribosome formation (Levitan and Webb, 1969; Weiss and Pitot, 1975; Reichman *et al.*, 1973). Mechanisms of resistance have not been studied in human tumor cells. In resistant animal tumors deletion of the initial activating enzyme, uridine-cytidine kinase, has been observed (Vesely *et al.*, 1970).

In clinical use 5-azacytidine does not appear to share cross-resistance with cytosine arabinoside, since responses to 5-azacytidine have been observed in patients resistant to the latter agent (McCredie *et al.*, 1973).

B. Pharmacokinetics in Humans

5-Azacytidine undergoes very rapid degradation following intravenous injection. Although the metabolic products have not been identified, it is likely that deamination by hepatic cytidine deaminase plays an important role, since 5-azacytidine is known to be a substrate for this enzyme (Chabner *et al.*, 1973). Because of the considerable nausea and vomiting associated with rapid intravenous administration of 5-azacytidine, the drug is frequently given as a continuous intravenous infusion. In this schedule, studies with [^{14}C]5-azacytidine have shown that approximately 13% of plasma radioactivity is associated with the intact parent compound (Israili *et al.*, 1976), although only limited pharmacokinetic information is available.

5-Azacytidine is quite labile in aqueous solution, undergoing spontaneous decomposition in neutral or alkaline solution with a half-life of approximately 4 hr (Israili *et al.*. 1976; Notari and DeYoung, 1975). Hydrolytic cleavage of the pyrimidine ring occurs with formation of N-formylamidino-ribofuranosylguanyl urea. The latter may again form the parent compound, but also further decomposes to ribofuranosylguanylurea, an inactive end product (Beisler, 1978). 5-Azacytidine is considerably more stable in buffered solutions, particularly in Ringer's lactate (pH 6.2), in which it has a half-life of 65 hr at 25°C and 94 hr at 20°C (Notari and De Young, 1975).

C. Clinical Toxicity

As mentioned previously, 5-azacytidine causes severe and prolonged nausea and vomiting when administered as a rapid bolus injection. In view of recent studies indicating (1) stability of the drug in buffered solutions and (2) its equal therapeutic efficacy when administered as a continuous infusion (Vogler *et al.*, 1976), the latter regimen is now employed routinely. The primary toxic effects of 5-azacytidine are exerted on the bone marrow. This agent produces a 7- to 14-day period of leukopenia and thrombocytopenia, although recovery of counts may be considerably prolonged in occasional patients. Transient temperature elevations not infrequently occur, as well as reversible abnormalities in liver function tests, myalgias, stomatitis, and rash (McCredie *et al.*, 1973; Vogler *et al.*, 1976; Bellet *et al.*, 1973).

IV. 5-FLUOROURACIL

Heidelberger *et al.* (1957) synthesized 5-fluorouracil (5-FU) as an analogue of thymine based on the observation that rat tumor cells more efficiently utilized the base uracil than did intestinal mucosa. It was reasoned that substitution of the atom fluorine for hydrogen in the 5 position would have only limited effect on the metabolism of uracil, since the molecular radius of fluorine was only slightly larger than the molecular radius of the hydrogen atom in the 5 position of uracil and might allow 5-FU to substitute for uracil and to inhibit the complex process of thymidylate synthesis (see Fig. 3). These predictions proved to be true, as the deoxynucleotide metabolite of 5-FU, 5-FdUMP, has since been demonstrated to be a potent inhibitor of thymidylate synthetase, and ultimately of DNA synthesis.

Since the introduction of 5-FU into clinical use, a wide spectrum of activity has been appreciated, primarily against adult solid tumors such as adenocarcinoma of the breast, colon, and ovary. However, this clinical activity has proved to be disappointing in most instances, since the response rates are generally in the range of 20–40% and complete, prolonged clinical remissions are unusual with single-agent therapy. This realization has led to a renewed examination of 5-FU pharmacokinetics, mechanism of action, and interaction with other agents, with the hope of identifying the means for augmenting its clinical action and placing clinical therapeutics on a more rational footing.

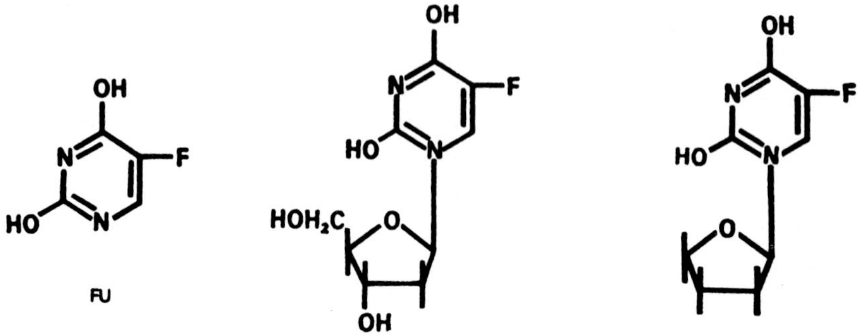

Fig. 3. Structure of fluorinated uracil analogues.

A. Mechanism of Action

Early observations on the action of 5-FU indicated that the drug blocked incorporation of formate into the methyl group of thymidine, an action consistent with inhibition of the thymidylate synthetase reaction (Bosch *et al.*, 1958). More recent work has shown a block of UdR incorporation into DNA, a finding consistent with the same site of action. The interaction of 5-FdUMP and thymidylate synthetase has been examined in detail by Santi *et al.* (1974), Pogolotti *et al.* (1976), Aull *et al.* (1974), and others and requires the presence of the folate cofactor—5,10-methylene tetrahydrofolate—in order to form the tightly bound terniary complex of enzyme, inhibitor, and cofactor. Sommer and Santi (1974) first isolated a peptide fragment of thymidylate synthetase to which is bound the inhibitor, indicating that a covalent bond can be formed under appropriate experimental conditions. Santi and co-workers (1974) have also shown that mammalian thymidylate synthetase binds two molecules of 5-FdUMP per molecule of enzyme; it is not known whether these two binding sites are equivalent in binding affinity or display cooperativity. The reversibility of the complex *in vivo* has not been determined as yet, although Myers *et al.* (1975), on the basis of assessment in nucleotide pool size changes, have provided evidence that the natural enzyme substrate, dUMP, may compete effectively with FdUMP for binding and may prevent inhibition of the enzyme.

The reversal of 5-FU cytotoxicity by thymidine in some tissue culture systems and the potent binding of 5-FdUMP to thymidylate synthetase support the conclusion that inhibition of this enzyme represents the primary and lethal biochemical lesion caused by this agent. However, 5-FU has also been shown to impair RNA maturation (Fig. 4), and in bacteria to alter the translation of RNA. These effects are felt to be a consequence of the formation of FUTP and its incorporation into RNA (Heidelberger, 1965; Wilkinson *et al.*, 1975). Further support for this concept has been provided by the demonstration of increased antitumor activity and host toxicity for the combination of 5-FU and thymidine in experimental animals. Martin *et al.* (1978) have shown that this combination leads to increased 5-FU incorporation into RNA, possibly by inhibiting 5-FU activation to FdUMP and increasing FUTP formation, although pharmacokinetic explanation for this enhanced toxicity of 5-FU–thymidine combinations are also possible (see below). Thus it is not clear at present to what degree these two actions of 5-FU, namely, inhibition of thymidylate synthetase and incorporation into RNA, are responsible for this drug's cytotoxicity.

B. Metabolism and Elimination

5-FU requires activation to the nucleotide level in order to exert either of its potentially cytotoxic actions. Several alternate pathways for this activation are available in mammalian cells, including direct transfer of a ribose phosphate by phosphoribosyl transferase to form FUMP, or a two-step reaction to this nucleotide involving nucleoside phosphorylase and uridine kinase. Further activation to FUTP occurs via a nucleotide monophosphate kinase and a nucleoside diphosphate kinase, whereas FdUMP formation requires the action of ribonucleotide reductase. All these enzymes have been identified in human tumor cells, although their activities are known to vary widely; resistance in murine tumors has

5 FUTP
1. Incorporated into RNA
2. Causes mis-translation, altered RNA processing
3. This action increased by thymidine

FdUMP
1. Inhibits thymidylate synthetase leading to block of DNA synthesis
2. This action reversed by thymidine

Fig. 4. Possible metabolic routes and active products of 5-fluorouracil (5-FU).

been associated with deletion of uridine kinase (Reichard *et al.*, 1962), nucleoside phosphorylase (Kasbekar and Greenberg, 1963), or uracil phosphoribosyl transferase (Reyes, 1969), or an increase in thymidylate synthetase activity (Baskin, *et al.*, 1975). However, on the basis of limited clinical studies available at this writing, it is not possible to implicate a single enzymatic mechanism for resistance to 5-FU. Factors other than specific enzyme changes in anabolic enzymes may determine sensitivity, including the ability of cells to generate competitive amounts of the natural substrate dUMP and the ability to utilize thymidine as a means of escaping the block in thymidylate synthesis. Further studies are clearly needed, and should be forthcoming now that it is possible to grow human colon tumors in athymic mice and to culture human tumor cells *in vitro*.

5-FU is eliminated primarily by hepatic metabolism, less than 20% appearing unchanged in the urine (Clarkson *et al.*, 1964). The initial degradative step consists of reduction of the pyrimidine ring by dihydrouracil dehydrogenase, an enzyme found predominantly in the mitochondrial fraction of liver, although a small fraction of activity was associated with other subcellular fractions (Smith and Yamada, 1971). The product, dihydro-5FU, is further degraded to carbon dioxide, urea, and F-β-alanine. Chaudhuri *et al.* (1958) speculated that the absence of this degradative pathway in sensitive tumors might account for the selective toxicity of 5-FU for these cells, but Cooper *et al.* (1972) demonstrated that inhibition of dihydrouracil dehydrogenase activity enhanced toxicity for both normal and tumor tissues; they concluded that 5-FU catabolism occurred primarily in the liver and that toxicity to peripheral tissues was primarily a function of availability of drug. Thymine, a degradation product of thymidine, inhibits catabolism of 5-FU. This effect may account for the increased toxicity of the thymidine–5-FU combination.

C. Pharmacokinetics

The pharmacokinetics of 5-FU has immediate relevance to the clinical use of this agent for several reasons: First, the drug is known to be highly schedule dependent, with markedly different patterns of toxicity for various routes and schedules of administration. Second, 5-FU is used by intra-arterial and intraperitoneal routes, as well as by oral and intravenous administration. Monitoring of drug levels would undoubtedly be of value in adjusting doses and schedules of administration. However, the routine monitoring of 5-FU in plasma has been hampered by the lack of a sensitive, specific, and rapid assay procedure, and in general available information is incomplete. The recent introduction of high-pressure liquid chromatography promises to provide a sensitive and specific means for drug assay, although the method is laborious compared to the simpler competitive binding assays routinely used for bleomycin, methotrexate, allopurinol, and other compounds (Sitar, 1977; Jones *et al.*, 1979).

The early phases of drug disappearance from plasma have been adequately defined. Following a single intravenous dose of 15 mg/kg, the drug is rapidly distributed into total body water, producing peak blood concentrations of 10^{-4} to $10^{-3} M$. Rapid hepatic metabolism produces a rapid decline in plasma concentrations with a half-life of approximately 20 min, although considerable variation has been noted (Sitar, 1977; Jones *et al.*, 1980; MacMillan *et al.*, 1978; Finn and Sadee, 1975). In the dose range of 10–15 mg/kg intravenously, drug levels remain above 1 μM for approximately 6 hr. The relationship between drug concentration and toxicity for target organs has not been defined, although gastrointestinal mucosa appears to be more sensitive than bone marrow. The later phases of drug elimination have been incompletely defined, although a slower terminal half-life is suggested by the data of Finn and Sadee (1975) using a mass fragmentographic assay. Approximately 20% of an intravenous dose is excreted unchanged in the urine.

Intravenously administered 5-FU penetrates peritoneal and cerebrospinal spaces well, with concentrations approaching those of plasma within 1–2 hr (Clarkson *et al.*, 1964). Levels in cerebrospinal fluid remain above 10^{-8} M for approximately 12 hr. Direct administration of drug into the peritoneal cavity is currently being explored as a possible therapeutic measure for intra-abdominal tumor or for hepatic metastasis; intraperitoneal drug is absorbed through the hepatic portal circulation and is almost completely metabolized and degraded in the liver before reaching the systemic circulation (Jones *et al.*, 1978). Thus a differential of 100- to 1000-fold is anticipated between the peritoneal and systemic concentrations, and peripheral tissues can be protected from toxicity.

5-FU has also received extensive clinical evaluation when given by the oral route of administration. However, pharmacokinetic studies have demonstrated considerable variability in drug absorption. Peak plasma concentrations are lower, but more prolonged, than when drug is given by the intravenous route (Cohen *et al.*, 1974). Clinical results with oral 5-FU have revealed a lower response rate and shorter durations of remission (Stolinsky *et al.*, 1975), and in the absence of reliable and routine pharmacological monitoring to assure adequate drug absorption this route of administration has limited utility at present.

Intrahepatic arterial infusion of 5-FU is widely used, with clear pharmacokinetic advantages as compared to systemic administration; high local concentrations of drug are achieved locally and limited compound escapes into the systemic circulation. Effective infusion regimens of 25–30 mg/kg per day produce plasma levels below 10^{-6} M (Jones *et al.*, 1979), usually with only mild stomatitis and no bone marrow toxicity as a consequence. Again, routine drug level monitoring would be very helpful in guiding dosage.

The kinetic profile of 5-FdUMP and 5-FUTP formation has not been examined in human tissues in relation to blood concentrations of 5-FU. On the basis of studies of murine bone marrow, gastrointestinal epithelium, and ascites tumor cells, Myers *et al.* (1975) concluded that free FdUMP persists in these tissues for different periods of time for each tissue examined. However, in all tissues the active nucleotide FdUMP persisted intracellularly for longer than the parent compound in plasma.

D. Dosage Schedule and Clinical Toxicity

A number of schedules of drug administration have been employed and are summarized in Table I. The 5-day loading schedule, as employed by Curreri *et al.* (1958), produced severe myelosuppression with unacceptable frequency and has been modified to the less toxic single, weekly dose schedule. Doses of 10–12 mg/kg per week are in general well tolerated, with only moderate and reversible myelosuppression. Dose modification in the presence of liver dysfunction is not routinely used and requires further pharmacological study. An alternative regimen employing continuous intravenous infusion for 5 days has produced an equivalent response rate with only mild stomatitis and gastrointestinal toxicity and infrequent myelosuppression (Seifert *et al.*, 1975). However, logistic problems (hospitalization or continuous drug infusion devices) have limited the use of this schedule.

Hepatic metastases are frequently the major or only site of disease in patients relapsing after primary bowel surgery for colonic carcinoma. Direct intrahepatic arterial infusion has been used in these patients, with response rates usually in excess of those reported for systemic therapy (35–85%); in addition, responses have been noted in patients who previously failed intravenous 5-FU (Burokev *et al.*, 1976). As mentioned previously, the toxicity of intrahepatic infusion primarily involves stomatitis and intestinal epithelial injury, although catheter-related

TABLE I

Schedule-Dependent Toxicity of 5-Fluorouracil

		Toxicity			
Schedule		Bone marrow	Gastro-intestinal	Oral mucositis	Other
1.	Single weekly dose	Major	Major	Minor	–
2.	Continuous I.V. infusion	Minor	Minor	Major	–
3.	Hepatic artery infusion	Minor	Minor	Minor	Catheter related

problems may be serious and include thrombosis of the extremity artery used for percutaneous catheterization, hemorrhage from the puncture site, infection, or accidental slippage of the catheter into the arterial supply of the small bowel, with resulting necrosis of the intestinal epithelium. The routine use of this procedure is also limited by the vascularity of the tumor (poorly vascularized tumors appear to be less responsive to arterial infusion of drug) (Burokev *et al.*, 1976) and by the accessibility of the feeding artery(s) to catheterization. Nonetheless, in selected patients, arterial perfusion can be an effective palliative approach to cancer treatment. Hepatic portal perfusion has also been employed, and has shown promising results in a randomized study compared to no treatment, for patients at high risk of hepatic metastasis following primary resection of colon cancer (Taylor *et al.*, 1977).

V. OTHER 5-FLUORO PYRIMIDINES

5-FUdR (5-fluorodeoxyuridine) (Fig. 3) has also received extensive clinical evaluation. Certain advantages in its metabolism (activation to 5-FdUMP requires only the single step, thymidine kinase) have prompted this investigation, but the clinical response rate appears to approximate that of 5-FU. The effective dose for 5-FUdR is much lower than 5-FU, possibly because of its lack of activity as a substrate for dihydrouracil dehydrogenase.

A second 5-fluoro analogue has recently been introduced in the United States after its development in the Soviet Union. Ftorafur, 1-(2-tetrahydrofuranyl)-5,5-fluorouracil (Fig. 3), is slowly converted to 5-FU and produces prolonged exposure of sensitive tissues to the active compound (Benvenuto *et al.*, 1978). The mechanism of this ftorafur → 5-FU conversion has not been clarified. The parent compound has a plasma half-life of 8.8 hr and readily penetrates the central nervous system, with equivalent or greater concentrations in the cerebrospinal fluid within 6 hr of administration (Benvenuto *et al.*, 1978). 5-FU levels in spinal fluid equal those of plasma at 6 hr and are somewhat lower than plasma levels thereafter. The parent compound is eliminated primarily by conversion to 5-FU and hydroxylated metabolites (3'- and 4'-OH ftorafur); less than 20% of the administered dose is recoverable in the urine. The pharmacokinetics of ftorafur are of particular interest in view of the different pattern of dose-limiting toxicity for this drug as compared to intravenous doses of 5-FU. Ftorafur in the range of 1.5 g/m² per day for 5 days produces diarrhea, cramps, vomiting, and mucositis as its primary toxicity, with only minimal myelosuppression (Hall *et al.*, 1977). This pattern of toxicity closely resembles the side effects of low-dose continuous infusion of 5-FU. Ftorafur also causes central nervous system changes, including altered mental status, cerebellar ataxia, and rarely coma; these effects resemble the toxicity of high-dose infusions of 5-FU into the carotid arterial system. The central nervous system toxicity has been attributed to the high concentrations of ftorafur and its derivative 5-FU in the spinal fluid.

In view of its lack of bone marrow suppression, the primary interest in ftorafur at present is based on its possible substitution for 5-FU in combination therapy regimens.

VI. 3-DEAZAURIDINE

A. Mode of Action

3-Deazauridine (Fig. 5), an analogue of the naturally occuring nucleoside uridine, was first synthesized by Robins and Currie (1968) and was later found to have antitumor activity against Ehrlich ascites and L1210 tumor cells (Bloch *et al.*, 1973). The primary action of this agent as the active triphosphate is inhibition of CTP synthetase (McPortland *et al.*, 1974). It is not incorporated into RNA or DNA (Wang and Bloch, 1972). Other actions of 3-deazauridine and its nucleotide 3-deazaUMP include inhibition of the enzymes cytidine deaminase and deoxycytidylate deaminase (Hande *et al.*, 1978), as well as inhibition of ribonucleotide reductase by 3-deazaUDP (Brockman *et al.*, 1973).

A number of interesting interrelationships have been found between the biochemical actions of 3-deazauridine and cytosine arabinoside. First, collateral sensitivity to 3-deazauridine has been found in L1210 cells resistant to cytosine arabinoside (Brockman *et al.*, 1973), a finding consistent with increased dependence of cytosine arabinoside-resistant tumors on the *de novo* pathway for CTP synthesis. Second, 3-deazauridine treatment augments the formation of ara-CTP in tumor cells (Mills-Yamamoto *et al.*, 1978); the mechanism of this effect is not known, although inhibition of the catabolic enzymes cytidine deaminase and deoxycytidylate deaminase by 3-deazauridine and its mononucleotide, respec-

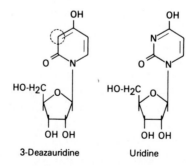

Fig. 5.   Structure of 3-deazauridine and uridine.

tively, may be responsible (Hande *et al.*, 1978). These observations have prompted clinical interest in 3-deazauridine as a potential antileukemic agent in combination with cytosine arabinoside. 3-Deazauridine is currently undergoing phase I trial in man.

B. Pharmacokinetics

Initial studies of 3-deazauridine in man have produced conflicting results on the major route of its elimination. Creaven *et al.* (1978) reported recovery of approximately 80% of an administered dose in urine within 48 hr of its administration by intravenous infusion. However, Benvenuto *et al.* (1980) found urinary excretion of less than 8% of a dose administered by bolus or continuous intravenous infusion. The latter were unable to identify any metabolites in urine, but did find the aglycone, 2,4-dihydroxypyridine, in plasma. The lack of urinary excretion of parent compound in man contrasts with reports of the disposition of 3-deazauridine in mice, in which greater than 50% of the drug is excreted unchanged in the urine (Cysyk *et al.*, 1978).

Other observations in the initial pharmacokinetic studies included a larger volume of distribution for patients receiving continuous infusion of the drug, a slower half-life of parent compound in plasma after constant infusion (21.4 hr) versus bolus administration (4.4 hr), and less than equivalent levels of drug in the cerebrospinal fluid [spinal fluid concentrations were 22 and 55% of plasma levels in two observations.

C. Toxicity and Schedule Dependency

The clinical toxicity and schedule dependency of this agent remain to be determined. A constant infusion schedule or multiple doses per day will be required to maintain drug concentrations above 1×10^{-5} M in view of the drug's rapid terminal half-life.

VII. PURINE ANALOGUES

The primary purine analogues currently in clinical use for cancer treatment are 6-mercaptopurine (6-MP) and 6-thioguanine (6-TG). These compounds are 6-thiol analogues of the naturally occurring 6-OH purine bases, hypoxanthine and guanine, respectively (Fig. 6), and were only two of a number of clinically useful purine analogues synthesized by Elion (1967) and colleagues. Others of this series, including the immunosuppressant azathioprine and the xanthine oxidase inhibitor allopurinol, are widely employed in the treatment of nonmalignant conditions. Both 6-MP and 6-TG are effective agents in the treatment of

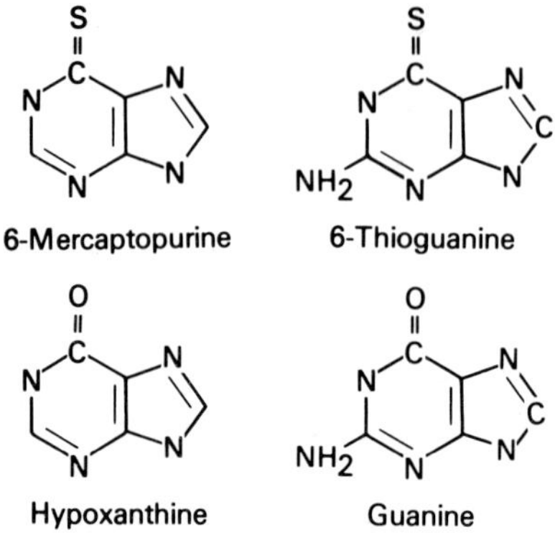

Fig. 6. Purine analogues and their physiologic counterparts.

acute leukemia in man, but have no established utility against solid tumors. 6-MP is primarily used as a maintenance agent after remission induction by vincristine, prednisone, and other agents in acute lymphocytic leukemia, whereas 6-TG is employed for remission induction and maintenance in acute nonlymphocytic leukemia. These two analogues have quite similar mechanisms of action, pharmacokinetic properties, and clinical toxicities, and thus will be considered jointly in the following discussion.

A. Mechanism of Action and Metabolism

In order to inhibit cell growth, both 6-MP and 6-TG must be activated to the ribonucleotide level by the enzyme hypoxanthine-guanine phosphoribosyl transferase (HG-PRT'ase) (Fig. 7). Deficiency of this enzyme has been associated with resistance to these analogues in experimental tumors but not in human leukemia cells. As nucleotides, these analogues exert several inhibitory actions on *de novo* purine biosynthesis. Both 6-MP-ribosephosphate and 6-TG-ribosephosphate inhibit the first enzyme in purine biosynthesis, phosphoribosylpyrophosphate (PRPP) amidotransferase, and in addition prevent conversion of inosine monophosphate (IMP) to either of the purine nucleotides, GMP or AMP, found in DNA and RNA (Brockman, 1963; LePage and Jones, 1961). However, more recent work indicates that incorporation of the analogues themselves into DNA may better account for the antitumor effects of these compounds, since the quantitative incorporation of both compounds, in the form of 6-TG deoxyribose phosphate, into DNA correlated strongly with cytotoxicity (Tidd and Paterson, 1974). A ratio of one 6-TG base per 1000 DNA nucleotides was required to produce toxic effects against cells in tissue culture. This finding is of clinical importance in that the simultaneous use of thiopurines with agents that inhibit DNA synthesis, such as ara-C, would prevent incorporation of these analogues into DNA and would antagonize their antitumor effect. This explanation for thiopurine toxicity, although supported by considerable experimental evidence, does not account for the observation that some resistant tumor cell lines have paradoxically increased incorporation of 6-thiopurine bases into DNA (Rosman *et al.*, 1974).

Although thiopurine resistance in murine tumor cells appears to be related to deletion of the activating enzyme, HG-PRT'ase, human leukemic cell resistance does not arise by this mechanism but instead has been attributed to an increase in the concentration of membrane-bound alkaline phosphatase activity. These phosphatase enzymes have been partially characterized by Lee and co-workers (1978), and appear to be distinct from the enzymes found in lower concentration in sensitive cells, showing greater heat lability and a higher pH maximum.

B. Pharmacokinetics and Elimination in Man

6-MP is well absorbed orally and is therefore an advantageous drug for maintenance therapy; 6-TG is absorbed erratically and thus is usually administered by intravenous infusion. Both compounds are rapidly and extensively metabolized in man, with plasma half-lives of 80–90 min for 6-TG (LePage and Whitecar, 1971) and 20–45 min for 6-MP (Loo *et al.*, 1968). The primary metabolic product of 6-MP is thiouric acid, a result of xanthine oxidase action. Both 6-MP and 6-TG also undergo desulfuration and alternatively methylation of the thiol group. In the case of 6-MP, the methylation product, 6-methyl MP, can be further metabolized to the ribonucleotide level, where it may exert inhibitory effects on ribosylamine phosphate formation (Hill and Bennett, 1969).

Allopurinol, a potent inhibitor of xanthine oxidase, is frequently used to prevent hyperuricemia in patients with acute leukemia and markedly prolongs the plasma half-life of 6-MP, enhancing toxicity of a given dose of this agent (Elion

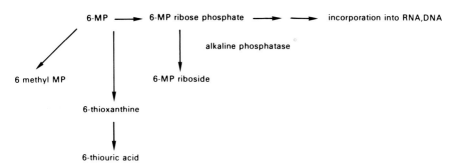

Fig. 7. Metabolism of 6-mercaptopurine. The primary degradative product, 6-thiouric acid, is produced by xanthine oxidase action in the liver. Anabolic steps leading to active phosphorylated derivatives occur within tumor cells.

et al., 1963). Therefore 6-MP dosage must be reduced to 25% of usual doses for patients receiving concurrent 6-MP and allopurinol. A similar enhancement of 6-TG toxicity by allopurinol has not been demonstrated, probably because conversion of 6-TG to 6-thiouric acid represents a minor degradative pathway for this analogue.

C. Clinical Toxicity

Both 6-MP and 6-TG exert their most important toxic effects on rapidly dividing cells and thus produce myelosuppression that reaches a maximum 7–14 days after treatment. In addition, both agents produce a reversible hepatotoxicity with elevation of alkaline phosphatase, transaminase, and occasionally clinical jaundice. Hepatotoxicity is less frequent with 6-TG than with 6-MP. Mucositis and gastrointestinal ulceration are infrequent side effects in patients receiving thiopurines as single agents.

VIII. ARABINOSYL ADENINE

9-β-D-Arabinofuranosyladenine (ara-A), although synthesized as a potential antitumor agent (Lee *et al.*, 1960), has found its major usefulness as an antiviral compound with activity against various DNA viruses, including those of the herpes group (Pavan-Langston *et al.*, 1975). Clinical interest in this compound and its monophosphate, ara-AMP, has been renewed with the introduction of inhibitors of adenosine deaminase, the primary enzyme responsible for degradation of ara-A to the inactive metabolite arahypoxanthine.

A. Mechanism of Action

Ara-A is activated to a triphosphate nucleotide, which inhibits DNA polymerase (Furth and Cohen, 1967) (Fig. 8). The major limitation to antitumor efficacy of this compound is its deamination to arahypoxanthine by adenosine deaminase, an enzyme found in high concentrations in many experimental (LePage *et al.*, 1976) and human (Smyth and Harrap, 1975) neoplasms, and particularly those of lymphoid origin. In the treatment of cells with high deaminase levels, the antitumor activity of ara-A is markedly potentiated by coadministration of a deaminase inhibitor, such as 2′-deoxycoformycin (LePage *et al.*, 1976; Cass and Au-Yeung, 1976). This combination may be curative in tumor strains such as L1210, which is highly resistant to ara-A alone. 2′-Deoxycoformycin currently undergoing initial clinical trials, prior to its use in combination with ara-A and other adenosine nucleoside analogues such as xylosyl, adenine, and 3′-deoxyadenosine.

Another mechanism of resistance to ara-A has been implicated by LePage

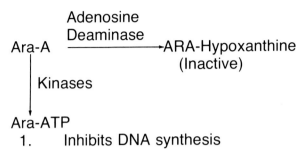

Fig. 8.   Metabolic pathways for arabinosyl adenine (ara-A).

(1978), who found decreased affinity of DNA polymerase for ara-ATP in a murine lymphoma cell line.

B. Pharmacokinetics

Following intravenous administration, ara-A is rapidly deaminated to arahypoxanthine (LePage *et al.*, 1973); almost 90% of an administered dose is recoverable in the urine, primarily as the metabolite, within 4 hr of administration. Initial clinical trial indicated only minimal myelosuppression (Bodey *et al.*, 1974), but correspondingly unimpressive antitumor effects, although these studies were limited by the inability to increase ara-A doses to toxic levels, because of the insolubility of the compound. Attention has how turned to ara-AMP, which is much more soluble, undergoes slow phosphorolysis in plasma, and yields steady high levels of the active compound ara-A (LePage *et al.*, 1975). Clinical trials of ara-AMP in combination with 2'-deoxycoformycin are awaited with interest.

IX. CONCLUSIONS

The nucleoside analogues represent an important group of very well-characterized antineoplastic agents. However, much remains to be learned and new analogues of clinical potential may be developed in the future.

REFERENCES

Aull, J. L., Lyon, J. A., and Dunlap, R. B. (1974). *Arch. Biochem. Biophys.* **165,** 805–808.
Band, P. R., Holland, J. F., Bernard, J., Weil, M., Walker, M., and Rall, D. (1973). *Cancer (Philadelphia)* **32,** 744–748.

Baskin, F., Carlin, S. C., Kraus, P., Friedkin, M., and Rosenberg, R. N. (1975). *Mol. Pharmacol.* **11**, 105–117.

Beisler, J. A. (1978). *J. Med. Chem.* **21**, 204–208.

Bellet, R. E., Mastrangelo, M. J., Engstrom, P. F., and Custer, R. P. (1973). *Neoplasma* **20**, 303.

Benvenuto, J. A., Lu, K., Hall, S. W., Benjamin, R. S., and Loo, T. L. (1978). *Cancer Res.* **38**, 3867–3870.

Benvenuto, J., Hall, S. W., Farquhar, D., Stewart, D. J., Benjamin, R. S., and Loo, T. L. (1979). *Cancer Res.* (39:349–352).

Bloch, A. J., Datschmann, B. L., Currie, B. L., Robins, R. K., and Robins, M. J. (1973). *J. Med. Chem.* **16**, 294–297.

Bodey, G. P., Gottlieb, J., McCredie, K. B., and Freireich, E. J. (1974). *Proc. Am. Assoc. Cancer Res.* **15**, 129.

Bosch, L., Habers, E., and Heidelberger, C. (1958). *Cancer Res.* **18**, 335–343.

Brewen, J. G., and Christie, N. T. (1967). *Exp. Cell Res.* **46**, 276.

Brockman, R. W. (1963). *Cancer Res.* **23**, 1191–1201.

Brockman, R. W., Shaddix, S. C., Williams, M., Laster, W. R., and Schabel, F. M., Jr. (1973). *Proc. Am. Assoc. Cancer Res.* **14**, 16.

Burgess, M. A., Bodey, G. P., Minow, R. A., and Gottlieb, J. A. (1977). *Cancer Treat. Rep.* **61**, 437–443.

Burokev, T., Samson, M., Correa, J., Fraile, R., and Vaitkevicius, V. K. (1976). *Cancer Treat. Rep.* **60**, 1277–1279.

Cass, C. E., and Au-Yeung, T. H. (1976). *Cancer Res.* **36**, 1486–1491.

Chabner, B. A., Drake, J. C., and Johns, D. G. (1973). *Biochem. Pharmacol.* **22**, 2763–2765.

Chang, P., Wiernik, P., Bachur, N., Stoller, R., and Chabner, B. (1977). *Proc. Am. Soc. Clin. Oncol.* **18**, 352.

Chaudhuri, N. K., Montag, B. J., and Heidelberger, C. (1958). *Cancer Res.* **18**, 318–328.

Chou, T. C., Arlin, Z., Clarkson, B. D., and Philips, F. S. (1977). *Cancer Res.* **37**, 3561–3570.

Chu, M. Y. (1971). *Biochem. Pharmacol.* **20**, 2057–2063.

Clarkson, B., O'Connor, A., Winston, L., and Hutchinson, D. (1964). *Clin. Pharmacol. Ther.* **5**, 581–610.

Cohen, J. L., Irwin, L. E., Marshall, C. J., Darvey, H., and Bateman, J. R. (1974). *Cancer Chemother. Rep.* **58**, 723–731.

Cooper, G. M., Dunning, W. F., and Greer, S. (1972). *Cancer Res.* **32**, 390–397.

Creavan, P. J., Rustum, Y. M., Slocum, H. K., and Mittleman, A. (1978). *In* "Current Chemotherapy" (W. Segenthaler and R. Lathy, eds.), pp. 1208–1210. Am. Soc. Microbiol., Washington, D.C.

Curreri, A. R., Ansfield, F. J., McIver, F. A., Waisman, H. A., and Heidelberger, C. (1958). *Cancer Res.* **18**, 478–484.

Cysyk, R. L., Gormley, P. E., D'Anna, M. E., and Adamson, R. H. (1978). *Drug Metab. Dispos.* **6**, 125–132.

Draharosky, B. D., and Kreis, W. (1970). *Biochem. Pharmacol.* **19**, 940–944.

Drake, J. C., Stoller, R. G., and Chabner, B. A. (1977). *Biochem. Pharmacol.* **26**, 64–66.

Elion, G. B. (1967). *Fed. Proc., Fed. Am. Soc. Exp. Biol.* **26**, 898–904.

Elion, G. B., Callahan, S., Nathan, H., Bieber, S., Rundles, R. W., and Hitchings, G. H. (1963). *Biochem. Pharmacol.* **12**, 85–93.

Ellison, R. R. (1968). *Blood* **32**, 507–523.

Finn, C., and Sadee, W. (1975). *Cancer Chemother. Rep.* **59**, 279–286.

Furth, J. J., and Cohen, S. S. (1967). *Cancer Res.* **227**, 1528–1533.

Hall, S. W., Valdivieso, M., and Benjamin, R. S. (1977). *Cancer Treat. Rep.* **61**, 1495–1498.

Hande, K. R., and Chabner, B. A. (1978). *Cancer Res.* **38**, 579–585.

Hande, K., Lewis, B., and Chabner, B. (1978). *Proc. Am. Assoc. Cancer Res.* **19**, 149.

Heidelberger, C. (1965). *Prog. Nucleic Acid Res.* **4**, 1–50.

Heidelberger, C., Chaudhuri, N. K., Dannenburg, P., Greisbach, L., Dashinsky, R., Schnitzer, R. J., Pleven, E., and Scheiner, J. (1957). *Nature (London)* **179**, 663–666.

Hill, D. L., and Bennett, L. L. (1969). *Biochemistry* **8**, 122–130.

Hiss, E. A., and Preston, R. J. (1978). *Biochim. Biophys. Acta* **478**, 1.

Ho, D. H. W., and Frei, E. (1971). *Clin. Pharmacol. Ther.* **12**, 944–954.

Israili, Z. H., Vogler, W., Mingioli, E. S., Pirkle, J. L., Smithwick, R. W., and Goldstein, J. H. (1976). *Cancer Res.* **36**, 1453–1461.

Jones, R. B., Myers, C. E., Guarino, A. M., Dedrick, R. L., Hubbard, S. M., and DeVita, V. T. (1978). *Cancer Chemother. Pharmacol.* **1**, 161–166.

Jones, R., Buckpitt, A., Londer, H., Myers, C., Chabner, B., and Boyd, M. (1979). *Bull. Cancer* **66**:75–78.

Kasbekar, D. K., and Greenberg, D. M. (1963). *Cancer Res.* **23**, 818–824.

Kreis, W., Woodcock, T., Tan, C., and Krakoff, I. H. (1977). *Proc. Am. Assoc. Cancer Res.* **18**, 226.

Kremer, W. B. (1975). *Ann. Intern. Med.* **82**, 684.

Lee, M. H., Huang, Y. M., and Sartorelli, A. C. (1978). *Cancer Res.* **38**, 2413–2423.

Lee, W. W., Benitez, A., Goodman, L., and Baker, B. R. (1960). *J. Am. Chem. Soc.* **82**, 2648–2649.

LePage, G. A. (1978). *Cancer Res.* **38**, 2314–2320.

LePage, G. A., and Jones, M. (1961). *Cancer Res.* **21**, 642–649.

LePage, G. A., and Whitecar, J. P., Jr. (1971). *Cancer Res.* **31**, 1627–1631.

LePage, G. A., Khalig, A., and Gottlieb, J. A. (1973). *Drug Metab. Dispos.* **1**, 756–759.

LePage, G. A., Naik, S. R., Katakkar, S. B., and Dhalig, A. (1975). *Cancer Res.* **35**, 3036–3040.

LePage, G. A., Worth, L. S., and Kimball, A. P. (1976). *Cancer Res.* **36**, 1481–1485.

Levitan, I. B., and Webb, T. E. (1969). *Biochim. Biophys. Acta* **182**, 491.

Li, L. H., Olin, E. J., Buskirk, H. H., and Reineke, L. M. (1970). *Cancer Res.* **30**, 2760–2769.

Loo, T. L., Luce, J. K., Sullivan, M. P., and Frei, E., III (1968). *Clin. Pharmacol. Ther.* **9**, 180–194.

McCredie, K. B., Bodey, G. P., Burgess, M. A., Gutterman, J. U., Rodriguez, V., Sullivan, M. P., and Freireich, E. J. (1973). *Cancer Chemother. Rep.* **57**, 319–323.

MacMillan, W. E., Wolberg, W. H., and Welling, P. G. (1978). *Cancer Res.* **38**, 3479–3482.

McPortland, R. P., Wang, M. C., Bloch, A., and Weinfeld, H. (1974). *Cancer Res.* **34**, 3107–3111.

Martin, D., Stolfi, R. L., and Spiegelman, S. (1978). *Proc. Am. Assoc. Cancer Res.* **19**, 221.

Mills-Yamamoto, C., Lauzon, G. J., and Paterson, A. R. P. (1978). *Biochem. Pharmacol.* **27**, 181–186.

Momparler, R. L. (1972). *Mol. Pharmacol.* **8**, 362–370.

Momparler, R. L., Chu, M. Y., and Fischer, G. A. (1968). *Biochim. Biophys. Acta* **161**, 481.

Myers, C. S., Young, R. C., and Chabner, B. A. (1975). *J. Clin. Invest.* **56**, 1231–1238.

Notari, R. E., and DeYoung, J. L. (1975). *J. Pharm. Sci.* **64**, 1148–1157.

Pavan-Langston, D., Buchanon, R. A., and Alford, C. A., Jr. (1975). "Adenine-Arabinoside: An Antiviral Agent." Raven, New York.

Pogolotti, A. L., Ivanetlich, K. M., Sommer, H., and Santi, D. V. (1976). *Biochem. Biophys. Res. Commun.* **70**, 972–978.

Rashbaum, S. A., and Cozzarelli, N. R. (1976). *Nature (London)* **264**, 679–680.

Reichard, P., Skold, O., Klein, G., Revesz, L., and Magnusson, P. H. (1962). *Cancer Res.* **22**, 235–243.

Reichman, M., Kaplan, D., and Penman, S. (1973). *Biochim. Biophys. Acta* **299**, 173–176.

Reyes, R. (1969). *Biochemistry* **8,** 2057–2062.
Robins, M. J., and Currie, B. L. (1968). *Chem. Commun.* **2,** 1547–1548.
Rosman, M., Lee, M. H., Creasey, W. A., and Sartorelli, A. C. (1974). *Cancer Res.* **34,** 1952–1956.
Rustum, Y. M., Priesler, H., Wrzosek, C., Wang, G., Rubenstein, J., and Kelly, E. (1978). *Proc. Am. Soc. Clin. Oncol.* **19,** 338.
Santi, D. V., McHenry, C. S., and Sommers, H. (1974). *Biochemistry* **13,** 471–480.
Seifert, P., Baker, L. H., Reed, M. L., and Vaitkevicius, V. K. (1975). *Cancer (Philadelphia)* **36,** 123–128.
Sitar, D. S. (1977). *Cancer Res.* **37,** 3981–3984.
Smith, A. E., and Yamada, E. W. (1971). *J. Biol. Chem.* **246,** 3610–3617.
Smyth, J. F., and Harrap, K. R. (1975). *Br. J. Cancer* **31,** 544–549.
Smyth, J. R., Robbins, A. B., and Leese, C. L. (1976). *Eur. J. Cancer* **12,** 567–573.
Sommer, H., and Santi, D. V. (1974). *Biochem. Biophys. Res. Commun.* **57,** 689–695.
Steuart, C. D., and Burke, P. J. (1971). *Nature (London), New Biol.* **233,** 109–110.
Stolinsky, D. C., Pugh, R. P., and Bateman, J. R. (1975). *Cancer Chemother. Rep.* **59,** 1031–1033.
Stoller, R. G., Coleman, C. N., Chang, P., Hande, K. R., and Chabner, B. A. (1975). *In* "Comparative Leukemia Research" (J. Clemmesen and Y. S. Yohn, eds.), Bibliotheca Haematologica, No. 43, pp. 531–533. Karger, Basel.
Stoller, R. G., Myers, C. S., and Chabner, B. A. (1978). *Biochem. Pharmacol.* **27,** 53–59.
Tattersall, M. H., Ganeshaguru, K., and Hoffbrand, A. V. (1974). *Br. J. Haematol.* **27,** 39–46.
Taylor, I., Brooman, P., and Rowling, J. T. (1977). *Br. Med. J.* **ii,** 1320–1322.
Tidd, D. M., and Paterson, A. R. P. (1974). *Cancer Res.* **34,** 738–746.
Vesely, J., Cihak, A., and Sorm, F. (1970). *Cancer Res.* **30,** 2180–2186.
Vogler, W. R., Miller, D. S., and Keller, J. W. (1976). *Blood* **48,** 331–337.
Von Hoff, D. D., Slavik, M., and Muggia, F. M. (1976). *Ann. Intern. Med.* **85,** 237–245.
Weiss, J. C., and Pitot, H. C. (1975). *Biochemistry* **14,** 316–326.
Wilkinson, D. S., Tlsty, T. D., and Hanas, R. J. (1975). *Cancer Res.* **35,** 3014–3020.

2
CYCLOPHOSPHAMIDE AND ANALOGUES
Michael Colvin

I. INTRODUCTION

Cyclophosphamide (Cytoxan) is the most widely used alkylating agent and probably the most frequently used antitumor drug of any type. The reasons for this popularity are its demonstrated activity against a variety of tumors, a relatively high therapeutic index, and the relative ease of administration. The drug exerts few, if any, direct biological effects and is enzymatically activated in the body. A considerable body of investigation has been directed toward the elucidation of the complex metabolic conversions that generate the chemicals responsible for the drug's biological activities. Despite the high therapeutic index and relative ease of administration of cyclophosphamide, the drug produces a number of toxicities, some of which are unique to this agent. For this reason patients receiving the drug must be carefully monitored to prevent or recognize and treat these toxic effects.

II. STRUCTURE AND METABOLISM

The structure of cyclophosphamide is shown in Fig. 1. As can be seen, the compound consists of the bischloroethylamino group of the nitrogen mustards

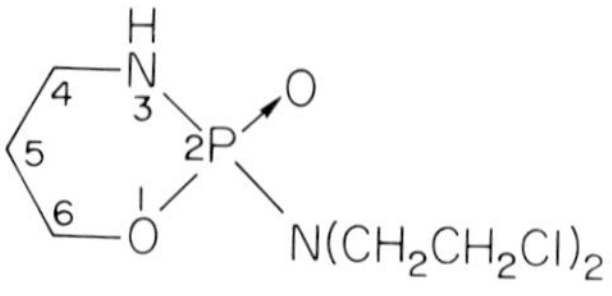

Cyclophosphamide

Fig. 1.   Structure of cyclophosphamide.

attached to the phosphorus of an unusual heterocyclic six-membered ring, oxazaphosphorine. The structure of this ring is responsible for the complex metabolic and chemical conversion that the drug undergoes *in vivo*. In recent years most of the important metabolites of cyclophosphamide have been identified and the chemical and biological activities of these metabolites investigated. The presently accepted metabolic scheme of cyclophosphamide is shown in Fig. 2. The parent compound is initially oxidized by the microsomal mixed function oxidases (Brock and Hohorst, 1963; Cohen and Jao, 1970) of the hepatic microsomes to produce 4-hydroxycyclophosphamide (IIa), which is probably in spontaneous equilibrium with the open ring aldophosphamide (IIb) (Connors *et al.*, 1974; Takamizawa *et al.*, 1973; Fenselau *et al.*, 1977). Both 4-hydroxycyclophosphamide and aldophosphamide are oxidized enzymatically, the former to 4-ketocyclophosphamide (VI) and the latter to carboxyphosphamide (VII) (Bakke *et al.*, 1971; Struck *et al.*, 1971). These two oxidation products are not significantly cytotoxic (Struck *et al.*, 1971) but are quantitatively important in that well over 50% of a dose of cyclophosphamide is excreted in the urine as carboxycyclophosphamide (the major metabolite) or 4-ketocyclophosphamide in several animal species (Bakke *et al.*, 1971; Struck *et al.*, 1971). The enzymes that carry out the oxidation of the initial oxidation products are located in the cytosol of the cell. It has been suggested that certain normal tissues may be protected from the effect of the drug by high levels of these inactivating enzymes (Cohen and Jao, 1970; Sladek, 1973).

The aldophosphamide that has escaped enzymatic oxidation may eliminate acrolein (IV) (Alarcon and Meienhofer, 1971) to form phosphoramide mustard (III) (Cohen and Jao, 1970; Colvin *et al.*, 1973). Since phosphoramide mustard has been demonstrated to have strong alkylating properties, whereas 4-hydroxycyclophosphamide and aldophosphamide do not, phosphoramide mustard probably represents the alkylating agent responsible for the biological activities of cyclophosphamide (Colvin *et al.*, 1976; Struck *et al.*, 1975). In at least some cell systems, however, 4-hydroxycyclophosphamide exhibits *in vitro* cytotoxicity at approximately one-tenth the concentration of phosphoramide mustard required for similar cytotoxicity (Colvin, 1974; Takamizawa *et al.*, 1973). Similarly, *in vitro* studies of nucleic acid cross-linking demonstrate that 4-hydroxycyclophosphamide produces cross-links at approximately one-fourth

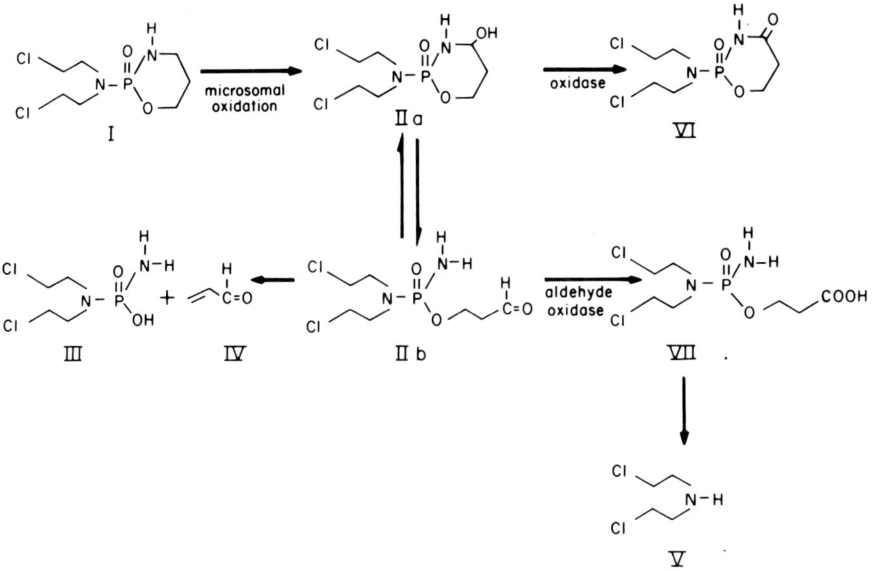

Fig. 2. Metabolic scheme of cyclophosphamide.

the levels of phosphoramide mustard required for a similar degree of cross-linking (Hilton, unpublished observations). These findings are consistent with the hypothesis that either 4-hydroxycyclophosphamide and/or aldophosphamide enter target cells more facilely than phosphoramide mustard and thus act as "transport forms" for phosphoramide mustard into the cell. Furthermore, in animal studies and in limited clinical trials (Nathanson et al., 1967), phosphoramide mustard does not produce certain characteristic effects of the parent drug. Phosphoramide mustard appears to have a lower therapeutic index than cyclophosphamide, exhibits relatively little immunosuppressive activity (Sensenbrenner et al., 1979), and does not produce alopecia (Feil and Lamoureux, 1974; Nathanson et al., 1967). These observations are consistent with the hypothesis that at least some of the characteristic effects of the parent compound are mediated by a metabolite occurring prior to phosphoramide mustard in the metabolic scheme.

III. CLINICAL PHARMACOLOGY

Thus far, studies of the clinical pharmacology of cyclophosphamide have been relatively few, since our knowledge of the key metabolites and techniques for quantitating them have been limited. Investigations using radioactive cyclophosphamide indicated that the plasma half-life of the parent compound in man varies from 2 to 10 hr, and these values have now been supported by measurement of

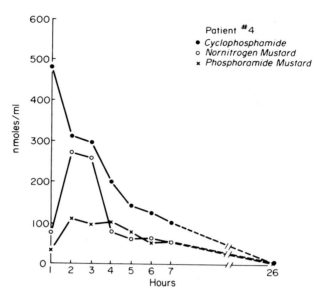

Fig. 3. Plasma levels of cyclophosphamide and metabolites.

plasma cyclophosphamide levels by mass spectrometric techniques (Jardine *et al.*, 1978; Jarman *et al.*, 1975). Prior to the chemical identification of the intermediate metabolic products, the activated metabolites in plasma and urine were estimated by means of the nitrobenzyl pyridine test for alkylating activity (Bagley *et al.*, 1973; Brock *et al.*, 1971). These measurements indicated that peak levels of "activated metabolites" occurred at 2–4 hr after a dose of the parent compound and the peak levels attained were variable between patients.

Recently Jardine and co-workers (1978) have used gas chromatography to measure plasma and urine levels of the parent compound and the metabolites phosphoramide mustard and nornitrogen mustard in patients receiving intravenous cyclophosphamide. The results from one patient receiving 75 mg/kg of cyclophosphamide are shown in Fig. 3. The plasma half-life of cyclophosphamide was 3.5 hr, and in the other patients studied the plasma half-life varied up to 7 hr, which is in agreement with the results obtained using less direct measurements of cyclophosphamide.

Most of the patients studied by Jardine and colleagues showed high initial levels of nornitrogen mustard (Fig. 3), which then declined rapidly. There was a marked variation in nornitrogen mustard levels between patients, however, and significant decomposition of other metabolites, especially carboxyphosphamide, to nornitrogen mustard was found to occur during storage and extraction of the samples. These findings suggest that the levels of nornitrogen mustard that were seen in these and in animal studies (Struck *et al.*, 1975) may be artifactually elevated by the *in vitro* decomposition of other metabolites. However, it seems

TABLE I

Urinary Excretion of Cyclophosphamide and Metabolites over 24-Hr Period[a]

	Excretion (mmoles)		
	Patient 2	Patient 3	Patient 4
Cyclophosphamide	2.8 (19.5)	5.4 (25.1)	2.0 (16.3)
Phosphoramide mustard	0.4 (2.8)	0.3 (1.2)	0.2 (1.8)
Nornitrogen mustard	1.4 (10.4)	2.4 (11.0)	1.8 (14.5)
Total	4.6 (32.7)	8.1 (37.3)	4.0 (32.6)

[a] Numbers in parentheses, percentage of dose.

likely that significant levels of nornitrogen mustard are present *in vivo* and may play a role in the biological effect of cyclophosphamide. Since nornitrogen mustard is a strong alkylating agent at low pH, but not under physiologic conditions, it may well contribute to the renal and bladder damage of cyclophosphamide.

Peak levels of phosphoramide mustard of 50–100 nmoles (15–30 μg)/ml were found in the patients studied by Jardine and colleagues. Peak levels of this compound occurred at 2–3 hr after the end of a 1-hr infusion of cyclophosphamide and were sustained for at least 2 hr before starting to decline. Since none of the other metabolites (except aldophosphamide) were found to decompose to phosphoramide mustard, the levels measured very likely represent the actual levels of this compound present in the plasma *in vivo*.

The quantities of cyclophosphamide, phosphoramide mustard, and nornitrogen mustard excreted during the first 24 hr after drug administration are shown in Table I and the time course of excretion of these compounds in the urine is shown in Fig. 4. The values of up to 25% of the parent compound excreted in the first 24 hr, and negligible quantities excreted thereafter are in agreement with previous studies in both man and animals. As can be seen, significant amounts of nornitrogen mustard, but only small amounts of phosphoramide mustard, are found in the urine. Previous studies (Bagley *et al.*, 1973; Struck *et al.*, 1971) have shown that the major route of excretion of cyclophosphamide and metabolites is the kidney. The majority (70–85%) of a dose of cyclophosphamide can be accounted for in animals by carboxyphosphamide (VII, 50–60%) and 4-ketocyclophosphamide (VI, ~10%) (Bakke *et al.*, 1971; Brock *et al.*, 1971), neither of which was measured in the study by Jardine and colleagues.

The plasma levels of phosphoramide mustard that have been described are within the levels that have been found to be cytotoxic to cells *in vitro* (Maddock *et al.*, 1966). Therefore it is probable that circulating phosphoramide mustard plays some role in the therapeutic and toxic effects of cyclophosphamide. How-

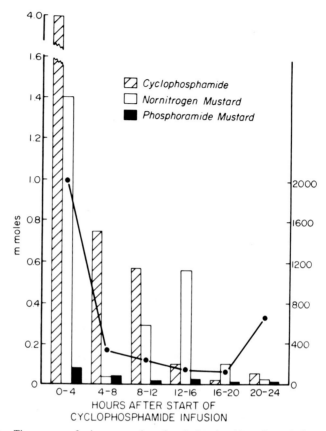

Fig. 4.   Time course of urinary excretion of cyclophosphamide and metabolites.

ever, because of the unique properties of the primary metabolites described earlier it will be important to quantitate levels of 4-hydroxycyclophosphamide and aldophosphamide in plasma after cyclophosphamide administration. Techniques for quantitating the primary metabolites have now been described (Fenselau *et al.*, 1977) and the application of these techniques to measuring plasma levels should further clarify the clinical pharmacology of cyclophosphamide.

Since cyclophosphamide is activated by hepatic microsomal enzymes, it is not surprising that drugs that stimulate or inhibit these enzymes can alter the pharmacokinetics of the drug. The effects of alterations in hepatic metabolism on the therapeutic and toxic effects of the drug appear to be complex, and conflicting reports from animal studies have appeared (Alberts and Daalen Wetters, 1976). It has been shown that the plasma half-life of cyclophosphamide can be shortened by the prior administration of a barbiturate (Jao *et al.*, 1972), and the variations in the plasma half-life of cyclophosphamide in man that have been reported may be due to the effects of other drugs on the hepatic microsomal enzymes. However, no firm evidence has been presented that the therapeutic index or toxicities of cyclophosphamide are altered in man as the result of the concomitant administration of other drugs.

Two reports have described elevated levels of cyclophosphamide metabolites in the plasma of patients with renal failure, and on this basis a reduction in dose has been recommended for such patients (Bagley *et al.*, 1973; Mouridsen and Jacobsen, 1975). However, it has not been established that these elevated metabolite levels are associated with increased toxicity, and one report indicates that it is possible to give full doses of cyclophosphamide to patients with severe renal impairment without an increase in the hematologic and other toxicities of the drug (Humphrey and Kvols, 1974).

IV. TOXICITIES

The most commonly encountered and serious toxicities of cyclophosphamide are listed in Table II. Probably the most consistently encountered toxicity is that of depression of the blood leucocyte count. The nadir of the leucocyte count usually occurs at 10–12 days after a dose of cyclophosphamide (Fig. 5), and recovery is usually complete by 21 days. The drug demonstrates a significant platelet sparing effect and depression of the platelet count is usually not seen, even at doses that produce significant depression of the leucocyte count. However, at doses above 50 mg/kg depression of the platelet count occurs and can be serious. Most patients can receive repeated doses of cyclophosphamide without showing a decreasing hematopoietic tolerance to the drug, indicating that the agent does not cause cumulative or irreparable damage to the bone marrow.

Although nausea and vomiting are not life threatening, these side effects are a significant source of discomfort and debilitation to patients. The degree of this side effect of cyclophosphamide is quite variable from patient to patient, with some patients suffering severe nausea and vomiting and others experiencing little

TABLE II

Toxicities of Cyclophosphamide

1.	Hematopoietic depression
2.	Nausea and vomiting
3.	Alopecia
4.	Hemorrhagic cystitis
5.	Water retention
6.	Cardiac damage
7.	Gonadal atrophy
8.	Carcinogenicity

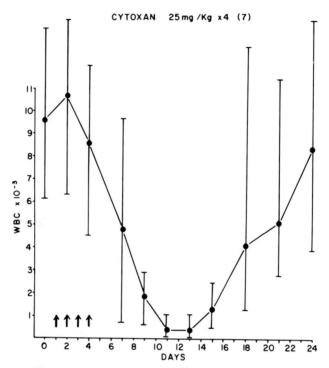

Fig. 5.   Leucocyte count after cyclophosphamide therapy.

discomfort even with high doses. It is important to remember that the onset of nausea and vomiting is usually delayed for several hours and may not be seen until 8 hr after the dose of drug.

Cyclophosphamide is unusual among the alkylating agents in that it produces alopecia, a distressing side effect to many patients. Some degree of hair fragility and loss occurs at modest doses, and at high doses, especially in combination with other agents, almost complete alopecia may occur. Regrowth of the hair always occurs, although the rate of regrowth varies between patients. Phosphoramide mustard does not produce alopecia in man or depilation in sheep (Feil and Lamoureux, 1974), suggesting that this effect is mediated by the lipophilic primary metabolites.

A unique and potentially serious toxicity that occurs in 10–20% of patients is sterile cystitis. The patient may present with dysuria and hematuria or with the abrupt onset of frank hematuria. The hematuria may be very severe, and in some instances has either been fatal or required cystectomy to prevent fatal bleeding. It is important to remember that this side effect may appear suddenly in patients who have been on daily oral cyclophosphamide for a long time without difficulty. Attention to adequate hydration and frequent emptying of the bladder will reduce the incidence of this problem, but even under these conditions a severe case of hemorrhagic cystitis may occur.

The bladder damage appears to be due to excretion of toxic metabolites into the bladder, and irrigation of the bladder with sulfhydryl reagents has been used to reduce the bladder damage (Primack, 1971). In mice systemic administration of N-acetylcysteine in conjunction with cyclophosphamide has been shown to prevent bladder damage, but not to reduce the lympholytic or antitumor effects of the drug (Botta *et al.*, 1973; Kline *et al.*, 1972), suggesting that systemic administration of an appropriate sulfhydryl reagent might be used to block this effect in patients.

Approximately 50% of patients who receive an acute dose of 50 mg/kg or greater of cyclophosphamide will show a syndrome of decreased urinary output, weight gain, increase in urine osmolality, and decrease in serum sodium and serum osmolality (DeFronzo *et al.*, 1973). The onset of this syndrome coincides with the peak excretion of alkylating metabolites in the urine, indicating that this effect may be due to a direct action of the metabolites on the renal tubules. The syndrome is self-limited, and by 12–16 hr after the dose of drug the fluid retention spontaneously reverses. Attempts to reverse the fluid retention immediately by vigorous diuretic therapy may lead to electrolyte imbalance.

At high doses of cyclophosphamide, cardiac damage may be seen. This syndrome is characterized in its most fulminant form by the rapid onset of intractable heart failure, leading to death in 10–14 days. High-dose patients who do not show the complete syndrome may have decreased electrocardiographic voltage and transient increase in heart size. Cardiac damage has been seen only in patients receiving doses of over 100 mg/kg during a 48-hr period and has been seen mainly in patients receiving very high doses in preparation for bone marrow transplantation. The histologic appearance of the heart in this syndrome is different from that of anthracycline damage, and there is no definite evidence for an additive effect of these two agents on the heart.

Cyclophosphamide, like other alkylating agents, may produce severe gonadal damage (Fairley *et al.*, 1972; Kumar *et al.*, 1972). Aspermia and amenorrhea are seen after prolonged therapy, and these effects are correlated with atrophy of the Sertoli cells in males and ovarian atrophy in females. These lesions are usually reversible, and both men and women have become the parents of normal children after documented gonadal damage from cyclophosphamide. Although the drug is teratogenic in animals, there have been several reports of a normal pregnancy and child despite cyclophosphamide therapy in the first trimester of pregnancy (Lergier *et al.*, 1974).

Cyclophosphamide is carcinogenic in animals, and the increasing number of reports of new tumors in patients treated with the drug make it certain that this complication occurs in man. Although most of the new tumors have been acute leukemias and reticulum cell sarcomas, a variety of second tumors have now been described. The occurrence of this complication makes it imperative to attempt to define the minimum effective therapy for responsive malignancies.

V. CLINICAL ACTIVITY AND DOSE SCHEDULES

The activity of cyclophosphamide against a wide spectrum of experimental animal tumors is reflected in the large range of human tumors with at least some degree of responsiveness to cyclophosphamide. Although the drug is perhaps most effective against lymphomas, it is used in the treatment of many solid tumors. In combination with other agents cyclophosphamide is widely used in the therapy of carcinoma of the breast, multiple myeloma, ovarian carcinoma, lung cancer, and sarcomas.

Cyclophosphamide may be administered in a wide variety of doses and schedules. The drug is active by mouth and is thought to be well absorbed from the gastrointestinal tract, although extensive bioavailability studies have not been carried out in man. The usual dosage by the oral route is 50–200 mg per day given either continuously or for 2-week periods. Animal studies and limited clinical experience indicate that intermittent high doses of cyclophosphamide may be given by mouth as effectively as parenterally, but the drug is seldom used in this manner.

A wide range of parenteral doses and schedules has also been used. A single dose of up to 25 mg/kg is usually well tolerated without serious hematologic depression, and single doses of up to 75 mg/kg may be given if severe leucopenia and thrombocytopenia can be tolerated. Doses above this level should be divided over at least two days to diminish acute toxicity to the bladder and heart. High single doses can be repeated every 3–4 weeks without cumulative toxicity.

VI. ANALOGUES

Although a great many analogues of cyclophosphamide have been synthesized and tested, only two have shown sufficient promise to receive significant clinical

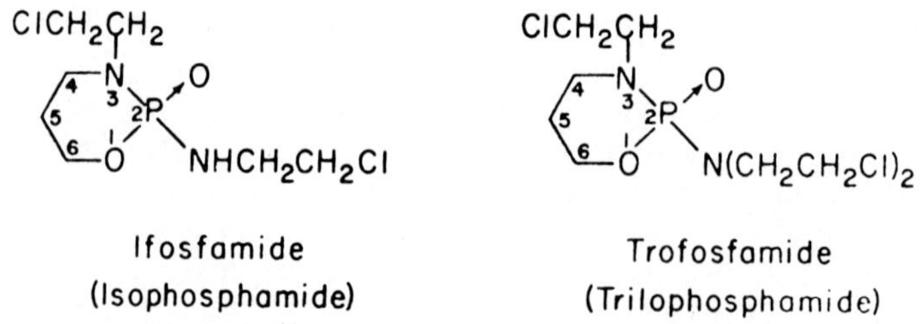

Ifosfamide
(Isophosphamide)

Trofosfamide
(Trilophosphamide)

Fig. 6. Structures of isophosphamide and trilophosphamide.

testing. These two analogues are trilophosphamide and isophosphamide, shown in Fig. 6. Trilophosphamide appears to be similar to cyclophosphamide in its effects but has been suggested to be better tolerated orally. Isophosphamide has been the more extensively used clinically of the two and has been claimed to be more effective against solid tumors, especially testicular tumors and carcinoma of the lung, than cyclophosphamide. However, the drug has not been compared directly with cyclophosphamide at equally toxic doses. The metabolism of isophosphamide and trophosphamide are analogous to that of cyclophosphamide. However, the oxidation of a chloroethyl side chain, which is a very minor pathway in cyclophosphamide metabolism, is quantitatively important in the metabolism of isophosphamide. Although isophosphamide exhibits considerably less hematopoietic toxicity than cyclophosphamide, the renal tubular toxicity is increased and appears to be the dose-limiting toxicity.

REFERENCES

Alarcon, R. A., and Meienhofer, J. (1971). *Nature (London), New Biol.* **233**, 250-252.

Alberts, D. S., and Daalen Wetters, T. (1976). *Cancer Res.* **36**, 2785-2789.

Bagley, C. M., Jr., Bostick, F. W., and DeVita, V. T., Jr. (1973). *Cancer Res.* **33**, 226-233.

Bakke, J. E., Feil, V. J., and Zaylskie, R. G. (1971). *J. Agric. Food Chem.* **19**, 788-790.

Botta, J. A., Jr., Nelson, L. W., and Weikel, J. H., Jr. (1973). *J. Natl. Cancer Inst.* **51**, 1051-1057.

Brock, N., and Hohorst, H.-J. (1963). *Arzneim.-Forsch.* **13**, 1021-1031.

Brock, N., Gross, R., Hohorst, H.-J., Klein, H. O., and Scheider, B. (1971). *Cancer (Philadelphia)* **27**, 1512-1529.

Cohen, J. L., and Jao, J. Y. (1970). *J. Pharmacol. Exp. Ther.* **174**, 206-210.

Colvin, M. (1974). *Proc. Am. Assoc. Cancer Res.* **15**, 70.

Colvin, M., Padgett, C. A., and Fenselau, C. (1973). *Cancer Res.* **33**, 915-920.

Colvin, M., Brundrett, R. B., Kan, M.-N. N., Jardine, I., and Fenselau, C. (1976). *Cancer Res.* **36**, 1121-1126.

Connors, T. A., Cox, P. J., Farmer, P. B., Foster, A. B., and Jarman, M. (1974). *Biochem. Pharmacol.* **23**, 115-129.

DeFronzo, R. A., Braine, H. G., Colvin, M., and Davis, P. J. (1973). *Ann. Intern. Med.* **78**, 861-869.

Fairley, K. F., Barrie, J. U., and Johnson, W. (1972). *Lancet* **i**, 568-569.

Feil, V. J., and Lamoureux, C. J. H. (1974). *Cancer Res.* **34**, 2596-2598.

Fenselau, C., Kan, M.-N., N., Subba Rao, S., Myles, A., Friedman, O. M., and Colvin, M. (1977). *Cancer Res.* **37**, 2538-2543.

Humphrey, R. L., and Kvols, L. K. (1974). *Proc. Am. Assoc. Cancer Res.* **15**, 84.

Jao, J. Y., Jusko, W. J., and Cohen, J. L. (1972). *Cancer Res.* **32**, 2761-2764.

Jardine, I., Fenselau, C., Appler, M., Kan, M.-N., Brundrett, R. B., and Colvin, M. (1978). *Cancer Res.* **38**, 408-415.

Jarman, M., Gilby, E. D., Foster, A. B., and Bondy, P. K. (1975). *Clin. Chim. Acta* **58**, 61-69.

Kline, I., Gang, M., and Venditti, J. M. (1972). *Proc. Am. Assoc. Cancer Res.* **13**, 29.

Kumar, R., Biggart, J. D., McEvoy, J., and McGeown, M. G. (1972). *Lancet* **i**, 1212-1214.

Lergier, J., Jimenez, E., Maldonado, N., and Veray, F. (1974). *Cancer (Philadelphia)* **34**, 1018-1022.

Maddock, C. L., Handler, A. H., Friedman, O. M., Foley, G. E., and Farber, S. (1966). *Cancer Chemother. Rep.* **50,** 629–639.

Mouridsen, H. T., and Jacobsen, E. (1975). *Acta Pharmacol. Toxicol.* **36,** 409–414.

Nathanson, L., Hall, T. C., Rutenberg, A., and Shadduck, R. K. (1967). *Cancer Chemother. Rep.* **51,** 35–39.

Primack, A. (1971). *J. Natl. Cancer Inst.* **47,** 223–227.

Sensenbrenner, L. L., Marini, J. J., and Colvin, M. (1979). *J. Natl. Cancer Inst.* **62,** 975–981.

Sladek, N. E. (1973). *Cancer Res.* **33,** 1150–1158.

Struck, R. F., Kirk, M. C., Mellett, L. B., El Dareer, S., and Hill, D. L. (1971). *Mol. Pharmacol.* **7,** 519–529.

Struck, R. F., Kirk, M. C., Witt, M. H., and Laster, W. R., Jr. (1975). *Biomed. Mass Spectrom.* **2,** 46.

Takamizawa, A., Matsumoto, S., Iwata, T., Katagiri, K., Tochino, Y., and Yamaguchi, K. (1973). *J. Am. Chem. Soc.* **95,** 985–986.

3
NITROSOUREAS
Philip S. Schein

I. INTRODUCTION

In 1959, 1-methyl-1-nitro-3-nitrosoguanidine (MNNG) was reported to have limited but reproducible antitumor activity aginst the murine L1210 leukemia. Although it was recognized that the therapeutic potential of this compound was insufficient to warrant extensive clinical trial, the observation formed the basis of the intensive evaluation of the N-nitroso containing compounds as antitumor agents that has since occurred. During the subsequent 20 years there has been a series of advances and structure–activity analyses that has resulted in the development of a class of drugs representing some of the most clinically useful therapeutic agents. Major contributions were made by Dr. Baker and co-workers at Stanford Research Institute. In a sequence of structure–activity studies they demonstrated that the nitroso group of the MNNG molecule was an essential requirement for antitumor activity and that substitution of a chloroethyl for the methyl group considerably enhanced this cytotoxicity. These findings led to the synthesis of 1-(2-chloroethyl)-1-nitrosourea (CNU), a drug that possesses curative activity for mice bearing the L1210 leukemia (Hyde et al., 1962). Concurrently, Dr. Montgomery and colleagues at the Southern Research Institute undertook a study of compounds with structural similarities to MNNG that would have the potential of releasing deazomethane. 1-Methyl-1-nitrosourea (MNU), was found to produce greater antitumor activity against the intraperitoneally implanted L1210 leukemia than MNNG (Skipper et al., 1961). In addition, MNU penetrated the blood–brain barrier and increased the life span of mice bearing intracranially implanted L1210 cells. This property was subsequently correlated with the lipid solubility of MNU. At the time this was an important finding, since the majority of clinically available anticancer drugs did not achieve cytotoxic concentration in the central nervous system. Furthermore, it had become recognized that the central nervous system was a pharmacologic sanctuary for leukemic cells and that meningeal leukemia was the cause of relapse from complete remission in one-half of cases with acute lymphocytic leukemia. Montgomery and Johnston proceeded to synthesize over 200 congeners of the original MNU molecule. This work led to the development and clinical use of a series of chloroethyl derivatives including 1,3-bis(2-chloroethyl)-1-nitrosourea (BCNU) (Schabel *et al.*, 1963), a compound with curative activity in mice implanted either intraperitoneally or intracranially with L1210 leukemia cells (Schabel *et al.*, 1963); substitution of a cyclohexyl group resulted in the synthesis of CCNU and eventually methyl-CCNU.

The original methylnitrosourea (MNU) has now undergone extensive clinical testing in the USSR and has been demonstrated to have useful activity for the treatment of lymphomas and small cell carcinoma of the lung (Emmanuel *et al.*, 1974). Streptozotocin consisting of MNU attached to the C-2 position of glucose was found to occur naturally as a product of the fermentation of *Streptomyces achromogenes;* this compound is a potent toxin for the pancreatic islet beta cell of rodents and higher animal species. It has been demonstrated that the diabetogenic activity of streptozotocin is mediated by a rapid reduction in pyridine nucleotides and that beta cell destruction and the associated reduction in NAD can be prevented by the use of pharmacological doses of nicotinamide (Schein *et al.*, 1973a). Recent work has suggested that the reduction in NAD can be correlated with a significant increase in the activity of poly-ADP ribose polymerase, a chromatin-associated enzyme that uses NAD as a substrate (Smulson *et al.*, 1977). Streptozotocin is now used in the treatment of islet cell carcinoma.

The major clinical emphasis has been directed toward the more active chloroethyl nitrosourea derivatives. They have established clinical antitumor activity for a broad range of human malignancies, including acute lymphocytic leukemia, lymphomas, myeloma, gliomas, and gastrointestinal neoplasms (Wasserman *et al.*, 1975). Unfortunately, these same agents produce delayed and cumulative bone marrow toxicity that seriously limits their clinical application.

II. DECOMPOSITION AND METABOLISM

Under physiologic conditions the nitrosoureas decompose spontaneously (Colvin *et al.*, 1976; Montgomery *et al.*, 1975). The chemical half-life of the individual compounds in phosphate buffered saline (pH 7.4) varies from 5 min to as long as 2 hr. In the process of degradation a number of alkylating moieties are formed of which alkyldiazohydroxide precursor and the chloroethyl carbonium ion are considered the most important. Organic isocyanates are also generated that may carbamoylate intracellular proteins. Thus there are two chemical activities, alkylation and carbamoylation (Wheeler et al., 1974). In addition to their spontaneous chemical dissociation, the nitrosoureas are now known to be metabolized by the liver microsomal mixed function oxidase system to more polar hydroxylated products that retain both the cyclohexyl ring structure and the cytotoxic nitrosoureido moiety (Reed and May, 1975). Current data indicate that the rate of metabolic hydroxylation of CCNU exceeds the rate of chemical dissociation (Walker et al., 1976) and that as a result it is probable that hydroxylated metabolites are the immediate precursors of the therapeutic and toxic moieties. Metabolism of CCNU produces compounds in which the chemical properties of the parent compound are significantly modified. Wheeler et al. (1977) have shown that all of the hydroxylated derivatives of CCNU are more water soluble, have higher alkylating activities, and in some cases have lower carbamoylating activities than CCNU.

III. MECHANISM OF ACTION

A. Alkylation

The relative alkylating activities of the nitrosoureas have been estimated in reactions with 4-(p-nitrobenzyl) pyridine (NBP) (Wheeler et al., 1974). There is an inverse linear relationship between the relative alkylating activity of each analogue and its respective chemical half-life (Panasci et al., 1977a, b). In addition, we have found an inverse linear correlation between the molar LD10 dose in mice and alkylating activity. However, there is no statistical relationship with the degree of bone marrow toxicity and relative alkylating activity in this species (Panasci et al., 1977a). Alkylation is widely accepted as the principal mechanism of nitrosourea antitumor activity. Cheng et al. (1972) and Schmall et al. (1973) have shown that the chloroethyl group of CCNU binds to nucleic acid and proteins, whereas the cyclohexyl group was extensively and almost exclusively bound to protein. We have recently confirmed these data in studies in which L1210 cells were incubated with radiolabeled CCNU and chlorozotocin. The degree of covalent binding of the respective chloroethyl groups to DNA was approximately proportional to their relative alkylating activities.

Ludlum et al. (1975) have reacted BCNU with the polynucleotides poly C, poly G, poly A, and poly U and were able to isolate several derivative nucleotides, including 3-(B-hydroxyethyl)CMP, 3, N⁴-ethano-CMP and 7-(B-hydroxyethly)CMP. Hilton et al. (1977) have shown that CCNU produces a concentration and time-dependent damage to L1210 DNA that is expressed as single-strand breaks on exposure to alkali. These studies have also suggested that the rate and extent of repair after CCNU alkylation is slow and incomplete when compared to the rapid repair following X-irradiation damage. Recently, Kohn (1977) has proposed that the single alkylating function of the chloroethyl nitrosoureas can cross-link DNA as determined by inhibition of alkali-induced strand separation. The reaction occurs in two steps, the initial chloroethylation of a nucleophilic site on the first strand, followed by the gradual displacement of Cl^- by a nucleophilic site on the opposite strand, resulting in an ethyl bridge.

B. Carbamoylation

A number of investigators have suggested an important biological role for the carbamoylating activity of isocyanates generated on decomposition of a nitrosourea. The contribution of carbamoylation to antitumor activity of toxicity has been largely inferred from *in vitro* studies. Among such reports the clinically active nitrosoureas BCNU, CCNU, and methyl-CCNU and their respective isocyanates have been shown to inhibit rat liver (Baril *et al.*, 1975) and human leukemia (Chuang *et al.*, 1976) DNA polymerase II. A reduction of nucleolar RNA processing by organic isocyanates has been reported by Kann and coworkers (1974a) and cyclohexyl isocyanates generated by CCNU were shown to bind to the lysine-rich H-1 histone fraction of L1210 cells (Woolley *et al.*, 1976). The demonstration that isocyanates can inhibit the repair of X-irradiation damage to DNA (Kann *et al.*, 1974b) is particularly important, since inhibition of repair processes could enhance the therapeutic effect of drugs causing alkylation damage but may also increase their carcinogenic potential and toxicity to normal tissues. We have investigated the effect of carbamoylating acitvity on the repair of DNA alkylation damage produced by the nitrosoureas themselves (Heal *et al.*, 1979). Two methylnitrosoureas were studied, streptozotocin—in which the cytotoxic moiety is attached to the C-2 position of a glucose carrier—and GNU, a C-1 substituted analogue. Streptozotocin has similar alkylating activity (100%) to GNU (92%), a comparable half-life, but widely differing carbamoylating activity (3% versus 42% for GNU). There was no statistical difference in the frequency of single-strand breaks produced in L1210 cells after a 2-hr exposure to a 0.5-cm concentration of either drug. After incubation with streptozotocin, full repair of these lesions was documented 8 hr after drug removal. In contrast, the repair of GNU-induced damage was not complete for 12 hr. The cytotoxicity of the two drugs for L1210 cells both *in vitro* using a colony cloning assay and *in vivo* in mice was not statistically different. Thus, although the carbamoylating activity of GNU can be correlated *in vitro* with a delay in repair of single-strand breaks, the antitumor activity of this drug both *in vitro* and *in vivo* is not significantly increased by either the carbamoylating activity or the delay in repair of alkylated lesions. Other reports have also questioned whether the *in vitro* effects of carbamoylation contribute significantly to nitrosourea cytotoxicity *in vivo*. Wheeler and Bowdon (1974) found that incubation of BCNU with intact L1210 cells reduced the total DNA ploymerase activity in cell free extracts of these cells. However, administration of BCNU to mice bearing L1210 in either the ascitic or solid tumor form did not alter the total DNA polymerase activity measured in tumor extracts (Wheeler and Bowdon, 1974). A prolongation of S phase in L1210 cells by cyclohexyl isocyanates has been demonstrated, but this was not associated with any antitumor activity in mice bearing L1210 cells (Bray *et al.*, 1971). Similarly, in an analysis of the biological effects of 17 nitrosoureas in mice, Wheeler found no correlation of carbamoylating activity with antitumor activity but suggested that it might play a role in toxicity *in vivo* (Wheeler *et al.*, 1974).

We have conducted a series of structure-activity analyses of methyl and chloroethyl nitrosoureas in an attempt to define a biological correlate for carbamoylation activity. Linear regression analyses of carbamoylating activity with lethal toxicity, granulocyte suppression, and antitumor activity failed to demonstrate a significant correlation (Panasci *et al.*, 1977a,b). The excellent antitumor activity of chlorozotocin, despite its negligible carbamoylating activity, suggests that this chemical reaction is not a major factor in antitumor activity.

IV. CLINICAL USE

The initial phase I trial of BCNU, conducted in 1962, demonstrated clinical activity in lymphomas. Unfortunately, the problem of delayed and cumulative bone marrow toxicity was not appreciated in animal toxicology studies, and the original schedule of frequent drug administration produced serious and lethal toxicity. In recognition of this inherent treatment-limiting toxicity, recently designed studies have employed intermittent schedules of treatment, to allow for full bone marrow recovery between each course. This represents an important limitation of this class of agents, which prevents the use of intensive courses and complicates the design of drug combinations. The most commonly employed dose schedules for the chloroethylnitrosoureas, when used as single agents, in previously untreated patients, include the following: BCNU, 150–200 mg/m² intravenously every 6–8 weeks; CCNU, 100–130 mg/m² orally every 6–8 weeks; methyl-CCNU, 150–200 mg/m² orally every 6–8 weeks (Wasserman *et al.*, 1975).

The chloroethylnitrosoureas have been demonstrated to possess a broad spectrum of activity against human malignancies. The major indications include gliomas, lymphoproliferative diseases, small cell carcinomas of the lung, melanoma, and gastrointestinal cancer (Wasserman *et al.*, 1975).

The use of nitrosoureas for gliomas represents an attempt to exploit the lipid solubility of most members of this class of antitumor agent. The reported response rates for BCNU and CCNU are 45% and 37%, respectively, whereas methyl-CCNU, at 23%, appears to be less active (Wasserman *et al.*, 1975). The Brain Tumor Study Group has carried out an important controlled randomized trial of nitrosourea chemotherapy for patients with glioblastoma who had undergone a "definitive" surgical resection (Walker and Gehan, 1976). Patients were randomized to receive one of four postoperative treatment options: (1) BCNU, 80 mg/m^2 per day on three successive days every 6–8 weeks; (2) radiation therapy (5000–6000 rads over 6–8 weeks); (3) a combination of BCNU plus radiation therapy; (4) best conventional care. An analysis of survival data for patients who received at least 5000 rads of irradiation or two courses of BCNU revealed the following: the median survival for conventional care was 17 weeks; this was contrasted with a 25-week median for BCNU, 37.5 weeks for radiation therapy, and 40.5 weeks for the combination. All forms of active therapy, including BCNU alone, provided a statistically better survival than conventional postoperative care. The difference between radiation therapy and the combined modality approach, however, is not significant. The survival at 18 months of followings for radiation therapy was 9% versus 18% for BCNU plus irradiation, a marginal improvement but achievement without appreciable additive toxicity (Walker and Gehan, 1976).

The principal indication for nitrosourea therapy in lymphoproliferative disorders is Hodgkin's disease. Five independent clinical trials of BCNU chemotherapy, following relapse from previous therapy, have shown an overall objective response rate of 47%, with a range of 34–55% (Anderson *et al.*, 1976; Selawry and Hansen, 1972). Responses usually occur early, within 2 weeks, and with a median duration of 4 months. The Cancer and Acute Leukemia Group B (CALGB) has tested the activity of three chloroethylnitrosoureas in patients with advanced previously treated Hodgkin's disease (Selawry and Hansen, 1972). In the initial trial BCNU, 200 mg/m^2, was compared with CCNU, 100 mg/m^2; the latter drug produced a 69% objective response, which was superior to that achieved with BCNU, 36% ($P = 0.02$). Methyl-CCNU proved inferior to CCNU in a subsequent clinical trial, having produced only a 15% response compared to one of 42% for CCNU.

The CALGB subsequently initiated a comparative trial of four regimens of combination chemotherapy for stage IIIB and IV disease, with substitutions of CCNU for the standard alkylating agent, nitrogen mustard, vinblastine, procarbazine, and prednisone (MVPP); CCNU, vinblastine, procarbazine, and prednisone (CCNU-VPP). The CCNU-containing combinations have produced complete remission rates that are either equivalent to MOPP or superior to it; this included patients without prior therapy as well as those with stage IIIA disease having relapsed after primary radiation therapy. In addition, the CCNU-containing programs have resulted in a significantly longer duration of complete remission. It is apparent that the nitrosoureas have an established role in the treatment of advanced Hodgkin's disease.

The National Cancer Institute has used BCNU as a maintenance therapy following induction of complete remission with the MOPP combination (Anderson *et al.*, 1976). Although BCNU appeared to delay the time to relapse (mean of 26 months versus 6 months for control), there was no significant effect following a two-year period of followup. The use of BCNU maintenance, 200 mg/m^2 every 3 months for 15 months, resulted in a higher incidence of serious complications and, in particular, bacterial infections. The results of this study do not support a role for nitrosourea maintenance chemotherapy for Hodgkin's disease.

The nitrosoureas have single-agent activity for lung cancer, specifically small-cell carcinomas of the lung; remission rates of 13–20% have been reported for CCNU and BCNU (Selawry and Hansen, 1972). These agents have been employed in many combination chemotherapy programs, notably the NCI-VA Medical Oncology Branch Study, where CCNU has been combined with cyclophosphamide and methotrexate, CMC (Cohen *et al.*, 1977). This regimen is reported to produce a 96% response, with 30% complete regressions, for a patient population with predominantly extensive disease. The median survival of this high-dose regimen is 10.5 months for all patients, and in excess of 20 months for cases that achieved a complete remission (range 13–48+ months) (Cohen *et al.*, 1977). One of the rationales for the incorporation of a lipid-soluble nitrosourea in a drug combination for small-cell carcinoma has been an attempt to prevent central nervous system relapse. The overall incidence of brain, spinal cord, or meninges involvement by small-cell carcinoma is estimated to be 40%, and as high as 60% in some series. Clinical trials employing nitrosoureas, without the addition of prophylactic cranial radiation, have clearly demonstrated that these agents make no impact on the incidence of CNS metastases (Bunn *et al.*, 1978).

All three chloroethylnitrosoureas have demonstrated single-agent activity for melanoma. The reported objective response rates of 12–26% are comparable to the activity of DTIC in this disease; and none of the nitrosoureas present a distinct advantage. Attempts to increase response rates by combining nitrosoureas with DTIC, vincristine, or cyclophosphamide have not been successful to date.

The nitrosoureas have been actively employed in the treatment of advanced gastrointestinal cancer. They have demonstrated only modest activity as single agents, with response rates of 8–18% in gastric cancer, 0–9% in pancreatic cancer, and 9–13% in advanced colorectal carcinoma (Wasserman *et al.*, 1975). Nevertheless combinations of nitrosoureas with 5-fluorouracil have in some studies resulted in response rates that were better than that achieved with either drug used alone. Kovach *et al.* (1974) have reported a 40% objective response with 5-fluorouracil (5-FU) plus BCNU in patients with advanced gastric cancer, with a significant improvement in survival at the 18-month period of followup. A trial of 5-FU plus methyl-CCNU conducted by the Eastern Cooperative Oncology Group has produced a similar response rate (Douglass *et al.*, 1976). Adriamycin, a drug with relatively high activity for gastric cancer, has now been successfully added to this regimen in studies conducted by the Gastrointestinal Tumor Study Group. A 33% response was recorded for patients with advanced pancreatic cancer treated with 5-FU plus BCNU, but without an apparent impact on survival (Kovach *et al.*, 1974). There had been great enthusiasm for the combination of 5-FU, methyl-CCNU, and vincristine for advanced colorectal cancer following the report of a 43% response rate in the initial controlled trial conducted at the Mayo Clinic (Moertel *et al.*, 1975). While two other randomized trials have confirmed the increased activity of this regimen, compared to 5-FU (Baker *et al.*, 1976), many studies have failed (Engstrom *et al.*, 1978). The current response rate for the 5-FU, methyl-CCNU, vincristine regimen at the Mayo Clinic has dropped to 27%. The role of methyl-CCNU for the treatment of colorectal cancer remains undecided at present. The current controlled trials of 5-FU plus methyl-CCNU as an adjuvant therapy for Dukes B_2 and C colon cancer will, it is hoped, produce a definitive answer within the next 2 years.

V. CLINICAL TOXICITIES

The clinical toxicity of the chloroethylnitrosoureas has been carefully analyzed (Wasserman *et al.*, 1975). Gastrointestinal toxicity in the form of nausea and vomiting is common to all agents, and occurs approximately 2–4 hr after administration. It can be partially controlled with antiemetics and is usually of short duration.

The most serious common toxicity is bone marrow depression, with nadir platelet and white blood counts occurring 4–5 weeks after single, drug doses, requiring 1–2 weeks for recovery. For the majority of patients, thrombocytopenia predominates. After repeated courses of treatment there is evidence of cumulative toxicity, and a resultant state of chronic bone marrow hypoplasia. Ancedoctal reports of presumed drug-related acute myelogenous leukemia have begun to appear in the literature, but at present carcinogenesis does not appear to be a clinically important problem.

Pulmonary fibrosis has been reported by several investigators, which resembles the syndrome produced by busulfan and cyclophosphamide. Hepatic toxicity has rarely been a clinically important problem. Recently, renal toxicity has been reported in some patients who have received nitrosoureas for periods of 18 months and longer. BCNU may cause burning and phlebitis at the injection site and occasionally will produce conjunctional flushing.

The chemotherapeutic agent most actively employed for the treatment of malignant islet cell tumors is streptozotocin, a naturally occurring methyl nitrosourea isolated from the fermentation cultures of Streptomyces achromogenes. A single dose of this compound in rodents, dogs, and monkeys is capable of producing a permanent diabetic state, an action mediated through the selective destruction of the pancreatic beta cell. Biochemically, the acute diabetogenic activity of streptozotocin has been related to the drug's ability to be selective uptake into islets and its ability to depress the concentrations of pyridine nucleotides, NAD, and NADH; this activity can be prevented in animals with pharmacological doses of nicotinamide (Schein, 1967) (Schein et al., 1973b) (Panasci et al., 1979).

In our series of 12 patients with metastatic islet cell carcinoma, treated with streptozotocin as a single agent, three patients acheived a complete clinical disappearance of tumor and hormone production. This included a patient with advanced malignant insulinoma who evidenced an objective response for one year after a single intravenous course at a daily dose of 500 mg/m^2 for five consecutive days (Schein et al., 1973b). Two patients with "pancreatic cholera" and islet cell carcinoma achieved a complete or near complete response to treatment with intraarterial streptozotocin (Kahn et al., 1975). Before therapy they had stool volumes from 2 to 8 liters per day and required 200–300 meq per day of supplemental potassium. After three to five doses of streptozotocin, 1.5 g/m^2 at weekly intervals, both stool volume and number and size of hepatic metastases decreased markedly. Partial remissions, averaging four months in duration, have been demonstrated in three additional patients with tumors that produced insulin, gastrin, or serotonin. Our results are in general agreement with data compiled by the Cancer Therapy Evaluation Branch of the National Cancer Institute, which analyzed the records of 52 patients treated with streptozotocin (Broder and Carter, 1973). In patients with functioning tumors, 60% were reported to have experienced a lessening in severity of hypoglycemia or hyperinsulinemia, and in 26% these hormonal parameters returned to normal levels. Three patients in whom the tumor was secreting multiple hormones, insulin, and gastrin, in addition to glucagon in one, have responded. Objective reduction of tumor mass had been reported in 48% of patients with functioning tumor; 17% were considered to have obtained a complete remission. Five of eight patients with islet cell carcinoma without demonstrable hormone secretion also had a reduction in tumor size. The median duration of objective remission was approximately one year. The median survival of patients who have responded to streptozotocin was 4.5 years compared to 1.5 years for nonresponders. The latter figure is similar to the median survival recorded prior to the advent of specific chemotherapy. Although streptozotocin is quite specific for the beta cell of the animal islet, it is of interest that this drug has proved an effective therapy for patients with non-beta-cell neoplasms. In addition to our cases with "pancreatic cholera" and serotonin secretion, there have been series of patients with pure gastrin-secreting (Zollinger-Ellison) non-beta-cell carcinomas that have similarly responded to treatment with streptozotocin.

The toxicity of streptozotocin is largely confined to acute nausea and vomiting, which occurs within hours after administration, and renal tubular damage (Schein et al., 1974). The later drug effect can be quite severe, resulting in a full Fanconilike syndrome and renal failure, which limits further treatment with this agent. It is of interest that the normal human beta cell appears to be resistant to the diabetogenic action of streptozotocin and only a rare case of overt diabetes has been reported. Of particular interest is the almost complete lack of bone marrow toxicity, in contrast to the severe depression in function produced by the chloroethylnitrosoureas. We have found that this drug can be safely and effectively administered intravenously at maximum weekly doses of 1.5 g/m^2, or a daily schedule of 0.5 g/m^2 for five consecutive days with courses repeated at 3–4-week intervals. The majority of remissions with streptozotocin have been reported after intravenous administration. However, there are several case reports of patients who, having failed to respond to intravenous streptozotocin, subsequently achieved an objective remission with intra-arterial treatment. Administration of the drug via the celiac axis does appear to offer the potential advantage of delivering high concentrations of drug to sites of disease while sparing the other peripheral tissues, in particular the kidney, the toxic effects of this agent. Because the intra-arterial route has not been proved to be more efficacious, intravenous administration still represents the standard method of drug delivery.

VI. DISCUSSION

What are the current directions in nitrosourea drug development? Structure-activity studies with the nonmyelosuppressive methylnitrosourea, streptozotocin, and its cytotoxic group MNU suggested that bone marrow toxicity could be reduced by attachment of the nitrosourea cytotoxic group to the carbon-2 position of glucose (Schein et al., 1978). To evaluate further the influence of the glucose carrier for the more active chloroethyl nitrosourea class, a new water-soluble compound, chlorozotocin, was synthesized for our studies by Johnston and co-workers. Chlorozotocin has alkylating activity that is two-fold greater than that produced by an equimolar concentration of BCNU but has negligible carbamoylating activity (Panasci et al., 1977b), probably the result of intramolecular carbamoylation. Using the L1210 leukemia model, chlorozotocin was demonstrated to have curative antitumor activity comparable to BCNU and CCNU at 50% of the molar dose. In addition, chlorozotocin was nonmyelosuppressive at the LD10 dose; this was confirmed by measurement of absolute peripheral neutrophil counts, bone marrow histology and DNA synthesis, and measurement of the marrow stem cells committed to granulocytomacrophage differentiation (CFU-C) (Schein *et al.*, 1976, 1978).

This relative bone-marrow-sparing property of chlorozotocin has now been confirmed clinically. During the phase I clinical trial of chlorozotocin, a dose of 120 mg/m² was demonstrated to be therapeutically active but did not produce myelopsuppressive toxicity in previously untreated cases or in patients who had less than six months of prior chemotherapy (Hoth *et al.*, 1978). Thrombocytopenia did occur at higher doses. In pharmacology studies, rapid intravenous administration of a 120 mg/m² dose of chlorozotocin produced a peak concentration in excess of 1×10^{-4} M, comparable to a 150 mg/m² dose of BCNU. After an initial distribution phase, the half-life of the prolonged phase of N-nitroso intact chlorozotocin was 7 min, compared to 9 min for BCNU. Both drugs remained at a concentration in excess of 1×10^{-5} M for a minimum of 10 min (Hoth *et al.*, 1978). It should be emphasized that at equimolar plasma concentrations, chlorozotocin has the potential of exposing the normal bone marrow, and the tumor, to twice the alkylating activity of BCNU. Nevertheless, chlorozotocin has been demonstrated to be significantly less myelosuppressive.

Seventy-one evaluable patients with advanced measurable malignancies have now been treated in an ongoing phase II trial utilizing 120 mg/m² I.V. every 6 weeks, with activity being demonstrated in melanoma and colon cancer as in the phase I study, patients with no prior therapy have not developed significant white blood cell platelet depression, and no cumulative toxicity has occurred with up to one year of treatment. If these data are confirmed in phase III trials, chlorozotocin may permit the use of intensive schedules of treatment that have heretofore proved impossible with existing nitrosourea agents.

REFERENCES

Anderson, T., DeVita, V. T., and Young, R. C. (1976). *Cancer Treat. Rep.* **60**, 761–767.
Baker, L. H., Vaitkevicius, V. K., and Gehan, E. (1976). *Cancer Treat. Rep.* **60**, 733–737.
Baril, B. E., Baril, E. F., Laszlo, J., and Wheeler, G. P. (1975). *Cancer Res.* **35**, 1–5.
Bray, D. F., DeVita, V. T., Adamson, R. H., and Oliverio, V. T. (1971). *Cancer Chemother. Rep.* **55**, 215–220.
Broder, L. E., and Carter, S. K. (1973). *Ann. Intern. Med.* **79**, 108.
Bunn, P. A., Nugent, J. L., and Matthews, M. J. (1978). *Semin. Oncol.* **5**, 314–322.
Cheng, C. J., Fujimura, S., Granberger, D., and Weinstein, I. B. (1972). *Cancer Res.* **32**, 22–27.
Chuang, R. Y., Laszlo, J., and Keller, P. (1976). *Biochim. Biophys. Acta* **425**, 453–468.
Cohen, M. H., Creaven, P. J., Fossieck, B. E., *et al.* (1977). *Cancer Treat. Rep.* **61**, 349–354.
Colvin, M., Brundhett, R. B., Cowens, W., Jardin, I., and Ludlum, D. B. (1976). *Biochem. Pharmacol.* **25**, 695–699.
Douglass, H. O., Lavin, P. T., and Moertel, C. G. (1976). *Cancer Treat. Rep.* **60**, 769–780.
Emmanuel, N. M., Vermel, E. M., Ostrovoskaga, L. A., and Korman, N. P. (1974). *Cancer Chemother. Rep.* **48**, 135–148.
Engstrom, P. F., MacIntyre, J., Douglass, H., and Carbone, P. C. (1978). *Proc. Am. Soc. Clin. Oncol.* **19**, 384.

Heal, J. M., Fox, P. A., and Schein, P. S. (1979). *Cancer Res.* **39,** 82-89.
Hilton, J., Bowie, D. L., Gutin, P. H., Zito, D. M., and Walker, M. D. (1977). *Cancer Res.* **37,** 2262-2266.
Hoth, D., Woolley, P., Green, D., Macdonald, J., and Schein, P. S. (1978). *Clin. Pharmacol. Ther.* **23,** 702-722.
Hyde, K. A., Acton, E., Skinner, W. A., Goodman, L., Greenberg, J., and Baker, B. R. (1962). *J. Med. Pharm. Chem.* **5,** 1-14.
Kahn, R., Levy, A., Gardner, J., Gorden, P., and Schein, P. S. (1975). *N. Engl. J. Med.* **292,** 941-945.
Kann, H. E., Kohn, K. W., and Lyles, J. M. (1974a). *Cancer Res.* **34,** 398-402.
Kann, H. E., Kohn, K. W., Widerlite, L., and Gullion, A. (1974b). *Cancer Res.* **34,** 1982-1988.
Kohn, K. W. (1977). *Cancer Res.* **37,** 1450-1454.
Kovach, J. S., Moertel, C. G., Schutt, A. J., Hahn, R. G., and Reitemeier, R. J. (1974). *Cancer (Philadelphia)* **33,** 563-567.
Ludlum, D. B., Kramer, B. S., Wang, J., and Fenselau, C. (1975). *Biochemistry* **14,** 5480-5485.
Moertel, C. G., Schutt, A. J., Hahn, R. G., and Reitemeier, R. J. (1975). *J. Natl. Cancer Inst.* **54,** 69-71.
Montgomery, J. A., James, R., McCaleb, G. S., Kirk, M. C., and Johnston, T. P. (1975). *J. Med. Chem.* **18,** 568-571.
Panasci, L. C., Fox, P. A., and Schein, P. S. (1977a). *Cancer Res.* **37,** 3321-3328.
Panasci, L. C., Green, D., Nagourney, R., Fox, P., and Schein, P. S. (1977b). *Cancer Res.* **37,** 2615-2618.
Panasci, L. C., Green, D., and Schein, P. S. (1979). *J. Clin. Investigation.*
Reed, D. J., and May, H. E. (1975). *Life Sci.* **16,** 1263-1270.
Schabel, F. M., Jr., Johnston, T. P., McCaleb, G. S., Montgomery, J. A., Laster W. R., and Skipper, H. E. (1963). *Cancer Res.* **23,** 725-733.
Schein, P. S., Cooney, D. A., and Vernon, M. L. (1967). *Cancer Res.* **27,** 2324-2332.
Schein, P. S., Cooney, D. A., McMenamin, M. G., and Anderson, T. (1973a). *Biochem. Pharmacol.* **22,** 2625-2631.
Schein, P. S., Kahn, R., Gorden, P., Wells, S., and DeVita, V. T. (1973b). *Arch. Intern. Med.* **132,** 555.
Schein, P. S., O'Connell, Blom, J., Hubbard, S., Magrath, I. T., Bergevin, P., Wiernik, P. H., Ziegler, J. L., and DeVita, V. T. (1974). *Cancer* **34,** 993-1000.
Schein, P. S., Panasci, L., Woolley, P. V., and Anderson, T. (1976). *Cancer Treat. Rep.* **60,** 801-805.
Schein, P. S., Bull, J. M., Doukas, D., and Hoth, D. (1978). *Cancer Res.* **38,** 257-260.
Schmall, B., Cheng, C. J., Fukimara, S., Gersten, N., Grunberger, D., and Weinstein, I. B. (1973). *Cancer Res.* **33,** 1921-1924.
Skipper, H. E., Schabel, F. M., Jr., Trader, M. W., Thomson, J. R. (1961). *Cancer Res.* **21,** 1154-1164.
Smulson, M. E., Schein, P. S., Mullins, G. W., and Sudhakar, S. (1977). *Cancer Res.* **37,** 3006-3012.
Walker, M. D., and Gehan, E. A. (1976). *Cancer Treat. Rep.* **60,** 713-716.
Walker, M. D., and Hilton, J. (1976). *Cancer Treat. Rep.* **60,** 725-728.
Wasserman, T. H., Slavik, M., and Carter, S. K. (1975). *Cancer (Philadelphia)* **36,** 1258-1268.
Wheeler, G. P., and Bowdon, B. J. (1968). *Cancer Res.* **28,** 52-59.
Wheeler, G. P., Bowdon, B. J., Grimsley, J., and Lloyd, H. H. (1974). *Cancer Res.* **34,** 194-200.
Wheeler, G. P., Johnston, T. P., Bowdon, B. J., McCaleb, G. S., Hill, D. L., and Montgomery, J. A. (1977). *Biochem. Pharmacol.* **26,** 2331-2336.
Woolley, P. V., Dion, R. L., Kohn, K. W., and Bono, V. H. (1976). *Cancer Res.* **36,** 1470-1474.

4

MITOMYCIN C—AN OVERVIEW
Stanley T. Crooke

I. INTRODUCTION

Mitomycin C is an antitumor antibiotic isolated from *Streptomyces caespitosus* in 1958 (Wakaki *et al.*, 1958). Although a review of the Japanese literature on mitomycin C in 1960 suggested that it was an active agent (Frank and Osterberg, 1960), the initial experience in the United States was quite poor (Jones, 1959). The initial clinical trials in the United States employed a series of dosage schedules and were characterized by serious myelosuppression and responses of very brief duration (Crooke and Bradner, 1976). Not until 1974, when the potential for Mitomycin C to induce delayed cumulative myelosuppression was adequately recognized, were more rational dose schedules developed (Baker *et al.*, 1974). Subsequently, although still highly toxic, and capable apparently of inducing only short-term remissions, mitomycin C has proved of increasing value in the treatment of various malignant diseases.

CANCER AND CHEMOTHERAPY, VOL. III

II. CHEMISTRY

Mitomycin C is isolated from *Streptomyces caespitosus* as blue-violet crystals (Wakaki *et al.*, 1958). It is closely related to mitomycin A and B and porfiromycin (Webb *et al.*, 1962). It has been purified by elution from an alumina column with hot methanol. It has a melting point greater than 300°C. In crystalline form, mitomycin C is stable for 4 hr at 100°C, but in solution it is less stable. It is soluble in water and organic solvents and when mixed with water forms a blue to gray solution. In solution it is inactivated by visible light, but not by ultraviolet light. It has a molecular weight of 334. The structures of mitomycin and porfiromycin are shown in Fig. 1 (Carter, 1968; Stevens *et al.*, 1965).

III. STRUCTURE–ACTIVITY RELATIONSHIPS

Mitomycin C is an alkylating agent (Phillips *et al.*, 1960; Schwartz, *et al.*, 1963). It has three potentially active groups—a quinone, a urethane, and an aziridine group—but requires activation by reduction of the quinone and subsequent loss of the methoxy group. A second alkylating group is probably developed at C-10, and a third is possibly at C-7. Figures 2 and 3 show the schema suggested by Iyer and Szybalski (1963, 1964). The proposed activation is rapid and the active intermediates are unstable; therefore DNA must be present during the reduction. Activation *in vivo* is NADPH dependent but can be performed in a cell-free system using isolated DNA and sodium hydrosulfite. When activated, mitomycin C is a bifunctional or trifunctional alkylating agent. Unlike the reactions proposed by Iyer and Szybalski, more recent studies have suggested that the hydroquinone mitomycin C intermediate is converted to another quinone by the loss of the carbamate and aziridine groups (Moore, 1977; Rao *et al.*, 1977; Bachur *et al.*, 1977).

Many structural analogues of mitomycin C have been synthesized in an effort to improve the therapeutic ratio. In general, these efforts have failed and, based on tumor screening methods, mitomycin C and porfiromycin are still considered the optimal members of this group. Certain generalizations can, however, be derived from these studies. These are

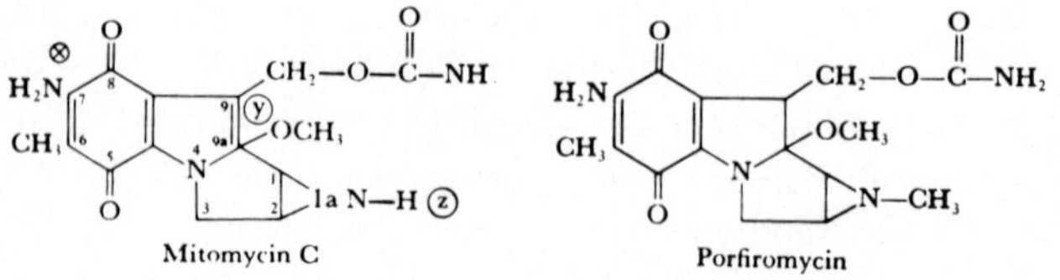

Mitomycin C   Porfiromycin

Fig. 1.   Structures of mitomycin and porfiromycin.

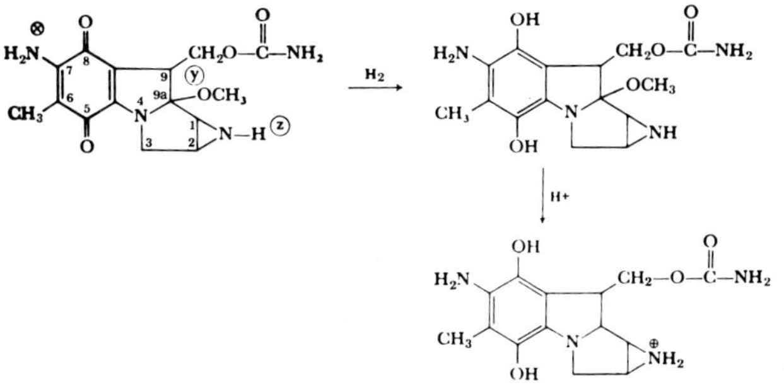

Fig. 2. Activation of aziridine ring.

(1) the aziridine ring is not essential for antibacterial activity, but is for antineoplastic activity,

(2) low quinone reduction potential enhances activity,

(3) increasing water solubility and decreasing lipophilic property results in enhanced antitumor activity,

(4) decreased binding to proteins results in increased activity,

(5) substitutions on positions x, y, or z have significant effects on activity (Fig. 1).

More recently a number of new analogues that are bifunctional alkylating agents, with low quinone reduction potential and relatively high lipophilicity, have been prepared. There are suggestions that some of these analogues and others may prove to be less myelosuppressant than mitomycin C (Remers, 1979).

IV. MOLECULAR PHARMACOLOGY

When activated, mitomycin C is an alkylating agent. Alkylation appears to occur preferentially at the O–6 position, and not the N–7 position of guanosine (Tomasz *et al.*, 1974; Lown *et al.*, 1976). Alkylation has been shown to increase as the pH decreases. Additionally, mitomycin C has been shown to produce cross-links in DNA, and this also occurs more rapidly at lower pH's (Iyer and Szybalski, 1963, 1964; Lown, 1979). Both processes have been shown to occur more extensively as the guanosine and cytosine content increases in the DNA (Goldberg, 1965).

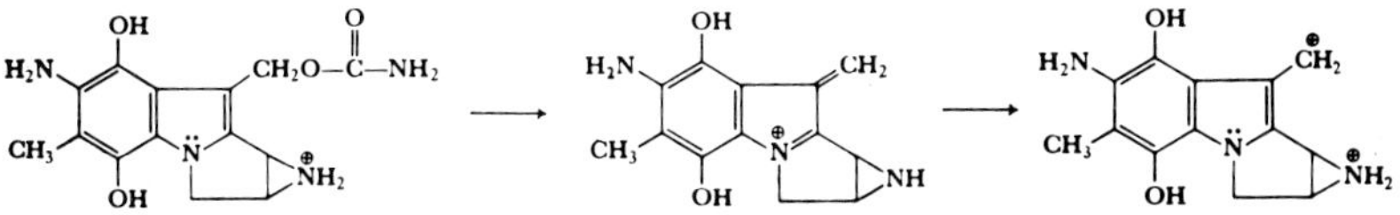

Fig. 3. Activation of C-10.

Mitomycin C has also been shown to degrade isolated purified DNA and intracellular DNA (Reich *et al.*, 1961; Wakaki, 1961). Although intracellular DNA degradation was initially ascribed to activation of exonucleases, more recently mitomycin C was shown to inhibit nuclease degradation of DNA (Goodman *et al.*, 1974) and to degrade DNA directly. The proposed mechanism involves the generation of free radicals and is shown in Fig. 4 (Lown, 1979). However, the importance of DNA degradation relative to alkylation and cross-linking in the mechanism of action of mitomycin C remains to be determined.

The most significant effect of the interactions of mitomycin C with DNA is the inhibition of *de novo* DNA synthesis (Reich *et al.*, 1961). Interestingly, repair DNA synthesis is apparently not inhibited by mitomycin C (Rauth *et al.*, 1970). Other effects such as inhibition of RNA synthesis have been shown to require much higher concentrations of mitomycin C. Moreover, it does not appear to affect DNA polymerase activity of nucleotide pools (Bach and Magee, 1962; Rauth *et al.*, 1970).

Morphologic manifestations of mitomycin C include nucleolar aberrations,

Proposed chemical mechanism of DNA degradation by reduced Mitomycin C

$$M + NADPH \xrightarrow{H^+} MH_2 + NADP^+ \qquad 1$$

$$MH_2 + O_2 \longrightarrow MH^{\cdot} + HO_2^{\cdot} \qquad 2$$

$$HO_2^{\cdot} \rightleftharpoons H^+ + O_2^{\cdot} \qquad 3$$

$$2O_2^{\cdot} + 2H^+ \xrightarrow{SOD} H_2O_2 + O_2 \qquad 4$$

$$2H_2O_2 \xrightarrow{Catalase} 2H_2O + O_2 \qquad 5$$

$$H_2O_2 + O_2^{\cdot} \longrightarrow OH^{\cdot} + OH^- + O_2(^1\Delta g + ^3\Sigma g) \qquad 6$$

$$ATP.Fe^{3+} + O_2^{\cdot} \longrightarrow ATP.Fe^{2+} + O_2 \qquad 7$$

$$ATP.Fe^{2+} + H_2O_2 \longrightarrow ATP.Fe^{3+} + OH^{\cdot} + OH^- \qquad 8$$

$$OH^{\cdot} + DNA \longrightarrow Strand\ Breakage \qquad 9$$

M = Mitomycin C
SOD = Superoxide Dismutase

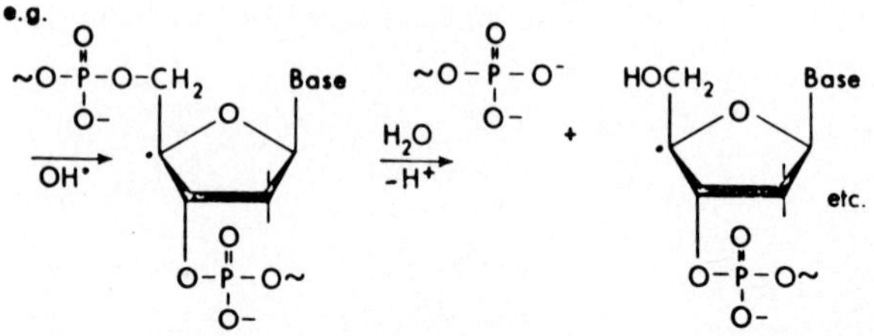

Fig. 4. Proposed chemical mechanisms of DNA degradation by reduced mitomycin C.

such as the formation of a compact configuration, segregation, and the induction of electron dense microspherules (Lapis and Bernhard, 1965; Daskal and Crooke, 1979). Two hours after incuation of cells with mitomycin C, ring-shaped nucleoli were observed, a phenomenon associated with complete inhibition of ribosomal RNA synthesis.

V. PHARMACOLOGY

Although mitomycin C is absorbed after oral administration, the dose required for activity and toxicity has been shown to be 3–12 times as large as an intraperitoneal dose in rodents (Bradner, 1968; Phillips *et al.*, 1960). Studies in human beings have shown that mitomycin C is absorbed erratically after oral administration. Peak serum concentrations of 0.4 μg/ml were associated with significant myelosuppression, but occurred at doses ranging from 22.5 to 45 mg/m^2, and it was concluded that absorption was too erratic to allow mitomycin C to be used orally (Crooke *et al.*, 1976). Mitomycin C is also absorbed after intraperitoneal and intrapleural administration but is not absorbed after intravesical administration of doses as high as 60 mg (Phillips *et al.*, 1960; Crooke *et al.*, 1978). Very little information is available concerning the distribution, metabolism, and elimination of mitomycin C in humans. The paucity of information is primarily due to the lack of a sensitive reproducible assay, a microbiological assay being the only assay available. However, it is known that mitomycin C is fairly widely distributed in animals, and that it is rapidly cleared from the serum. It has been reported that the rate of clearance is inversely proportional to the peak serum concentration, suggesting nonlinear pharmacokinetics (Fujita, 1971). Urinary excretion was shown to be due to glomerular filtration, but to be too small to account for the rapid serum clearance of mitomycin C. Moreover, the percentage of a dose recovered in the urine increased with increasing doses, suggesting that metabolism is the primary route of clearance and that the metabolic systems are relatively saturable (Fujita, 1971).

The metabolism of mitomycin C is important in two respects. It is activated enzymatically (it undergoes "lethal synthesis"), and it is inactivated enzymatically. That *in vivo* activation is necessary was shown by the lack of activity *in vitro* in the absence of appropriate reducing substances (Fujita, 1971). *In vivo* the activity of mitomycin C is dependent on a reducing system utilizing NADPH but does not require ATP, nicotinamide, or Mg^{2+}, localized to the micorsomal fraction and inhibited by oxygen. A second system that is less active and requires ATP and Mg^{2+} has also been described (Schwartz, 1962). It was subsequently suggested that *in vivo* activation by reduction was related to "unmasking" the fused aziridine ring (Schwartz *et al.*, 1963). The chemical scheme of activation, reproduced in the section on structure–activity relationships, is compatible with these observations.

Several tissues from man and dog have been shown to inactivate mitomycin C. Liver, spleen, kidney, brain, and heart were shown to be most active, and the inactivation was more rapid in anaerobic conditions. Homogenates of tumors sensitive to mitomycin C were less effective inactivators of mitomycin than homogenates of tumors insensitive to the drug (Fujita, 1971; Schwartz, 1962).

VI. CLINICAL EFFECTS

A. Dosage Schedules

Initial clinical trials used daily dose schedules. The first suggestion that an intermittent schedule might have therapeutic advantages was based on studies in mice with Ehrlich ascites tumors that showed that intermittent therapy was more effective, at equivalent levels of toxicity, than daily administration (Hata et al., 1961; Sokoloff et al., 1959, 1960). In mice with L1210 leukemia the effectiveness of mitomycin C given every 2, 3, or 4 days was approximately equal to daily dosing, but if given every 7 days, it was markedly less effective (Kojima et al., 1972). These studies suggest that treatment scheduling may be important in terms of activity and toxicity and that the optimum schedule may vary, depending on the type and stage of the tumor being treated.

Clinical studies also suggested that intermittent therapy might be an improvement (Shimada et al., 1956). In 1964 a schedule of intermittent doses of 20–50 mg repeated at several-week intervals was compared to a schedule of daily doses and found to result in an equivalent response rate but in less hematopoietic toxicity (Kenis et al., 1964; Kenis and Stryckmans, 1972). In a study of 106 patients, an overall response rate of 22%, associated with significantly less hematopoietic toxicity than with other regimens (see Table I), was obtained using 50 mg in two divided doses over a 6-day period, followed by 20–30 mg repeated at 6-week intervals (Godfrey and Wilber, 1972). Bolus injections of either 20 or 22.5 mg/m^2 administered every 6–8 weeks have been studied. A 37% response rate and manageable but significant hematologic toxicity were reported. A dose of 20 mg/m^2 was found to be as effective as 22.5 mg/m^2 and probably less toxic. The data suggested that the severity of hematologic toxicity increased with increasing numbers of courses (Baker et al., 1974). One study in which mitomycin C was given weekly at 0.125 mg/kg to patients with a variety of malignancies has been reported. The response rate was 9.25% of 54 patients, and it was not felt that hematopoietic toxicities were significantly reduced (Hum et al., 1974).

The results of a study on a small number of children suggest that single doses of mitomycin C given intermittently may produce less hematopoietic toxicity than intermittent administration of 4–5-day courses. However, neither schedule produced a significant response rate and both were toxic (Sutow et al., 1971).

More recent studies employing mitomycin C as a single agent and in combinations have confirmed the advantages of the high-dose intermittent schedule. Thus, the preferred regimen for mitomycin C when given as a single agent is 20 mg/m² I.V. every 6–8 weeks. After two full courses, subsequent doses are usually reduced to 10 mg/m² (Baker and Vaitkevicius, 1979).

B. Toxicities

The most significant toxicity of mitomycin C is delayed, cumulative myelosuppression (Crooke and Bradner, 1976). The incidence and severity of myelosuppression are dose related. At a dose of 20 mg/m² every 6–8 weeks, approximately 50% or 70% of the patients treated experienced leukopenia or thrombocytopenia, respectively. The nadirs for platelets and leukocytes occur approximately 5–6 weeks after a dose, and recovery is usually observed within 2 weeks of the nadir. Anemia is frequent but usually not so severe as leukopenia or thrombocytopenia. Patients who have been exposed to prior myelosuppressant chemotherapy or radiotherapy to the pelvis experience more severe myelosuppression and should receive lower doses of mitomycin C (Crooke and Bradner, 1976).

Other toxicities include severe cellulitis at injection sites if extravasation occurs (Moertel et al., 1968) and gastrointestinal disturbances consisting of anorexia, ausea, vomiting, and diarrhea, which are usually mild (Carter, 1968; Crooke and Bradner, 1976). Alopecia, stomatitis, and rashes occur infrequently. Occasionally patients have experienced hepatic dysfunction concomitant with mitomycin C therapy (Barbier et al., 1968).

It has been suggested that mitomycin C is a pulmonary toxin. The low and unpredictable incidence, the difficulty in eliminating other possible causes, and the multiplicity of interdigitating factors result in uncertainty relative to the effects of mitomycin C on the lung. However, approximately 10 cases of pulmonary dysfunction associated with mitomycin C (Martino et al., 1979; Samson et al., 1978; Orowell et al., 1978) have been reported. In all cases pulmonary fibrosis was observed at autopsy and accompanied by vasculitis, hyperplasia, and evidence of inflammation; nonspecific phenomena associated with numerous pulmonary toxins. The presentation is typical of any toxin-inducing diffuse interstitial pneumonitis. No predisposing factors or dose–response relationships have been detected, nor is the incidence known. However, the current data suggest that, like other alkylating agents, mitomycin C may be pulmonary toxic.

Similarly, mitomycin C has been suggested to be nephrotoxic. Again, diagnostic difficulties, multiple other causes and exacerbating factors, and a low incidence have resulted in difficulties in determining the nature of this toxic potential. The clinical presentation reported is typical of progressive renal dysfunction and the pathologic lesions typical of acute tubular necrosis. Moreover, this toxicity appears to be total dose related, since the incidence of renal dysfunction was higher in patients who received doses of 100 mg or more. Thus it appears likely that nephrotoxicity is a chronic, total-dose-related toxicity associated with mitomycin C (Liu *et al.*, 1971; Ratanatharathorn *et al.*, 1979).

C. Clinical Antitumor Activity

As a single agent employed in a variety of dosage schedules, mitomycin C has demonstrated significant activity against a number of malignancies. Presented in Table I are data derived from an earlier review demonstrating that mitomycin C has demonstrated activity against several solid tumors, and it has also demonstrated activity against the leukemias (Crooke and Bradner, 1976). More recent studies employing high-dose intermittent therapy have shown that mitomycin C induces an approximate 25% response rate in patients with adenocarcinoma and large-cell carcinoma of the lung (Samson *et al.*, 1979), and it has also demonstrated activity against squamous cell carcinoma of the rectum (Buroker *et al.*, 1979).

Mitomycin C has also been shown to be active in various combinations. Some of the more interesting recent combinations have employed mitomycin C in combination with adriamycin and in some cases 5-fluorouracil. In these combinations mitomycin C is employed in attenuated doses (usually approximately 10 mg/m² every 8 weeks), and the dose of adriamycin is also reduced. Mitomycin C and adriamycin in combination have been reported to be active against adenocarcinoma of the lung and stomach as first-line therapy and in patients with breast cancer who have failed primary chemotherapy with non-adriamycin-containing regimens (Morgan, 1979; Comis *et al.*, 1979). Furthermore, similar results have

TABLE I

Comparison of Recent Results with Data of Moore
***et al.* (1968)**

Tumor site or type	Response rate %	
	Moore *et al.*	Recent data
Breast	35.7	33.3
Stomach	31.2	26.0
Colorectal	20.0	18.0
Lung	18.5	12.0
Head and neck	15.3	24.3
Melanoma	14.8	13.3

been reported with the 5-fluorouracil-containing regimens in gastric, pancreatic cancers and adenocarcinoma of the lung (Schein *et al.*, 1979; Panettiere and Heilbrun, 1979).

Another interesting new series of combinations is based on combining bleomycin with mitomycin C. This combination in which relatively low doses of both agents are employed sequentially (bleomycin 5 U daily days 1–7, then mitomycin C 10 mg on day 8) was reported to produce remissions in 90% of the patients studied with disseminated squamous cell carcinoma of the cervix (Miyamoto, 1979). Also reported to be active is a combination employing vincristine in addition to bleomycin and mitomycin C. In this study full doses of mitomycin C were employed with two other agents. The response rate varied, depending on the dosage schedule of bleomycin, but was greater than 40% for all arms of the study (Baker and Vaitkevicius, 1979).

In addition, very promising results have been reported when mitomycin C was administered intravesically for the treatment of recurrent superficial bladder cancers. Using a schedule of 20 mg three times weekly for 8 weeks, Mishina and Watanabe (1979) reported a 44% complete response rate in patients with superficial bladder cancers. In a phase I–II study performed in the United States, patients with recurrent superficial bladder cancers not amenable to surgical therapy have been treated with 20, 25, 30, or 40 mg instilled intravesically every week for 8 weeks. The results obtained for each dose are shown in Table II. In this study no systemic absorption, systemic toxicities, or significant local toxicities were observed. Moreover, complete remissions have proved to be quite prolonged and responses have been observed in patients who failed prior intravesical chemotherapy (Crooke *et al.*, 1978; Bracken and Johnson, 1979).

TABLE II

Response Rate by Dose of Mitomycin C

Dose (mg/wk)	No. patients eval/ent.	Patient response no. (%)	Complete response no. (%)	Response rate (% complete response + partial response)
20	15/15	3 (20)	5 (33)	53%
25	10/10	1 (10)	6 (60)	70%
30	8/15[a]	2 (25)	3 (38)	63%
40	5/5[a]	3 (60)	2 (40)	100%
Total	38/45[a]	9 (24)	16 (42)	66%

[a] To date.

VII. CONCLUSIONS

Mitomycin C is an antitumor antibiotic that has demonstrated a relatively broad spectrum of activity against a variety of malignancies. However, its utility is limited by the rapid emergence of resistance and severe myelotoxicity. With the development of the high-dose intermittent schedule of administration, mitomycin C has proved of greater value, and as a consequence a number of aspects of mitomycin C are currently undergoing extensive research.

REFERENCES

Bach, M. K., and Magee, W. E. (1962). *Fed. Proc. Fed. Am. Soc. Exp. Biol.* **21,** 463.
Bachur, N. R., Gordon S. L., and Gee, M. V. (1977). *Mol. Pharmacol.* **13,** 901–910.
Baker, L. H., and Vaitkevicius, V. K. (1979). *In* "Mytomycin C: Current Status and New Developments" (S. K. Carter and S. T. Crooke, eds.), pp. 77–82. Academic Press, New York.
Baker, L. H., Caoli, F. M., Izbicki, R. M., Opipari, M. I., and Vaitkevicius, V. F. (1974). *Proc. Am. Assoc. Cancer Res.* **15,** 182.
Barbier, R. J., Manester, J., and Jacobs, E. (1968). *Digestion* **1,** 229–232.
Bracken, R. B., and Johnson, D. E. (1979). *In* "Mitomycin C: Current Status and New Developments" (S. K. Carter and S. T. Crooke, eds.), pp. 205–211. Academic Press, New York.
Bradner, W. T. (1968). *Cancer Chemother. Rep.* **52,** 389–391.
Buroker, T., Nigro, N., Considine, B., and Vaitkevicius, V. K. (1979). *In* "Mitomycin C: Current Status and New Developments" (S. K. Carter and S. T. Crooke, eds.), pp. 183–188. Academic Press, New York.
Carter, S. K. (1968). *Cancer Chemother. Rep., Part 3* **1,** 99–114.
Comis, R. L., Ginsberg, S. J., and Crooke, S. T. (1979). *In* "Mitomycin C: Current Status and New Developments" (S. K. Carter and S. T. Crooke, eds.), pp. 83–89. Academic Press, New York.
Crooke, S. T., and Bradner, W. T. (1976). *Cancer Treat. Rev.* **3,** 97–115.
Crooke, S. T., Henderson, M., Samson, M., and Baker, L. H. (1976). *Cancer Treat. Rep.* **60,** 1633–1636.
Crooke, S. T., Johnson, D. E., and Bracken, R. B. (1978). *Proc. Am. Soc. Clin. Oncol.* **19,** 321.
Daskal, Y., and Crooke, S. T. (1979). *In* "Mitomycin C: Current Status and New Developments" (S. K. Carter and S. T. Crooke, eds.), pp. 41–60. Academic Press, New York.
Frank, W., and Osterberg, A. E. (1960). *Cancer Chemother. Rep.* **9,** 114–119.
Fujita, H. (1971). *Jpn. J. Clin. Oncol.* **12,** 151.
Godfrey, T. E., and Wilber, D. W. (1972). *Cancer (Philadelphia)* **29,** 1647–1652.
Goldberg, I. H. (1965). *Am. J. Med.* **39,** 722–752.
Goodman, M. F., Bessman, M. J., and Bachur, N. R. (1974). *Proc. Natl. Acad. Sci. U.S.A.* **71,** 1193–1196.
Hata, T., Hossenlopp, C., and Takita, H. (1961). *Cancer Chemother. Rep.* **13,** 67–77.
Hum, G. J., Bogdon, D. L., and Bateman, J. R. (1974). *Oncology* **30,** 236–243.
Iyer, V., and Szybalski, W. (1963). *Proc. Natl. Acad. Sci. U.S.A.* **50,** 355–362.
Iyer, V., and Szybalski, W. (1964). *Science* **145,** 55–58.
Jones, E. (1959). *Cancer Chemother. Rep.* **2,** 3–7.
Kenis, Y., and Stryckmans, P. (1972). *Cancer Chemother. Rep.* **56,** 151.

Kenis, Y., Stryckmans, P., and Leburn, J. (1964). *Proc. Int. Symp. Chemother. Cancer, New York,* pp. 182-196.

Kojima, R., Goldin, A., and Mantel, N. (1972). *Cancer Chemother. Rep., Part 2* **3,** 111-119.

Lapis, K., and Bernhard, W. (1965). *Cancer Res.* **25,** 628-643.

Liu, K., Mittelman, A., Sproal, E. E., and Elias, E. G. (1971). *Cancer (Philadelphia)* **28,** 1314-1320.

Lown, J. W. (1979). *In* "Mitomycin C: Current Status and New Developments" (S. K. Carter and S. T. Crooke, eds.), pp. 5-26. Academic Press, New York.

Lown, J. W., Begleiter, A., Johnson, D., and Morgan, A. R. (1976). *Can. J. Biochem.* **54,** 110-119.

Martino, S., Baker, L. H., Pollard, R. J., Correa, J. J., and DeMattia, M. D. (1979). *In* "Mitomycin C: Current Status and New Developments" (S. K. Carter and S. T. Crooke, eds.), pp. 231-242. Academic Press, New York.

Mishina, T., and Watanabe, H. (1979). *In* "Mitomycin C: Current Status and New Developments" (S. K. Carter and S. T. Crooke, eds.), pp. 193-203. Academic Press, New York.

Miyamoto, T. (1979). *In* "Mitomycin C: Current Status and New Developments" (S. K. Carter and S. T. Crooke, eds.), pp. 163-171. Academic Press, New York.

Moertel, C. G., Reitemier, R. J., and Hahn, R. G. (1968). *J. Am. Med. Assoc.* **204,** 1045-1048.

Moore, G. E., Bross, I. D. J., Ausman, R., Nadler, S., Jones, R., Slack, N., and Rimm, M. (1968). *Cancer Chemother. Rep.* **52,** 675-680.

Moore, H. W. (1977). *Science* **197,** 527-532.

Morgan, L. R. (1979). *In* "Mitomycin C: Current Status and New Developments" (S. K. Carter and S. T. Crooke, eds.), pp. 101-111. Academic Press, New York.

Orowell, E. S., Kiessling, P. J., and Patterson, J. R. (1978). *Ann. of Intern. Med.* **89,** 352-355.

Panettiere, F. J., and Heilbrun, L. (1979). *In* "Mitomycin C: Current Status and New Developments" (S. K. Carter and S. T. Crooke, eds.), pp. 145-157. Academic Press, New York.

Phillips, F. S., Schwartz, H. S., and Sternberg, S. S. (1960). *Cancer Res.* **20,** 1354-1361.

Rao, G. M., Lown, J. W., and Plambech, J. A. (1977). *J. Electrochem. Soc.* **124,** 195-198.

Ratanatharathorn, V., Baker, L. H., Cadnapaphornchai, P., and Rosenberg, B. F. (1979). *In* "Mitomycin C: Current Status and New Developments" (S. K. Carter and S. T. Crooke, eds.), pp. 219-229. Academic Press, New York.

Rauth, A. M., Barton, B., and Lee, C. P. Y. (1970). *Cancer Res.* **30,** 2724-2729.

Reich, E., Shatkin, A. J., and Tatum, L. (1961). *Biochim. Biophys. Acta* **53,** 132-149.

Remers, W. A. (1979). *In* "Mitomycin C: Current Status and New Developments" (S. K. Carter and S. T. Crooke, eds.), pp. 27-32. Academic Press, New York.

Samson, M. K., Comis, R. L., Baker, L. H., Ginsberg, S., Fraile, R. J., and Crooke, S. T. (1978). *Cancer Treat. Rep.* **62,** 163-165.

Samson, M. K., Fraile, R. J., Leichman, L. P., and Baker, L. H. (1979). *In* "Mitomycin C: Current Status and New Developments" (S. K. Carter and S. T. Crooke, eds.), pp. 121-127. Academic Press, New York.

Schein, P. S., Macdonald, J. S., Smith, F. P., Hoth, D. F., and Woolley, P. V. (1979). *In* "Mitomycin C: Current Status and New Developments" (S. K. Carter and S. T. Crooke, eds.), pp. 133-143. Academic Press, New York.

Schwartz, H. S. (1962). *J. Pharmacol. Exp. Ther.* **136,** 250-258.

Schwartz, H. S., Sedergren, J. E., and Phillips, F. S. (1963). *Science* **142,** 1181-1183.

Shimada, N., Ishii, R., Sato, Y., Toba, Q. J., Kuwana, K., Fukui, M., Noguchi, T., Kubouchi, K., and Takeishi, T. (1956). *Chemotherapy (Tokyo)* **4,** 305.

Sokoloff, B., Nakabayashi, K., Enomoto, K., Miller, T. R., Bicknell, A., Bird, L., Trauner, W., Niswonger, J., and Renninger, G. (1959). *Growth* **23,** 109-136.

Sokoloff, B., Fujisawa, M., Enomoto, K., Sadhof, C. C., Miller, T. R., McConnell, B., Nakabayashi, K., Renninger, G., and Trauner, W. (1960). *Growth* **24**, 1-27.

Stevens, C. L., Taylor, K. G., Munk, M. F., Marshall, W. S., Noll, K., Shah, G. D., Shah, L. G., and Uzu, K. (1965). *J. Med. Chem.* **8**, 1-10.

Sutow, W. W., Wilber, J. R., Viettia, T. J., Vuthibhagdee, P., and Watanabe, W. (1971). *Cancer Chemother. Rep.* **55**, 285-289.

Tomasz, M., Mercado, C. M., Olson, J., and Chatterjie, N. (1974). *Biochemistry* **13**, 4878-4887.

Wakaki, S. (1961). *Cancer Chemother. Rep.* **13**, 79-86.

Wakaki, S., Marumo, H., Tamioka, K., Shimizu, G., Kato, E., Kamada, H., Kudo, S., and Fujimoto, Y. (1958). *Antibiot. Chemother. (Washington, D.C.)* **8**, 228.

Webb, J. S., Cosulich, D. B., Mowat, J. H., Patrick, J. B., Broschard, R. W., Meyer, W. E., Williams, R. P., Wolf, C. F., Fulmor, W., and Pidacks, C. (1962). *J. Am. Chem. Soc.* **84**, 3185-3187.

5

OTHER ALKYLATING AGENTS
Steven D. Reich

I. INTRODUCTION

Alkylating agents with antitumor activity belong to a class of compounds that undergo chemical reactions leading to the addition by covalent bonding of organic carbon to biologically important molecules. The cytotoxicity of these agents under physiologic conditions was first reported in the late nineteenth century (Ross, 1974). Because of their vesicant action several alkylating agents were investigated, and sulfur mustard was developed as a poison gas that was used during World War I. In the 1930s sulfur mustard was shown to have antitumor activity in experimental animals and was employed clinically in the treatment of a solid tumor by direct injection into the tumor (Connors, 1975). However, toxicity was significant enough to forestall larger-scale clinical investigations. During the years prior to World War II, derivatives and analogues of sulfur mustard were synthesized and the nitrogen mustards were extensively studied. These agents were known to have suppressive effects on bone marrow and lymphoid tissue, and the suggestion was made that they might be effective therapy for disorders of white cells such as lymphoma and leukemia. Although clinical trials began in 1942 (Calabresi and Parks, 1975), secrecy restrictions prevented publication of results until after the war. Because temporary remissions were induced in patients with lymphosarcoma and Hodgkin's disease (Rhoads, 1946), the search was intensified for alkylating agents with antitumor activity that would not adversely affect normal proliferating tissues.

Several thousand alkylating agents have been synthesized or discovered. These agents can be divided into several classes, including 2-chloroethylamines, alkyl alkanesulfonates, aziridines, triazines, nitrosoureas, and epoxides (Fig. 2). Only a few of these compounds have reached clinical trials and even fewer are commercially available. Compounds belonging to the 2-chloroethylamine class are commonly known as the "classical alkylating agents" or as the "nitrogen mustards." Mechlorethamine (nitrogen mustard, NH_2, and Mustargen) is the

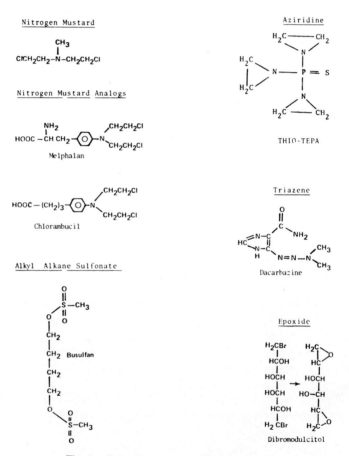

Fig. 1. Structures of selected alkylating agents.

parent compound for this group. Cyclophosphamide (Cytoxan, Endoxan) is a nitrogen mustard that was originally synthesized to be a tumor-specific alkylating agent. Although not tumor specific, cyclophosphamide has found a place in cancer chemotherapy because of its broad spectrum of action with tolerable toxicities and its stability in aqueous solutions. Because of the extensive literature on mechlorethamine and cyclophosphamide, these agents are often discussed separately from the other nitrogen mustards. The nitrosoureas are alkylating agents with several other mechanisms of action, so these compounds are often discussed as a group. Mitomycin C (mutamycin) is an alkylating agent belonging to the aziridine class. Because mitomycin C is a fermentation product produced by *Streptomyces caespitosus*, this drug is often classified as an antitumor antibiotic. Other alkylating agents are often "lumped together" and discussed under the heading of "Other Alkylating Agents." This heading includes chlorambucil (Leukeran) and melphalan (Alkeran, L-sarcolosyin, L-Phenylalanine mustard, L-PAM), which are nitrogen mustards; busulfan (Myleran), which is an alkyl alkanesulfonate; thio-TEPA (triethylenetriphosphoramide), which is an aziridine; and dacarbazine (DTIC-Dome, imidazole carboxamide), which is a triazene. These compounds are commercially available for clinical use. The epoxides such as dibromomannitol and dibromodulcitol have been used clinically and have antitumor, alkylating activity, but these agents are still investigational. The structures of selected alkylating agents are shown in Fig. 1.

II. MECHANISM OF ACTION

The alkylating agents with antitumor activity share the property of being able to form covalent bonds with a variety of chemical groups on essential cellular molecules under physiologic conditions. The reaction proceeds through the formation of carbonium ion intermediates or of transition complexes with target molecules usually having phosphate, amino, sulfhydyl, hydroxyl, carboxyl, imidazole, or other nucleophilic groups. The nucleophilic substitution step may follow second-order kinetics (S_{N2}), with the rate dependent on concentrations of both the alkylating agent and substrate or first-order kinetics (S_{N1}) where the rate-limiting step is solvent-assisted ionization of the alkylating agent with subsequent rapid reaction of the resulting ion with substrate (Price, 1975). In the majority of cases, alkylation proceeds through a second-order nucleophilic substitution. Basic aliphatic nitrogen mustards, aziridines, and epoxides alkylate by S_{N2} mechanisms. However, the less basic aromatic nitrogen mustards and the sulfur mustards require longer periods of time to generate unstable, active ions and so appear to follow first-order kinetics (S_{N1}), which is independent of the concentration of nucleophilic centers. These differences in mechanism may explain differences in biological effects between aliphatic and aromatic nitrogen mustards (Connors, 1975).

The alkylating agents can react with a variety of cellular components, including DNA, RNA, protein, and phospholipids. However, reaction with DNA appears to be the prime event leading to either cell death or its inability to reproduce. Correlations between DNA alkylation and lethality have been made for bacteriophage systems (Ludlum, 1975) but have not been firmly established for mammalian cells. The strongly nucleophilic 7-nitrogen of guanine, a purine base, appears to be the most susceptible group on DNA to the alkylating agents. Other areas for nucleophilic attack are the 0-6 and the N-3 positions of guanine, the N-1 and N-3 positions of adenine, and the N-3 position of cytosine (Calabresi and Parks, 1975; Ludlum, 1975). Esterification of the phosphate backbone of DNA may also occur (Ludlum, 1975). These minor reactions with DNA vary according to alkylating agent and may explain to some extent the differences among classes of alkylating agents or even among agents within a class.

Most of the biologically active, alkylating agents are at least bifunctional, which means that there are at least two groups on the molecule capable of alkylation. Although monofunctional agents are capable of producing irreversible damage to DNA, agents that are bifunctional can cause greater damage by interstrand or intrastrand cross-links. Linking of a DNA strand with an adjacent protein is also possible.

Although the alkylating agents appear to have a common mechanism of action, there are differences in toxicity and efficacy of these agents as antitumor drugs. Some of these differences are explained by pharmacokinetic factors that influence the amount of drug delivered to the target site. The stability of the compound in aqueous solution, protein binding, metabolism, and excretion all play a role in determining the amount of active drug delivered to the target cell. The cell permeability, the intracellular concentration and distribution of nucleophilic centers, the ability of the cell to repair damage of various types, and other factors combine to determine the effect of individual alkylating agents. In general, cells that are resistant to one alkylating agent will be resistant to other alkylating agents as well as other drugs that cross-link DNA such as cisplatin (Rosenberg, 1973). However, experimentally and clinically it has been shown that tumor cells resistant to one alkylating agent are sensitive to another. This may be related to transport across cell membranes. Mechlorethamine uptake into neoplastic cells *in vitro* was shown to be mediated by an active transport system that also acts in the transport of choline (Brockman, 1974). The structural analogues of mechlorethamine, such as chlorambucil, melphalan, and cyclophosphamide, did not inhibit the uptake of nitrogen mustard, which suggests a different transport mechanism for these drugs.

III. OTHER ALKYLATING AGENTS

A. Clinically Useful Alkylating Agents of the "Other Category"—General Considerations

Once it was known that mechlorethamine was clinically useful in the treatment of neoplastic disease, the search began for other alkylating agents with greater specificity for tumor cells. The methyl group of mechlorethamine was replaced by other groups to act as "carriers" for the rest of the molecule in which resided the alkylating activity. Melphalan was synthesized by replacing the methyl group with L-phenylalanine, which is an amino acid essential to melanin synthesis. The compound was expected to have activity against maligant melanoma. Clinically the drug had little activity against melanoma but had sufficient activity against multiple myeloma to warrant its commercial availability. Since aromatic rings attached to the nitrogen of nitrogen mustards have electron-withdrawing capacity, the rate of carbonium ion formation is greatly reduced. A compound such as chlorambucil therefore would be expected to be more stable than mechlorethamine. Chlorambucil has a long serum half-life and is stable enough to be orally effective.

Compounds containing ethylenimine groups were screened for antitumor activity, since this group resembles the ethylenimonium ion formed by the nitrogen mustards. Triethylenemelamine (TEM), a compound used for improving the finish of rayon fabrics, was shown to have activity. A closely related compound, triethylenethiophosphoramide (thio-TEPA), was synthesized and introduced clinically in the early 1950s. Thio-TEPA has fewer toxicities than mechlorethamine with an equivalent antitumor spectrum in animals (Calabresi and Welch, 1966).

Other types of alkylating agents besides the nitrogen mustards were synthesized or discovered. A large group of esters of alkanesulfonic acids were synthesized as alkylating agents. The alkyl–oxygen bonds undergo fission and react with intracellular molecules. Busulfan is a symmetrical methanesulfonic acid ester with four methylene groups between the esters. Increasing or decreasing the number of methylene groups in this molecule decreases the activity of the compound. These compounds have different spatial relationships from the nitrogen mustards and produce intrastrand but not interstrand cross-links of DNA (Fox, 1975).

During the investigation of compounds in the biosynthetic pathway to purine ribonucleotides an intermediate in the transformation of 5- aminoimidazole- 4- carboxamide (AIC) to 2-azahypoxanthine was synthesized. This intermediate, 5-diazoimidazole-4-carboxamide, was shown to have antitumor activity (Shealy *et al.*, 1961). Several other derivatives were synthesized as potential inhibitors of purine biosynthesis and dacarbazine [5-(3,3-dimethyl-1-triazeno)-imidazole-4-carboxamide] was found to be active with acceptable toxicity in animal systems so it was brought to clinical trials (Oliverio, 1975). Although dacarbazine may have significant antimetabolite activity, it has been shown to have alkylating activity with attack at the 7-nitrogen position of guanine (Skibba *et al.*, 1970).

Although the alkylating agents have a diverse background, their activities are similar. In fact, the clinical spectrum of disease treated by a specific alkylating agent is not due so much to its antitumor specificity as it is to the historical develoment of the drug. Chlorambucil, for example, is effective in the treatment of chronic myelogenous leukemia but has not been adequately evaluated against busulfan, which is considered the drug of choice in this disease (Livingston and Carter, 1970). Pharmacokinetic considerations were also important in determining which drugs were evaluated in patients with specific tumors. High, intermittent, intravenous doses of cyclophosphamide seemed appropriate for patients with Burkitt's lymphoma, which is a fast-growing tumor, whereas a relatively nontoxic daily oral dose of busulfan appeared to be appropriate for patients with chronic myelogenous leukemia.

The toxicities associated with the alkylating agents are similar, although important differences occur. All alkylating agents, if given in sufficient dosage, will cause bone marrow depression, which is manifested by peripheral white blood cell count depression. The red cell series and megakaryocytes are affected to varying degrees. Gastrointestinal symptoms, especially nausea and vomiting, are common with most of the alkylating agents. The incidence and severity of gastrointestinal symptoms are variable. About 75% of patients receiving dacarbazine have significant vomiting, whereas this symptom is minimal or absent in patients receiving standard doses of chlorambucil or busulfan. The reproductive system is affected by most alkylating agents. These effects are similar to those produced by X-irradiation. Amenorrhea of several months' duration sometimes follows therapy with alkylating agents. Spermatogenesis is impaired as well. Busulfan affects the early stage of spermatogenesis and the aziridines and aliphatic nitrogen mustards affect later stages (Calabresi and Parks, 1975). Melphalan and chlorambucil had little effect on male fertility in rats even when given at high doses (Jackson, 1959). Alopecia is variable with the alkylating agents. Melphalan is sometimes used in place of oral cyclophosphamide because melphalan infrequently produces alopecia.

A number of alkylating agents have been shown to cause immunosuppression but the biological mechanism of this phenomenon is not known. Cyclophosphamide appears to have the greatest effect on the immune system. Lymphocytes are relatively sensitive to the cytotoxic effects of cyclophosphamide but relatively resistant to those of busulfan, and this observation may account for the differences in ability of these drugs to cause myelosuppression (Calabresi and Parks, 1975).

Alkylating agents are mutagenic in a variety of biological systems (Loveless, 1966). Monofunctional alkylators are active mutagens but often lack cytotoxic properties. Alkylating agents are also carcinogenic in animal systems and apparently in humans as well (Rosner, 1978). Both monofunctional and polyfunctional agents are carcinogens in experimental systems. Although the nitrosoureas and triazianes are the most potent, the other agents have the potential to cause cancer if administered for long periods of time. All the commercially available alkylating agents have been shown to be teratogenic in animal studies when reproduction studies have been done. The evidence suggests that polyfunctional alkylating agents are teratogenic in humans as well, but it should be noted that some patients have normal pregnancies and offspring while receiving chemotherapy with alkylating agents (DiPaolo, 1969).

Since the activity and the toxicity of alkylating agents and X-irradiation are similar, it is usually advisable not to use these drugs concurrently with radiotherapy or other radiomimetic drugs. Dosage reductions are recommended when alkylating agents are given to patients with depressed bone marrow function secondary to concurrent or previous cytotoxic therapy, radiotherapy, or disease status. The effects on the reproductive system and the teratogenic risk of alkylating agents should be taken into account when younger patients are considered for therapy. The carcinogenic risks of these drugs may be important considerations in patients with an expected survival of several years. However, the potential benefits derived from the alkylating agents used with care and understanding outweigh the potential harm they may cause.

B. Specific Drugs

1. Melphalan

Melaphalan is approved for use in the treatment of multiple myeloma. Therapy is usually instituted once progressive, symptomatic disease is identified. The overall response rate is about 42%, but the recorded objective responses range from 15 to 78%, depending on the dose and schedule used and the criteria employed for defining response (Livingston and Carter, 1970). Corticosteroids were observed to increase response rates of alkylating agents and to prolong the survival of patients who were considered in a good risk category but not for those patients in a poor risk category (Costa et al., 1973).

The usual dosage of melphalan is 6 mg (three tablets) once a day for 2–3 weeks. A rest period is given until white blood cell and platelet counts have risen, sometimes requiring up to 4 weeks. A maintenance dose of 2 mg daily is then instituted. Several other dosage schedules have been employed, including higher loading doses for shorter periods of time or lower doses for longer periods of time (Livingston and Carter, 1970), but no clear-cut advantage of any schedule has been shown.

Beneficial responses of various other tumors to melphalan have been reported (Livingston and Carter, 1970; Greenwald, 1973), and the current literature (Carter *et al.*, 1977; Silver *et al.*, 1977) lists the major nonapproved indications for the drug as breast carcinoma, ovarian carcinoma, and testicular seminomas. However, melphalan is usually not used as therapy against metastatic breast carcinoma or testicular seminoma. Although melphalan has a 23% response rate against breast cancer, other agents or combination of agents have higher response rates (Broder and Tormey, 1974). The drug was used in several studies of postoperative adjuvant chemotherapy of breast carcinoma because of its mild toxicity, oral administration route, and lack of alopecia, and an increase in relapse-free survival in premenopausal women was found (Young *et al.*, 1977). The current trend is to use chemotherapy, usually in combinations without melphalan, as adjuvant therapy in patients with breast carcinoma. Testicular carcinoma is not often treated with melphalan, since other regimens (Samuels, 1975; Einhorn *et al.*, 1976) produce higher response rates with a larger percentage of long-term survivors. Alkylating agents, including melphalan, are considered the primary therapy for metastatic ovarian carcinoma, since response rates of 40–50% have been reported (Carter *et al.*, 1977).

Good to excellent results have been reported for the treatment of polycythemia vera (Laszlo, 1968) and for perfusion therapy of malignant melanoma (Irvine and Luck, 1966). Bone marrow suppression with subsequent decreases in peripheral red and white blood cells and platelet counts is the major toxicity associated with melphalan. The incidence and severity of myelosuppression is dependent on the dose and schedule employed. Nausea and vomiting are rare except when oral doses of greater than 20 mg are taken. A smaller initial dosage in patients with renal dysfunction has been suggested (Speed *et al.*, 1964).

2. Chlorambucil

Chlorambucil is approved for the palliative treatment of chronic lymphocytic leukemia and maligant lymphomas, including lymphosarcoma, giant follicular lymphoma, and Hodgkin's disease. Other drugs, usually in combination chemotherapeutic regimens, have replaced chlorambucil in the treatment of the lymphomas with unfavorable histologic types and Hodgkin's disease (Salmon, 1977; Medical Letter, 1978). The drug's main use is in the therapy of patients with chronic lymphocytic leukemia (CLL). Since complete remissions are rare and patients may do well for years without any therapy, it is sometimes difficult to determine the best time to institute therapy. Patients with active disease in whom anemia, thrombocytopenia, hypermetabolism, and enormous lymph node and spleen enlargement are present may be treated with a chronic schedule of chlorambucil with or without steroids (Carter *et al.*, 1977). Chlorambucil can be considered as single-agent therapy for the lymphomas with favorable histology; namely, nodular well and poorly differentiated lymphocytic, nodular mixed lymphocytic-histocytic, and well-differentiated lymphocytic lymphoma. Although patients who received combination chemotherapy had a greater complete response rate in a randomized study, patients treated with single-agent alkylating agent had about the same survival after 3 years (Portlock et al., 1976).

Chlorambucil has been shown to have significant activity in patients with ovarian carcinoma, with response rates reported between 40 and 60% (Greenwald, 1973). Although considered by some to be the drug of choice for ovarian carcinoma, chlorambucil and the other alkylating agents may be replaced by newer combinations containing cisplatin. Waldenstran's macroglobulinemia also appears to respond well to chlorambucil (Greenwald, 1973), but as is the case for ovarian carcinoma, the drug is not approved for this indication.

The usual dosage of chlorambucil is 0.1–0.2 mg/kg body weight daily for 3–6 weeks. This usually amounts to 4–10 mg (two to five tablets) a day.

Patients who receive greater than 6.5 mg/kg in a single course have a higher risk of developing severe neutropenia (Galton et al., 1961). White blood cell counts may continue to fall for 10 days after cessation of therapy.

The major toxicity of chlorambucil is myelosuppression, but this may not be a problem at therapeutic dose levels. The drug is relatively free from gastrointestinal side effects or other evidence of toxicity. There have been, however, reports of hepatotoxicity secondary to the drug (Koler and Fosgren, 1958; Ambronin et al., 1962).

3. Busulfan

Busulfan is the drug of choice for chronic myelogenous leukemia (Medical Letter, 1978), and this disease is the only approved indication for the drug. Chronic myelogenous leukemia (CML) is a disorder of the hematopoietic stem cell. The median survival of patients with CML is 3.5 years (Carter et al., 1977) with death due to an accelerated phase known as "blast crisis." Bufulfan is used for palliation of symptoms during the chronic phase of the disease, since blast crisis is refractory to this drug and all other therapy. Treatment with bulsulfan in a retrospective review showed a significant prolongation of survival compared to other therapies, but prospective studies have not shown an effect on the onset of blast crisis (Kardinal et al., 1976). The effect of treatment in the retrospective study may have been due to selection of patients with less aggressive disease in the busulfan group.

Polycythemia vera is another myeloproliferative disorder responsive to busulfan. The disease is manifested by high blood volume, plasma viscosity, and an increased level of circulating platelets. Although indolent disease can be treated by phlebotomy, most cases are treated with myelosuppressive therapy in the form of radioactive compounds, irradiation, or chemotherapy. The most commonly used drugs are the alkylating agents. Busulfan, chlorambucil, melphalan, and cyclophosphamide all give response rates around 80% (Carter *et al.*, 1977). Busulfan is most commonly used, but melphalan and chlorambucil are about as effective and may be less toxic (Laszlo and Huang, 1977).

The recommended therapy for CML is the oral administration of 4–8 mg (two to four tablets) daily, depending on the initial white count and severity of the disease. Therapy is continued until the white blood cell count falls below 10,000 cells/μl. When the white blood cell count rises to 50,000 cells/μl, therapy is restarted. An alternate dosing schedule is 4–6 mg daily until the white count is between 10,000 and 20,000 cells/μl. This level of white cells is maintained by daily doses, usually 2 mg of busulfan. For the treatment of polycythemia vera, the drug is given daily at doses needed to maintain red blood cell, white blood cell, and platelet counts within a normal range.

The major toxic effect of busulfan is dose-related myelosuppression, which requires discontinuation of therapy in less than 10% of patients (Greenwald, 1973). Aplastic anemia has been reported with higher than usual doses of busulfan (Wilkinson and Turner, 1959). Gastrointestinal disturbances are uncommon and often mild and include nausea, vomiting, diarrhea, cheilosis, and glossitis. Disturbances in reproductive function, as with other alkylating agents, include amenorrhea, sterility, and gynecomastia.

Several syndromes associated with long-term busulfan therapy have been described. Skin hyperpigmentation may occur with prolonged therapy. This condition has been associated with digestive disorders, fatigue, muscular weakness, and weight loss in a few patients, simulating adrenocortical insufficiency. However, laboratory tests failed to demonstrate decreased steroid levels in several of these patients (Kyle *et al.*, 1961). Two other patients on chronic busulfan therapy developed a syndrome suggestive of adrenal insufficiency, and endocrinologic studies suggested a diminished reserve for adenocorticotrophic hormone (Vivacqua *et al.*, 1967).

Cytologic dysplasia manifest by large, atypical epithelial cells in multiple organs such as lung, breast, pancreas, kidneys, adrenals, bladder, and cervix has been reported by several investigators (Greenwald, 1973) in patients receiving long-term therapy. This is probably a reaction to alkylating agents in general and may not be a specific toxicity of busulfan.

A pulmonary syndrome associated with prolonged use of busulfan has been observed in some patients (Rosenow, 1972). The symptoms include cough, dyspnea, and fever. The chest X-ray shows a diffuse interstitial and intra-alveolar process. Histologic examination of the lung shows an organizing fibrinous edema with bizarre, atypical cells that are possibly type II granular pneumocytes. The process of intra-alveolar fibrosis may be reversible by stopping the drug and administering corticosteroids, but patients with this disorder frequently die of restrictive pulmonary disease. A similar lung syndrome may be seen occasionally with cyclophosphamide therapy.

4. Thio-TEPA

Thio-TEPA is indicated for palliation of a variety of neoplastic diseases, including adenocarcinoma of the breast and ovary, metastatic lymphomas, and bronchogenic carcinoma, and for control of intracavitary effusions secondary to diffuse or localized neoplastic disease of various serosal cavities. However, new agents and combination chemotherapeutic regimens have replaced thio-TEPA as therapy for most of these diseases. The current major use for this drug is in the therapy of patients with malignant pleural or peritoneal effusions and superficial bladder cancers. Although activity is significant in ovarian carcinoma for thio-TEPA, it is no better than other alkylating agents, such as chlorambucil, melphalan, or cyclophosphamide (Carter *et al.*, 1977; Greenwald, 1973). Since most clinicians have a greater familiarity with these drugs, the popularity of thio-TEPA has decreased. The use of the thio-TEPA in the treatment of malignant effusions was once popular and considered reasonably effective, especially in pleural effusions secondary to ovarian or breast carcinoma (Greenwald, 1973). However, it is less effective for pleural effusions than mechlorethamine, which is more often used (Greenwald *et al.*, 1978). Thio-TEPA is probably a good choice of agents for malignant ascites, since it causes minimal irritation and less loculation of fluid (Silverberg, 1969).

Intravesical thio-TEPA is of value in the treatment of well- or moderately differentiated superficial bladder tumors but of little benefit once the tumor has invaded muscle (Murphy, 1977). Favorable results have been obtained using intravesical thio-TEPA prophylactically against superficial bladder tumors (Veenema *et al.*, 1969). Thio-TEPA is absorbed through the bladder epithelium; consequently, systemic toxicity, as well as local irritation can result. The promising results reported for the bladder instillation of mitomycin C and the lack of serious side effects with this antitumor antibiotic (Crooke *et al.*, 1977) make mitomycin C the prime rival to thio-TEPA therapy of superficial bladder tumors.

Although thio-TEPA is indicated for the palliative therapy of bronchogenic carcinoma, the drug is rarely used for therapy of this disease.

The drug is usually administered intravenously for systemic therapy, but it can also be given intramuscularly or directly into the tumor, since it is not irritating to tissues. Different dosage schedules have been recommended (Greenwald, 1973), but usually involve an initial loading dose of 50–75 mg divided into five consecutive days. Lower doses are suggested for patients with previous chemotherapy, those undergoing extensive radiotherapy, or those who are debilitated or who have chronic cardiovascular or renal disease or surgical shock. After a rest period of 1 or 2 weeks, maintenance therapy is instituted at 1–4-week intervals with 30 mg or less. For superficial bladder carcinoma, 60 mg of thio-tepa is added to 30–60 ml of distilled water and then instilled into the bladder by catheter and retained for 2 hr. The usual course of treatment is once a week for 4 weeks.

Bone marrow suppression is the main toxicity of thio-TEPA. Recovery of blood counts is usually seen within 30 days from cessation of therapy, but prolonged leukopenia or thrombocytopenia is not rare (Greenwald, 1973). Mild nausea, vomiting, headache, and anorexia are seen occasionally, and alopecia and allergic reactions are rare.

5. Dacarbazine

Dacarbazine is indicated for the treatment of metastatic malignant melanoma. The drug has been extensively studied in this disease, and an overall response rate of 25% with a complete response rate of 5% has been reported (Comis and Carter, 1974). This response rate is the highest of any single agent. Other alkylating agents are not very active against melanoma. Mechlorethamine has no clinical activity. The activity of cyclophosphamide is variable but has an overall response rate of 16%. Melphalan and chlorambucil produce responses in less than 10% of patients with malignant melanoma, although melphalan given by isolated perfusion appears more active (Carter et al., 1977).

Dacarbazine is employed in combination chemotherapeutic regimens in the treatment of Hodgkin's disease, neuroblastoma, and sarcomas. For Hodgkin's disease a combination (ABVD) of doxorubicin (Adriamycin), bleomycin, vinblastine, and dacarbazine was shown not to be cross-resistant with the standard therapy of late-stage Hodgkin's disease (Santoro et al., 1977). When the standard combination (MOPP) of mechlorethamine, vincristine, prednisone, and procarbazine was used alternating with the dacarbazine combination, a response rate of 100% with 100% 2-year survival was obtained for patients with stage IV Hodgkin's disease (Bonadonna et al., 1977). Another study using ABVD in slightly different doses did not show such encouraging results in the treatment of patients with stage IV Hodgkin's disease who failed MOPP therapy (Clamon et al., 1977).

Adult soft tissue sarcomas are usually resistant to chemotherapy. Doxorubicin is the single agent of choice in this disease, with an overall response rate of 27% (Carter et al., 1977). Dacarbazine was shown to have a 17% response rate as a single agent, but when combined with doxorubicin a 42% response rate was obtained (Gottlieb et al., 1975). When cyclophosphamide and vincristine were added to the combination (CYVADIC), an overall response rate of 55% was obtained, with 14% complete responders (Gottlieb et al., 1975). Attempts to duplicate these results have not always been successful (Giuliano et al., 1977).

Dacarbazine has been studied in children with various solid tumors. The drug was shown to have minimal but definite activity as a single agent for the treatment of advanced neuroblastoma and rhabdomyosarcoma (Finklestein et al.,

1975). The response rate for dacarbazine of 23% in neuroblastoma is less than that of 40% for combination therapy with cyclophosphamide and vincristine (Evans, 1972) or of 40% for doxorubicin as a single agent (Tan *et al.*, 1975), but it is high enough to suggest investigations using dacarbazine in combination therapy.

The usual dosage employed is 250 mg/m^2 per day for 5 days administered by intravenous injection and repeated every 3 weeks. Another dosage schedule is 2 mg/kg (about 60 mg/m^2) per day for 10 days. This schedule gave a statistically better response rate in melanoma than 4.5 mg/kg per day for 10 days (Nathanson *et al.*, 1971).

The most serious toxicity with dacarbazine is hematopoietic depression involving primarily white blood cells and platelets, although a mild anemia may sometimes occur. Bone marrow depression may be severe and life-threatening at high doses, but when given at a dose of 250 mg/m^2 per day for 5 days, less than 5% of patients will have white blood cell counts below 3000/μl or platelet counts below 50,000/μl (Luce *et al.*, 1970). The maximum nadir in counts occurs around 3 weeks after the last dose of dacarbazine with full recovery usually by 5 weeks after therapy. Bone marrow depression is somewhat delayed in comparison with the classical alkylating agents. Anorexia, nausea, and vomiting will occur to some degree in over 90% of patients treated with dacarbazine. The vomiting lasts 1–12 hr with the initial doses, but a tolerance develops to later doses. Diarrhea is rarely caused by the drug. A flulike syndrome with malaise, muscle aching, and weakness and fever to 40°C occurs in about 2% of patients. Facial parethesias have been reported to be common with dacarbazine administration (Moertel *et al.*, 1970). They occur 15–30 min after injection and persist for only a few minutes. Facial flushing may accompany the parethesias in less than 10% of patients. A few case reports of neurologic complications involving the central nervous system as manifest by seizures and delayed dementia have appeared in the literature (Paterson and McPherson, 1977). Liver and renal toxicities have also been reported, but it is not clear if they were due to drug or disease. Extravasation of the drug during intravenous injection may result in tissue damage and pain. Arm pain may be caused by too rapid injection of undiluted drug.

C. Investigational Agents

The search for new alkylating agents with greater tumor specificity continues. Derivatives of mannitol that behave as alkylating agents, probably by epoxide intermediates, have reached clinical trials. Dianhydrogalactitol, which is probably the active metabolite of dibromomannitol and dibromodulcitol, has undergone phase I and II trials in the United States (Carter, 1978; Carter and Slavik, 1976) and Europe (Mathé and Van Putten, 1978). The drug in experimental studies appears to have good penetration into the brain. Activity has been noted in bronchogenic carcinoma, renal cell carcinoma, and gastrointestinal tumors. Studies to determine if activity is greater than other alkylating agents have not been performed. The major toxicity of this drug is myelosuppression.

Attempts to link nitrogen mustards or other alkylating moieties to tumor-specific steroid carriers resulted in a variety of compounds (Muggia et al., 1978). Estramustine phosphate (Estracyt), a nitrogen mustard covalently linked to an estradiol, and prednimustine, a corticosteroid linked to chlorambucil, are two drugs undergoing clinical trials. Estramustine has activity against prostatic cancer and advanced melanoma, and prednimustine exerts effects on leukemia, lymphoma, breast carcinoma, and melanoma (Mathé and van Putten, 1978; Lopez et al., 1978). The role of these agents in the standard therapy of these diseases is yet to be determined.

Peptichemio is a novel compound thought to be an alkylating agent (Mathé and Van Putten,1978). It is a mixture of six peptides and has activity against neuroblastoma, cervical cancer, laryngeal carcinoma, and chronic myelogenous leukemia blast crisis (Mathé and Van Putten,1978). Activity has also been seen in lung, gynecologic, and bladder carcinomas and advanced neuroblastoma in children (Otten and Maurus, 1978). Peptichemio may be the prototype for a new class of compounds that are peptides with alkylating activity.

Yoshi 864 (1-propanol, 3,3'-iminodi-, dimethanesulfonate (ester) hydrochloride) was initially synthesized in Japan in the mid-1960s as an alkylating agent with no cross-resistance to mechlorethamine. A phase II study done by the Central Oncology Group showed an overall response rate of 11% with minimal toxicity. Sufficient activity was seen in chronic myelogenous leukemia, lymphomas, and carcinomas of the ovary and bladder to warrant further studies of the drug in combination with other drugs in these tumors (Altman et al., 1978). Toxicity consisted of bone marrow depression in about 50% of patients. Only 20% of patients had nausea and vomiting. About 10% of patients experienced somnolence, lethargy, or drowsiness. The future of this drug will be determined by further trials.

IV. CONCLUSIONS

The alkylating agents comprise a large class of compounds, some of which have significant antitumor activity. The goal of alkylating agent research is to synthesize or discover compounds that have greater toxicity to tumor cells than to normal proliferating cells. Currently, the clinically useful agents, for the most part, lack this specificity. However, thousands of alkylating agents are known and probably thousands more will be tested in antitumor screening systems. Even though tumor-specific alkylating agents have not been found, the alkylating agents as a group have added immensely to the benefits derived from chemotherapy by patients with cancer.

REFERENCES

Altman, S. J., Metter, G. E., Nealon, T. F., Weiss, A. J., Ramirez, G., Madden, R. E., Fletcher, W. S., Strawitz, J. G., and Multhauf, P. M. (1978). *Cancer Treat. Rep.* **62**, 389-395.

Ambronin, G. D., Deliman, R. M., and Shanbrom, E. (1962). *Gastroenterology* **42**, 401-410.

Bonadonna, G., Fossati, V., and DeLena, M. (1977). *Proc. Am. Soc. Clin. Oncol.* **19**, 363.

Brockman, R. W. (1974). *In* "Handbook of Experimental Pharmacology: Antineoplastic and Immunosuppressive Agents" (A. C. Sartorelli and D. G. Johns, eds.), Vol. 38, Part 1, pp. 352-410. Springer-Verlag, Berlin and New York.

Broder, L. E., and Tormey, D. C. (1974). *Cancer Treat. Rev.* **1**, 183.

Calabresi, P., and Parks, R. E., Jr. (1975). *In* "The Pharmacological Basis of Therapeutics" (L. S. Goodman and A. Gillman, eds.), 5th ed., pp. 1254-1307. Macmillan, New York.

Calabresi, P., and Welch, A. D. (1965). *In* "The Pharmacological Basis of Therapeutics" (L. S. Goodman and A. Gillman, eds.), 3rd ed., pp. 1345-1393. Macmillan, New York.

Carter, S. K. (1978). *Cancer Chemother. Pharmacol.* **1**, 15-24.

Carter, S. K. and Slavik, M. (1976). *Cancer Treat. Rev.* **3**, 43-60.

Carter, S. K., Bakowski, M. T., and Hellman, K. (1977). "Chemotherapy of Cancer," Wiley, New York.

Clamon, G., Corder, M., and Sheets, R. (1977). *Proc. Am. Soc. Clin. Oncol.* **19**, 329.

Comis, R. L., and Carter, S. K. (1974). *Cancer Treat. Rev.* **1**, 285.

Connors, T. A. (1975). *In* "Handbook of Experimental Pharmacology: Antineoplastic and Immunosuppressive Agents" (A. C. Sartorelli and D. G. Johns, eds.), Vol. 38, Part 2, pp. 18-34. Springer-Verlag, Berlin and New York.

Costa, G., Engle, R. L., Jr., Schilling, A., Carbone, P., Kochwa, S., Nachman, R. L., and Glidewell, O. (1973). *Am. J. Med.* **54**, 589-599.

Crooke, S. T., Johnson, D. E., and Bracken, R. B. (1977). *Proc. Am. Soc. Clin. Oncol.* **19**, 321.

DiPaolo, J. A. (1969). *Ann. N.Y. Acad. Sci.* **163**, 801-812.

Einhorn, L. H., Furnas, B. E., and Powell, N. (1976). *Proc. Am. Soc. Clin. Oncol.* **17**, 240.

Finklestein, J. Z., Albo, V., Ertel, I., and Hammond, D. (1975). *Cancer Chemother. Rep.* **59**, 351-357.

Fox, B. W. (1975). *In* "Handbook of Experimental Pharmacology: Antineoplastic and Immunosuppressive Agents" (A. C. Sartorelli and D. G. Johns, eds.), Vol. 38, Part 2, pp. 35-46. Springer-Verlag, Berlin and New York.

Galton, D. A. G., Wiltshaw, E., Szur, I., and Dasie, J. V. (1961). *Br. J. Hematol.* **7**, 73-98.

Giuliano, A. E., Larkin, K. L., Eilber, F. R., and Morton, D. L. (1977). *Proc. Am. Soc. Clin. Oncol.* **19**, 359.

Gottlieb, J. A., Baker, L. H., O'Bryan, R. M., Sinkovics, J. G., Hoogstraten, B., Quagliana, J. M., Rivkin, S. E., Bodey, G. P., Rodriguez, V. T., Blumenschein, G. R., Saiki, J. H., Coltman, C., Jr., Burgess, M. A., Sullivan, P., Thigpen, P., Bottomley, R., Balcerzak, S., and Moon, T. E. (1975). *Cancer Chemotherap. Rep.,Part 3* **6**, 271-282.

Greenwald, D. W., Phillips, C., and Bennett, J. M. (1978). *J. Surg. Oncol.* **10**, 361-368.

Greenwald, E. S. (1973). "Cancer Chemotherapy." Medical Exam. Publ. Co., Flushing, New York.

Irvine, W. T., and Luck, R. J. (1966). *Br. Med. J.* **i**, 770-774.

Jackson, H. (1959). *Pharmacol. Rev.* **11**, 135-172.

Kardinal, C. G., Bateman, J. R., and Weiner, J. (1976). *Arch. Intern. Med.* **136**, 305-313.

Koler, R. D., and Fosgren, A. L. (1958). *J. Am. Med. Assoc.* **167**, 316-317.

Kyle, R. A., Schwartz, R. S., Oliner, H. L., and Dameshek, W. (1961). *Blood* **18**, 497-510.

Laszlo, J. (1968). *Blood* **32**, 506.

Laszlo, J., and Huang, A. T. (1977). *Curr. Probl. Cancer* **2**(1), 1-42.

Livingston, R. B., and Carter, S. K. (1970). "Single Agents in Cancer Chemotherapy." IFI/Plenum, New York.

Lopez, R., Karkakousis, C. P., Didolkar, M. S., and Holyoke, E. D. (1978). *Cancer Treat. Rep.* **62**, 1329-1332.

Loveless, A. (1966). "Genetic and Allied Effects of Alkylating Agents." Pennsylvania State Univ. Press, University Park.

Luce, J. K., Thurman, W. G., Isaacs, B. L., and Talley, R. W. (1970). *Cancer Chemother. Rep.* **54**, 119-124.

Ludlum, D. R. (1975). *In* "Handbook of Experimental Pharmacology: Antineoplastic and Immunosuppressive Agents" (A. C. Sartorelli and D. G. Johns, eds.), Vol. 38, Part 2, pp. 6-17. Springer-Verlag, Berlin and New York.

Mathé, G., and Van Putten, L. M. (1978). *Cancer Chemother. Pharmacol.* **1**, 5.

Medical Letter (1978). *Cancer Chemother.* Sept. 22.

Moertel, C. G., Reitemeier, R. J., Hahn, R. G., and Schutt, A. J. (1970). *Cancer Chemother. Rep.* **54**, 471-473.

Muggia, F. M., Lippman, M., and Henson, J. C. (1978). *Cancer Treat. Rep.* **62**, 1239-1286.

Murphy, G. P. (1977). *N.Y. State J. Med* **77**, 1889-1895.

Nathanson, L., Wolter, J., Horton, J., Colsky, J., Shnider, B. I., and Schilling, A. (1971). *Clin. Pharmacol. Ther.* **12**, 955-962.

Oliverio, V. T. (1975). *In* "Cancer Medicine" (J. F. Holland and E. Frei, III, eds.), pp. 806-817. Lea & Febiger, Philadelphia, Pennsylvania.

Otten, J., and Maurus, R. (1978). *Cancer Treat Rep.* **62**, 1015-1019.

Patterson, A. H. G., and McPherson, T. A. (1977). *Cancer Treat. Rep.* **61**, 105-106.

Portlock, C. S., Rosenberg, S. A., Glatstein, E., and Kaplan, H. S. (1976). *Blood* **47**, 747-756.

Price, C. C. (1975). *In* "Handbook of Experimental Pharmacology: Antineoplastic and Immunosuppressive Agents" (A. C. Sartorelli and D. G. Johns, eds.), Vol. 38, Part 2, pp. 1-5. Springer-Verlag, Berlin and New York.

Rhoads, C. P. (1946). *J. Am. Med. Assoc.* **131**, 656-658.

Rosenberg, B. (1973). *Naturwissenschaften* **60**, 399-406.

Rosenow, E. C., III (1972). *Ann. Intern. Med.* **77**, 977-991.

Rosner, F. (1978). *Ca* **28**, 57-59.

Ross, W. C. J. (1974). *In* "Handbook of Experimental Pharmacology: Antineoplastic and Immunosuppressive Agents" (A. C. Sartorelli and D. G. Johns, eds.), Vol. 38, Part 1, pp. 33-51. Springer-Verlag, Berlin and New York.

Salmon, S. E. (1977). *In* "Current Medical Diagnosis and Treatment" (M. A. Krupp and M. J. Chatton, eds.), pp. 968-981. Lange Med. Publ., Los Altos, California.

Samuels, M. L. (1975). *Proc. Am. Assoc. Cancer Res.* **16**, 112.

Santoro, A., Monfardini, S., and Bonadonna, G. (1977). *Proc. Am. Soc. Clin. Oncol.* **19**, 363.

Shealy, Y. F., Struck, R. F., Holum, L. B., and Montgomery, J. A. (1961). *J. Org. Chem.* **26**, 2396-2401.

Silver, R. T., Lauper, R. D., and Jarowski, C. I. (1977). "A Synopsis of Cancer Chemotherapy." Dun-Donnelly, New York.

Silverberg, I. (1969). *Oncology* **24**, 26-30.

Skibba, J. L., Johnson, R. O., and Bryan, G. T. (1970). *Proc. Am. Assoc. Cancer Res.* **11**, 73.

Speed, D. E., Galton, D. A. G., and Swan, A. (1964). *Br. Med. J.* **i,** 1664-1669.

Tan, C., Rosen, G., and Ghavini, F. (1975). *Cancer Chemother. Rep., Part 3* **6,** 259-266.

Veenema, R. J., Dean, A. L., Jr., Uson, A. C., Roberts, M., and Longo, F. (1969). *J. Urol.* **101,** 711-715.

Vivacqua, R. J., Haurani, F. I., and Erslen, A. J. (1967). *Ann. Intern. Med.* **67,** 380-387.

Wilkinson, J. F., and Turner, R. L. (1959). *Prog. Hematol.* **2,** 225-238.

Young, R. S., Lippman, M., DeVitta, V. T., Bull, J., and Tormey, D. (1977). *Ann. Intern. Med.* **86,** 784-798.

6

THE VINCA ALKALOIDS AND
SIMILAR COMPOUNDS
William A. Creasey

I. THE VINCA ALKALOIDS

A. Introduction

The vinca alkaloids are dimeric indole derivatives (Fig. 1) isolated from the Madagascan periwinkle plant, *Vinca rosea* Linn., or more correctly, *Catharanthus roseus* G. Don. Of about 70 naturally occurring alkaloids, nine are cytotoxic (Svoboda and Blake, 1975; Creasey, 1979), but only four of these—vinblastine (Velban, VLB), vincristine (Oncovin, VCR), vinleurosine, and vinrosidine—have been used in the clinic. Two semisynthetic derivatives of vinblastine—vinglycinate (4-N, *N*-dimethylaminoacetyl desacetyl-vinblastine) and vindesine (desacetylvinblastine amide)—have also reached clinical trial. All are available

CANCER AND CHEMOTHERAPY, VOL. III

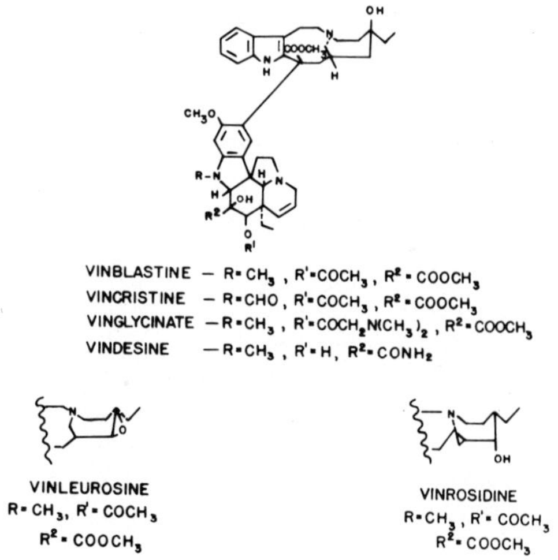

VINBLASTINE — $R = CH_3$, $R' = COCH_3$, $R^2 = COOCH_3$
VINCRISTINE — $R = CHO$, $R' = COCH_3$, $R^2 = COOCH_3$
VINGLYCINATE — $R = CH_3$, $R' = COCH_2N(CH_3)_2$, $R^2 = COOCH_3$
VINDESINE — $R = CH_3$, $R' = H$, $R^2 = CONH_2$

VINLEUROSINE
$R = CH_3$, $R' = COCH_3$
$R^2 = COOCH_3$

VINROSIDINE
$R = CH_3$, $R' = COCH_3$
$R^2 = COOCH_3$

Fig. 1. Structures of the vinca alkaloids.

as their sulfate salts. Vinrosidine, despite promising activity against experimental tumors and suggestion of a synergistic interaction with vincristine (Johnson *et al.*, 1963), had unacceptable human toxicity without therapeutic benefit (Gailani *et al.*, 1966).

Vinleurosine resembled vinblastine in its general actions but was somewhat inferior to that alkaloid in its clinical activity (Mathé *et al.*, 1965). In addition, vinleurosine had the disadvantage of producing a shocklike syndrome unless given by slow intravenous infusion. This effect probably stemmed from its autonomic and/or hypoglycemic actions (Svoboda and Blake, 1975).

Vinglycinate received some study, in part because of apparent activity in disease that was resistant to vinblastine; it is doubtful that this claim was substantiated. In the clinic, vinglycinate was active against Hodgkin's disease, lymphosarcoma, and bronchogenic carcinoma (Armstrong *et al.*, 1967). Thus its activity resembled that of vinblastine, but a 10-fold higher molar dose was required, making treatment economically unfeasible. In contrast, the molecular modifications that produced vindesine led to a compound distinctively different from vinblastine but of similar potency, as we shall see. Thus, at the present time, vinblastine and vincristine are the two alkaloids of established clinical value, whereas vindesine is being actively studied and may finally earn an accepted place in cancer chemotherapy.

In the remainder of this section we shall concentrate on these three widely used alkaloids.

B. Toxicology

1. Hematologic Effects

The three vinca alkaloids differ markedly in their toxicology (Table 1). For both vinblastine and vindesine, leukopenia is the most frequently encountered side effect, occurring in more than 30% of patients receiving these medications. The granulocyte nadir occurs between 5 and 9 days after drug, with essentially complete recovery by 14–21 days. Vincristine only rarely causes leukopenia, and then it is more transient, usually clearing up within a week. Anemia is generally uncommon, but in a series of six patients treated with vindesine at the Children's Hospital of Philadelphia, three required transfusions or had hemoglobin levels below 7 g%. Thrombocytopenia has not been characteristic of therapy with either vinblastine or vincristine; indeed thrombocytosis has often been reported (Robertson and McCarthy, 1969). However, the early clinical trials with vindesine have reported a significant incidence of this toxic symptom (Currie et al., 1976; Bodey and Freireich, 1976; Blum and Dawson, 1976; Mathé et al., 1978; Wong et al., 1977). In our limited experience with this alkaloid we have not encountered thrombocytopenia. It is thus apparent that clarification of the toxicology of vindesine awaits more detailed reports of the studies now in progress.

2. Neurologic Effects

As can be seen from Table I, vincristine is first and foremost a neurotoxin. Vindesine produces a somewhat lower incidence of neurologic sequelae, whereas

TABLE I

Human Toxicity of the Vinca Alkaloids

Percent incidence	Vinblastine	Vincristine	Vindesine
>30	Leukopenia	Neurotoxicity	Leukopenia
10–30	Nausea	Constipation	Neurotoxicity
	Anorexia	Hoarseness	Hair loss
	Vomiting		
5–10	Hair loss	Hair loss	Nausea
	Neurotoxicity	Muscle weakness	Vomiting
			Constipation
<5	Stomatitis	Abdominal pain	Abdominal pain
	Diarrhea	Muscle cramp	Cellulitis
	Constipation	Depression	Chills, fever
	Phlebitis	Phlebitis	Phlebitis

therapy with vinblastine is seldom accompanied by significant manifestations of this type. Early symptoms include tingling of the fingertips and numbness to be followed by frequently painful paresthesias. Loss of deep tendon reflexes, such as the Achilles reflex, is an early diagnostic indication of neurotoxicity. Diffuse muscle weakness, clumsiness, uncoordinated movements, and foot drop occur later; in experimental animals these effects may progress to hind limb paralysis. Neuromuscular deficit in specialized functions may result in diplopia and hoarseness. Jaw pain is a useful indicator of impending severe neuropathy and the need to withhold drug. The vinca alkaloids show some CNS depressant action (Svoboda and Blake, 1975), so depression is not an unexpected finding.

Physiologic, pathologic, and biochemical studies have demonstrated reduced nerve conduction velocities (McLeod and Penny, 1969), axonal degeneration and demyelination (Gottschalk et al., 1968), and inhibition of rapid axonal transport (Ochs and Worth, 1975; Dahlstrom et al., 1975). These phenomena offer a satisfactory basis for the observed neuropathies.

3. Gastrointestinal Effects

Nausea and vomiting are common findings with vinblastine and vindesine, and although diarrhea may occur, constipation is a much more common and troublesome side effect, especially during therapy with vincristine. Since constipation may be very severe and paralytic ileus also may develop, measures to prevent or alleviate the condition, such as the use of stool softeners, must be instituted before vincristine therapy commences.

4. Miscellaneous Side Effects

Hair loss is common with all three alkaloids but is somewhat more frequent with vincristine and vindesine. Recovery may occur despite continued therapy, but is likely to be slow. A headband inflated to arterial pressures and worn for about 15 min may reduce the severity of this side effect. Phlebitis usually results from local irritation and extravasation during injection, as these compounds are highly irritating agents capable of causing severe local necrosis. Great care to ensure that the needle is well seated in the vein is essential. A rare toxicity that has received attention is inappropriate secretion of antidiuretic hormone with hyponatremia, reported in patients receiving vincristine (Slater et al., 1969). It probably arises from a more generalized interference with secretory and phagocytotic processes that accompanies disorganization of the microtubule system. Since, as we shall see later, there is a major biliary component to the excretion pattern of these alkaloids, dose reduction should be considered in any patients with impaired liver function to prevent escalation of toxicity. This is especially true if the regimen of combined chemotherapy in which the vinca alkaloid is being used includes another agent, such as adriamycin, that is largely cleared through the bile. It should also be pointed out that children may generally tolerate more vincristine than adults, but the drug is not generally used in infants below the age of 24-30 months, in whom myelinization and neuronal migration is not complete.

Further discussion of the toxicity and biological actions of these drugs may be found in the reviews of Johnson *et al.* (1963), De Conti and Creasey (1975), and Creasey (1979).

C. Clinical Pharmacokinetics

Detailed knowledge of the pharmacokinetics of the vinca alkaloids was only acquired over the last few years, when radiolabeled alkaloids became available, and new methodologies, such as radioimmunoassay and high-pressure liquid chromatography, were applied to the problem. The intention here is to outline the main features of vinca alkaloid pharmacokinetics in humans, using animal data only to expand on the discussion. Data are derived from the work of several laboratories.

1. Plasma Pharmacokinetics

Early information on the plasma levels of the vinca alkaloids has been summarized elsewhere (Creasey, 1975; De Conti and Creasey, 1975). These measurements for the most part were performed by bioassay using growth inhibition of KB or L cells in culture.

Recent pharmacokinetic analyses of data obtained by radioimmunoassay (Owellen *et al.*, 1977a,b; Dyke and Nelson, 1977) are consistent with a three-compartment model giving plasma clearance curves that are triphasic with the pharmacokinetic parameters listed in Table II. It should be noted that whereas vinblastine and vindesine resemble each other, vincristine has longer half-lives for all three phases, particularly the terminal γ phase. The extremely rapid initial phase represents sequestration of drug by the cells. Studies with labeled

TABLE II

Pharmacokinetic Data for the Vinca Alkaloids[a]

Parameter	Vinblastine	Vincristine[b]	Vindesine
$t_{1/2}\alpha$, hr	0.105 (0.014)	0.038 (0.017)	0.074 (0.049)
$t_{1/2}\beta$, hr	3.24 (1.03)	0.822 (0.273)	1.74 (0.403)
$t_{1/2}\gamma$, hr	144 (15.2)	24.3 (11.1)	28.8 (3.70)
$V_d\gamma$, liter/kg	11.0 (0.60)	8.11 (4.02)	35.1 (9.40)
Clearance, liter/kg/hr	0.053 (0.003)	2.252 (0.100)	0.855 (0.333)

[a] Data derived from Dyke and Nelson (1977).

[b] ± Standard deviation.

vindesine in rats (Culp *et al.*, 1977) and with tritiated vinblastine in dogs (Creasey *et al.*, 1975) indicate that many tissues, including blood cells, are capable of rapidly accumulating levels of drug that are 10–100 times greater than those in the plasma. This may reflect both binding of drug by intracellular tubulin and the presence of a carrier-mediated mechanism for transport that has been demonstrated for vincristine in many tumor cells (Bleyer *et al.*, 1975). Whatever the mechanism, concentrations of the alkaloids within the blood cells may so greatly exceed those in the coincident plasma that the leukocytes and platelets, which compose only a very small fraction of the total blood volume, may contain nearly half the total drug content of the blood (Table III). Indeed, it has been suggested that bound, unmetabolized drug in these elements may constitute a significant reservoir for the body (Hebden *et al.*, 1970).

In the plasma about 75% of total alkaloid may be associated with proteins, particularly the α and β-globulin fractions (Donigian and Owellen, 1973; Owellen *et al.*, 1977a,b).

2. Retention and Excretion

In conformity with the longer half-life of vincristine, estimates of total body load show that this alkaloid persists very much longer in the body than do the other two drugs. At 48 hr the tissues still contain over 50% of the administered dose of vincristine. Nelson has suggested that such data make a twice weekly dose of vinblastine or vindesine more rational from a pharmacokinetic viewpoint than once weekly doses. He also considered it likely that the greater neurologic toxicity of vincristine is a reflection of the more prolonged retention of this alkaloid. However, since the neurologic toxicity of the more rapidly eliminated vindesine is comparable to that of vincristine, and myelotoxicity also varies among the drugs in a manner that does not reflect pharmacokinetic features, it is clear that the latter alone do not determine toxicity. There undoubtedly is a correlation ($r = 0.959$) between drug clearance, on the one hand (Table II), and clinical dose, on the other (2.0, 7.0, and 12.0 mg/70 kg for vincristine,

TABLE III

Distribution of [³H] Vinblastine in Blood Elements[a]

Time (min)	Percent of whole blood content			
	Plasma	Erythrocytes	Leukocytes	Platelets
5	43.0	24.4	7.4	25.2
90	39.5	22.5	15.6	23.1

[a] Data derived from Owellen *et al.* (1977a,b).

TABLE IV

Cumulation Excretion of Vinblastine[a]

	Percent of administered dose			
	Dogs		Humans	
Days	Urine	Stools	Urine	Stools
1	6.5	15.0	10.5	2.0
2	8.0		12.0	5.5
3	10.0		13.0	10.0
6	12.5	26.0	15.0	11.0
9	14.5	33.0		

[a] Data from dogs derived from Creasey *et al.* (1975); human data from Owellen *et al.*, (1977a,b).

vindesine, and vinblastine, respectively), so it would appear that although overall tolerance is related to pharmacokinetics, the incidence of a specific toxic symptom is not.

Excretion of vinblastine is divided between urine and stools in both dogs and humans, but it appears that biliary excretion ultimately predominates in dogs (Table IV), and probably humans. At early times material in the urine consists predominantly of unchanged drug and desacetyl vinblastine, itself an active antitumor agent, but later other breakdown products come to predominate (Table V). Unchanged vinblastine accounts for only a small fraction of the material excreted in the stools. The pattern for vinblastine applies also to vincristine and

TABLE V

Percent Composition of Urinary Excretion Products of Vinblastine[a]

Time	Desacetyl-vinblastine	Vinblastine
Humans, hr		
8	3.2	66.7
16	7.3	53.7
24	5.3	42.8
40	9.7	26.2
Dogs, days		
1	10.5	60.0
4	18.0	50.3
6	6.0	11.3
9	–	1.8

[a] Data for humans from Owellen *et al.* (1977a,b); for dogs from Creasey *et al.* (1975).

TABLE VI

**Cumulative Urinary Excretion of Vincristine and
Vindesine**[a]

	Percent of administered dose	
Time (hr)	Vincristine	Vindesine
4	6	4
12	9	13
24	10	32

[a] Data derived from Owellen *et al.* (1977a,b).

vindesine, but as might be expected from the data discussed earlier, urinary excretion of vincristine occurs at a much slower rate (Table VI). There is also evidence of less metabolic breakdown of vincristine.

D. Clinical Use

1. Spectra of Activity

The vinca alkaloids have been employed against a wide range of neoplastic diseases. However, the tumors against which they are effective represent a small percentage of total nonoperable cancer (Table VII). In particular, success has been most evident with leukemias, lymphomas, and childhood tumors. Favorable responses in breast, ovarian, and testicular carcinomas are more recent findings, generally obtained with combinations that include one or more vinca alkaloids. Another point about Table VII is that there are clear differences between the alkaloids in terms of their spectra of activity. This is most clearly evident on comparing vinblastine and vincristine. Vinblastine has not been of any value in the therapy of leukemias, for example, whereas it is here that vincristine has been most effective. Typical therapeutic dosages of these drugs are as follows: vinblastine, 6–8 mg/m²; vincristine, about 1.4 mg/m² in adults and 2 mg/m² in children; and vindesine, 4–6 mg/m². In present chemotherapy these alkaloids are, however, no longer used as single agents, but rather constitute important components of a large number of multiple drug protocols. Before dealing with examples of the use of vinca alkaloids it is appropriate to review the topic of combination chemotherapy.

2. Principles of Combination Chemotherapy

The criteria used in the derivation of chemotherapy regimens appear in Table VIII. The first criterion is toxicologic, of which the most important consideration

TABLE VII

Tumors Most Responsive to the Vinca Alkaloids

Disease	Vinblastine	Vincristine	Vindesine
Acute lymphoblastic leukemia		+	+
Acute myelocytic leukemia		+	+
Breast carcinoma		+	
Burkitt's lymphoma	+	+	
Ewing's sarcoma		+	+
Hodgkin's disease	+	+	+
Neuroblastoma		+	
Non-Hodgkin's lymphoma	+	+	+
Ovarian carcinoma	+		
Reticulum cell sarcoma		+	
Retinoblastoma		+	
Rhabdomyosarcoma		+	
Squamous and renal cell carcinoma			+
Testicular carcinoma	+	+	
Wilms' tumor		+	

is avoidance of overlapping toxicities. If each drug inflicts a metabolic insult on a tumor and on a particular normal tissue system such as the bone marrow, addition of another drug with the same actions will increase both antitumor effect and toxicity, and dose reduction will be needed. On the other hand, if the toxicities differ, the tumor will receive a double insult, and each normal tissue will have a tolerable toxicity. Vincristine has been a particularly valuable agent in this connection because its neurotoxicity does not overlap with the side effects of most other drugs that are commonly myelosuppressive. Vinblastine, on the other hand, with leukopenia as its limiting side effect, is not so readily adapted to multiple drug regimens. Attempts to use antidotes in the manner of the methotrexate–citrovorum system have not been successful. The only agent that has been used clinically is glutamate, which, in massive doses that cause gastrointestinal distress, may reduce cellular uptake of the vinca alkaloids if it precedes the drug.

Biochemical criteria for the use of vinca alkaloids in combination are not so well

TABLE VIII

Criteria for Combination Chemotherapy

Toxicologic	Nonoverlapping toxicities, use of antidotes
Biochemical	Increased selective inhibition of biosynthetic pathways by sequential, concurrent, and complementary inhibition
Pharmacologic	Modified transport, metabolism, protein binding, and excretion
Cell cycle kinetic	Use of phase specificity and scheduling recruitment from G_0

established. Since they are known to inhibit the biosynthesis of nucleic acid, protein, and phospholipid and to interfere with respiration, it might be possible to find other agents to potentiate these effects. An approach that involves mathematical modeling of possible biochemical perturbations might be of value here. It is possible that clinical advantage is already being taken of such interactions in the prednisone–vincristine combination. Corticosteroids may initiate degradation of RNA in sensitive cells (Ambellan and Hollander, 1966), whereas vincristine as an inhibitor of RNA biosynthesis (Creasey, 1975) may thus exert what is known as complementary inhibition.

Among the pharmacologic criteria, transport is one that has been exploited. Vincristine inhibits the part of the carrier-mediated transport system for methotrexate that is responsible for efflux of the drug from cells; this leads to intracellular accumulation of the antifolate. This combination has been used in the clinic.

Finally, cell cycle kinetic considerations provide another basis for rational use of the vinca alkaloids (Clarkson, 1974). These drugs block proliferating cells in mitosis, causing an accumulation of mitotic figures (C mitosis), but are actually preferentially lethal to cells in the DNA synthetic S phase. Since alkylating agents show somewhat enhanced kill of cells in mitosis and since their action often leads to recruitment of cells into cycle with need for DNA synthesis, there are clearly at least two potential interactions between vinca alkaloids and alkylating agents that might enhance cytotoxicity. Mitotic arrest itself may produce some degree of partial synchrony as surviving cells recover from the blockade and enter S phase, where they are sensitive to antimetabolites. Thus the lethal action of the latter agents might be enhanced by the availability of a relatively greater proportion of sensitive cells.

3. Treatment Protocols

In the therapy of acute lymphoblastic leukemia, combinations involving vincristine have become the first-line treatment with a high incidence of complete long-term remissions and apparent cure of nearly 60% (Pinkel, 1978). These types of "total therapy" involve three stages.

An initial rigorous induction phase serves to bring about complete remission. Early work, before the days of complex schedules, showed that vincristine, especially in conjunction with prednisone, produced a high incidence (80%) of remissions that were, however, of relatively brief duration, necessitating other approaches to maintain the remission. The vincristine–prednisone combination is still the basis of the induction regimens. Cranial irradiation or intrathecal methotrexate were added to take care of leukemic cells sequestered within the central nervous system and relatively inaccessible to drugs by reason of the blood–brain barrier. Additional drugs, such as L-asparaginase, daunorubicin, or methotrexate, may be included in the induction stage.

The introduction of a second stage of consolidation or intensification therapy was intended to expose those cells surviving induction, perhaps less than 10^9 leukemic cells, to intensive therapy, a concept based on cell kill kinetics in the L1210 mouse leukemia. Its value in the clinic over using a continuous level of maintenance therapy is still uncertain. Drugs used for maintenance therapy are typically those that when used as single agents may not have produced as high an incidence of complete remissions as the vincristine–prednisone combination, but they did have a more long-lasting action.

It is no longer possible to distinguish the treatment protocols on the basis of incidence of remission, which in all cases is in excess of 90%. The critical parameter is the duration of unmaintained disease-free survival. In Table IX some features of several of the more recent protocols are outlined. Optimal long-term therapy regimens have yet to be defined, and it is quite possible that patients may be exposed needlessly to a multiplicity of drugs when fewer would be as effective. The increasing numbers of long-term survivors of intensive cyto-toxic therapy, who were treated at an early age when development was not yet complete, raises the prospect of chronic toxic hazards that are at present not completely understood. Thus attention to devising regimens without such hazards is becoming imperative.

Another disease that has responded to combination chemotherapy schedules that include the vinca alkaloids is Hodgkin's disease (Lacher, 1978). The basic approach to this lymphoma originally developed by DeVita and co-workers (1970) was the MOPP regimen which has come to be the basis for a range of other strategies. MOPP is the abbreviation derived from the initials of mechlorethamine (nitrogen mustard), Oncovin (vincristine), prednisone, and procarbazine; the doses and schedules are outlined in Table X. With this regimen the complete response rate reached 81%. Other regimens have substituted cyclophosphamide for nitrogen mustard (COPP), vinblastine for vincristine (MVPP), or thio-TEPA and vinblastine for nitrogen mustard and vincristine (TVPP). The ABVD regimen of Bonadonna et al. (1975) uses adriamycin, bleomycin, vinblastine, and DTIC, as indicated in Table X. Complete response rates range up to 90% with these regimens, but it is more important that more than 60% of those who achieve remission have more than 5 years of relapse-free survival. The need now is to devise protocols that do not show cross resistance to MOPP-type regimens to use on nonresponding or relapsing patients.

As with acute lymphoblastic leukemia, long-term sequelae of intensive chemotherapy are of increasing concern. Indeed, with Hodgkin's disease they are better defined and include, on the one hand, secondary neoplasms associated with treatment and/or disease and, on the other, aseptic necrosis of the femoral heads.

While the vinca alkaloids have not been particularly successful as single agents in the treatment of solid tumors, recent combinations that include these drugs have shown promise. The most impressive responses have been observed in patients with testicular cancers treated with vinblastine and bleomycin in combi-

TABLE IX

Examples of the Combination Chemotherapy of Acute Lymphoblastic Leukemia

Study	Induction	Consolidation	Maintenance	Percent complete remission	Follow-up
Simone et al. (1975), St. Jude	VCR, Pred CNS prophylaxis	MTX, 6MP CYT, Pred	6MP + MTX VCR + Pred	89	64–71 months remission
Clarkson (1974), Memorial- L2	VCR, Pred DNR, MTX CNS prophylaxis	Ara-C, 6TG L-Asp, BCNU	6TG + CYT HU + DNR MTX + BCNU Ara-C + VCR	98	70% 5-yr survivors
Furman et al. (1976), Farber	VCR, Pred L-Asp CNS prophylaxis	VCR, ADR 6MP, Pred	VCR, ADR 6MP, Pred	91	20–23 months remission

TABLE X

Examples of Protocols Used for Hodgkin's Disease

| Regimen | Components | Percent responses | |
		Complete	Partial
MOPP—DeVita *et al.* (1970)	Nitrogen mustard, 6 mg/m² days 1 and 8	81	14
	Vincristine 1.4 mg/m² days 1 and 8		
	Procarbazine, 100 mg/m²/day × 14		
	Prednisone, 40 mg/m²/day × 14 cycles 1 and 4 only		
	Six 2-week cycles—14 days on, 14 days off		
ABVD—Bonadonna *et al.* (1975)	Adriamycin 25 mg/m² days 1 and 14	70	18
	Bleomycin, 10 mg/m² days 1 and 14		
	Vinblastine, 6₂mg/m² days 1 and 14		
	DTIC, 150 mg/m² days 1–5		
	Six courses q 28 days		
TVPP—Lacher (1978)	Thio-TEPA, 15 mg/kg days 1 and 8	90	10
	Vinblastine, 0.1 mg/kg days 1 and 8		
	Procarbazine, 75 mg/kg/day × 14		
	Prednisone, 50 mg/day × 14		
	Restart cycle every 3 weeks for 6 months		
	Maintenance by induction regimen q 3 months for 3 years		

nation (Samuels *et al.*, 1976) or with these two drugs plus *cis*-diammine dichloroplatinum (II) (Einhorn and Furnas, 1977). Complete remissions occur in almost 70% of the patients treated, and from the number of moderately long-term survivors being reported it is probable that these combinations have curative potential.

In this brief review it obviously has been impossible to cover all clinical aspects of the vinca alkaloids, but some idea has been conveyed of the overall value of these drugs.

II. THE PODOPHYLLOTOXIN DERIVATIVES

A. Introduction

The podophyllotoxin derivatives VM-26 and VP-16 (actually, VP-16-213), whose structures appear in Fig. 2, are synthetic modifications of natural agents

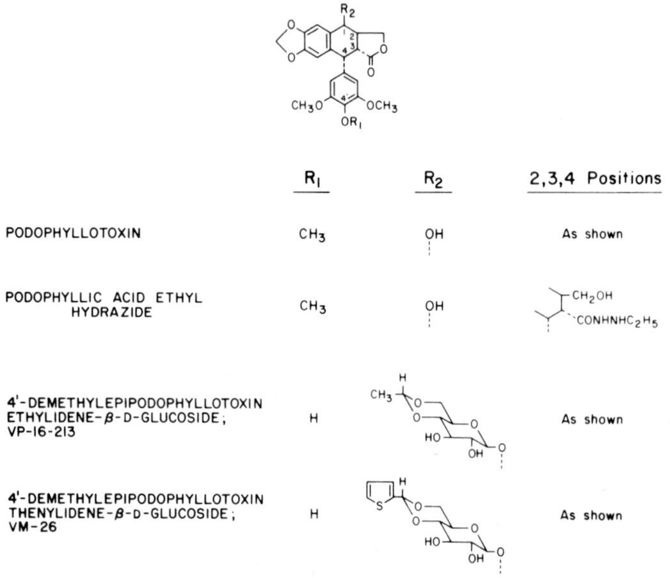

	R_1	R_2	2,3,4 Positions
PODOPHYLLOTOXIN	CH_3	OH	As shown
PODOPHYLLIC ACID ETHYL HYDRAZIDE	CH_3	OH	CH_2OH / $CONHNHC_2H_5$
4'-DEMETHYLEPIPODOPHYLLOTOXIN ETHYLIDENE-β-D-GLUCOSIDE; VP-16-213	H		As shown
4'-DEMETHYLEPIPODOPHYLLOTOXIN THENYLIDENE-β-D-GLUCOSIDE; VM-26	H		As shown

Fig. 2. Structures of the podophyllotoxin derivatives.

found in the resin of the may apple, *Podophyllum peltatum,* Linn. This material was traditionally used to treat warts and more recently was found effective as a topical agent for condylomata acuminata. The pharmacology of the podophyllotoxin derivatives has been reviewed (Creasey, 1977). Although the derivatives in general resemble the vinca alkaloids in producing mitotic arrest (Krishan *et al.,* 1975), apparently through interaction at the same site to which another antimitotic, colchicine, binds (Wilson, 1975), VM-26 and VP-16 exert an effect on the G_2 phase of the cell cycle (Misra and Roberts, 1975) and do not appear to inhibit the assembly of microtubules *in vitro* because of steric hindrance from the bulky glycosidic substituents (Loike *et al.,* 1978). An additional effect of VM-26 and VP-16, as well as of other podophyllotoxin derivatives with a 4'-hydroxy group, is to cause intracellular degradation of DNA (Loike and Horowitz, 1976). The podophyllotoxins also inhibit the biosynthesis of nucleic acids.

B. Toxicology

The most frequent side effects of VM-26 or VP-16 are nausea and vomiting, with occasional diarrhea. Myelosuppression, giving rise to both leukopenia and thrombocytopenia, is the dose-limiting toxicity. Other common toxic effects are alopecia and pruritis.

C. Clinical Pharmacokinetics

Allen and Creaven (1975) compared the pharmacokinetics of VM-26 and VP-16 in patients receiving these drugs. Data for VM-26 fit a triphasic pattern with a β half-life of 11–38 hr, whereas VP-16 plasma decay kinetics were biexponential with a β half-life of around 8–11 hr; the β phase is the chief phase of elimination. Both drugs were extensively bound to plasma proteins. After 72 hr, 30–45% of the administered dose of both drugs was excreted in the urine, but only 9% was present as unchanged VM-26 compared with 29% for VP-16.

D. Clinical Use

A wide range of tumors have responded to the podophyllotoxins in significant numbers of patients (Table XI). In addition, responses have been reported in Wilms' tumor, acute lymphoblastic leukemia, neuroblastoma, liposarcoma, embryonal testicular carcinoma, and carcinoma of the breast. The results in the latter disease, as well as in head and neck cancer, soft tissue sarcomas, melanoma, and colorectal cancers, have been rather discouraging. Introduction of VP-16 into multidrug regimens for treating oat cell or small cell carcinoma of the lung has been reported (Eagan *et al.*, 1977; Cohen *et al.*, 1977). Oldham *et al.* (1978) have used VP-16 as consolidation therapy for this disease following induction by adriamycin, cyclophosphamide, and vincristine. This program may have curative potential when the disease is limited. It is evident that more exploration is required to establish the roles of VM-26 and VP-16 in the armamentarium of cancer chemotherapy.

TABLE XI

Tumors Most Responsive to VM-26 and VP-16[a]

Disease	Percent responses	
	VM-26	VP-16
Hodgkin's disease	36	23
Reticulum cell sarcoma	42	22
Lymphosarcoma	30	19
Bladder cancer	19	20
Brain cancer	33	0
Small-cell lung cancer		42
Acute nonlymphocytic leukemia	14	37
Ovarian cancer		15

[a] Data derived from Rozencweig *et al.* (1978)

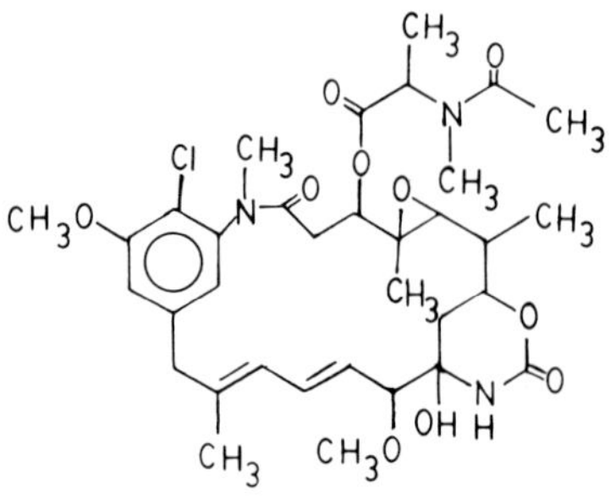

MAYTANSINE

Fig. 3.   Structure of maytansine.

III. MAYTANSINE

A. Introduction

Maytansine is an ansa macrolide (Fig. 3), derived from the East African shrubs *Maytenus ovatus* and *M. Serrata,* that shows antitumor activity (Kupchan *et al.,* 1972). The drug is included in this chapter because of resemblances to the vinca alkaloids in its mechanism of action. Thus it is an inhibitor both of DNA biosynthesis and of mitosis (Wolpert-Defilippes *et al.,* 1975a,b). Studies of its interaction with rat brain tubulin indicate that it binds more avidly with this protein than does vincristine and may react both at the vinca alkaloid site and at some other site for which vincristine does not compete (Mandelbaum-Shavit *et al.,* 1976). Like other antimitotics, it inhibits tubulin polymerization as a result of this interaction (Remillard *et al.,* 1975).

B. Clinical Trials

As a result of its interesting mode of action and impressive activity against experimental tumors, maytansine has been given clinical trial. The phase I studies (Cabanillas *et al.,* 1978; Chabner *et al.,* 1978; Blum and Kahlert, 1978) have disclosed a few responses in non-Hodgkin's lymphoma, acute lymphocytic leukemia, breast carcinoma, ovarian carcinoma, melanoma, and head and neck cancer that are encouraging for further studies. Gastrointestinal toxicity is dose limiting (≥ 0.5 mg/m^2), and consists of nausea, vomiting, diarrhea, and occasional stomatitis. Weakness and other evidence of neurologic toxicity, rare myelosuppression, alopecia, and abnormal liver function tests were also reported. Unless the drug was diluted in a volume greater than 250 ml, superficial phlebitis occurred at the injection site.

REFERENCES

Allen L. M., and Creaven, P. J. (1975). *Eur. J. Cancer* **11**, 697–707.

Ambellan, E., and Hollander, V. P. (1966). *Cancer Res.* **26**, 903–909.

Armstrong, J. G., Dyke, R. W., Fouts, P. J., Hawthorne, J. J., Jansen, C. J., Jr., and Peabody, A. M. (1967). *Cancer Res.* **27**, 221–227.

Bleyer, W. A., Frisby, S. A., and Oliverio, V. T. (1975). *Biochem. Pharmacol.* **24**, 633–639.

Blum, R. H., and Dawson, D. M. (1976). *Proc. Am. Assoc. Cancer Res.* **17**, 108.

Blum, R. H., and Kahlert, T. (1978). *Cancer Treat. Rep.* **62**, 435–438.

Bodey, G. P., and Freireich, E. J. (1976). *Proc. Am. Assoc. Cancer Res.* **17**, 128.

Bonadonna, G., Zucali, R., Monfardini, S., DeLena, M., and Uslenghi, C. (1975). *Cancer (Philadelphia)* **36**, 252–259.

Cabanillas, F., Rodriguez, V., Hall, S. W., Burgess, M. A., Bodey, G. P., and Freireich, E. J. (1978). *Cancer Treat. Rep.* **62**, 425–428.

Chabner, B. A., Levine, A. S., Johnson, B. L., and Young, R. C. (1978). *Cancer Treat. Rep.* **62**, 429–433.

Clarkson, B. (1974). *In* "Handbook of Experimental Pharmacology: Antineoplastic and Immunosuppressive Agents" (A. C. Sartorelli and D. G. Johns, eds.), Vol. 38, Part 1, pp. 156–193. Springer-Verlag, Berlin and New York.

Cohen, M. H., Broder, L. E., Fossieck, B. F., Ihde, D. C., and Minna, J. D. (1977). *Cancer Treat. Rep.* **61**, 489–490.

Creasey, W. A. (1975). *In* "Handbook of Experimental Pharmacology: Antineoplastic and Immunosuppressive Agents" (A. C. Sartorelli and D. G. Johns, eds.), Vol. 38, Part 2, pp. 670–694. Springer-Verlag, Berlin and New York.

Creasey, W. A. (1977). *In* "Cancer—A Comprehensive Treatise" (F. F. Becker, ed.), Vol. 5, pp. 379–425. Plenum, New York.

Creasey, W. A. (1979). *In* "Antibiotics" (F. Hahn, ed.), Vol. 5, pp. 414–438. Springer-Verlag, Berlin and New York.

Creasey, W. A., Scott, A. I., Wei, C. C., Kutcher, J., Schwartz, A., and Marsh, J. C. (1975). *Cancer Res.* **35**, 1116–1120.

Culp, H. W., Daniels, W. D., and McMahon, R. E. (1977). *Cancer Res.* **37**, 3053–3056.

Currie, V., Wong, P., Tan, R., Tan, C., and Krakoff, I. (1976). *Proc. Am. Assoc. Cancer Res.* **17**, 174.

Dahlstrom, A., Heiwall, P. O., Haggendal, J., and Saunders, N. R. (1975). *Ann. N.Y. Acad. Sci.* **253**, 507–516.

De Conti, R. C., and Creasey, W. A. (1975). *In* "The Catharanthus Aklaloids" (W. I. Taylor and N. R. Farnsworth, eds.), pp. 237–278. Dekker, New York.

DeVita, V. T., Serpick, A. A., and Carbone, P. P. (1970). *Ann. Intern. Med.* **73**, 881–895.

Donigian, D. W., and Owellen, R. J. (1973). *Biochem. Pharmacol.* **22**, 2113–2119.

Dyke, R. W., and Nelson, R. L. (1977). *Cancer Treat. Rev.* **4**, 135–142.

Eagan, R. T., Carr, D. T., Lee, R. E., Frytak, S., Rubin, J., and Coles, D. T. (1977). *Cancer Treat. Rep.* **61**, 93–95.

Einhorn, L. H., and Furnas, B. (1977). *J. Clin. Hematol. Oncol.* **7**, 662–671.

Furman, L., Camitta, B. M., Jaffe, N., Sallan, S. E., Cassady, J. R., Traggis, D., Leavitt, P., Nathan, D. G., and Frei, E., III (1976). *Med. Pediatr. Oncol.* **2**, 157–166.

Gailani, S. D., Armstrong, J. G., Carbone, P. F., Tan, C., and Holland, J. F. (1966). *Cancer Chemother. Rep.* **50**, 95–103.

Gottschalk, P. G., Dyck, P. J., and Kiely, J. M. (1968). *Neurology* **18**, 875–882.

Hebden, H. F., Hadfield, J. R., and Beer, C. T. (1970). *Cancer Res.* **30**, 1417–1424.

Johnson, I. S., Armstrong, J. G., Gorman, M., and Burnett, J. P., Jr. (1963). *Cancer Res.* **23,** 1390-1427.

Krishan, A., Paika, K., and Frei, E., III (1975). *J. Cell Biol.* **66,** 521-530.

Kupchan, S. M., Komoda, Y., Court, W. A., Thomas, G. J., Smith, R. M., Karim, A., Gilmore, C. J., Haltiwanger, R. C., and Bryan, R. F. (1972). *J. Am. Chem. Soc.* **94,** 1354-1356.

Lacher, M. J. (1978). *In* "Cancer Chemotherapy III—The Forty-Sixth Hahnemann Symposium" (I. Brodsky, S. B. Kahn, and J. F. Conroy, eds.), pp. 363-382. Grune & Stratton, New York.

Loike, J. D., and Horowitz, S. B. (1976). *Biochemistry* **15,** 5443-5448.

Loike, J. D., Brewer, C. F., Sternlicht, H., Gensler, W. J., and Horowitz, S. B. (1978). *Cancer Res.* **38,** 2688-2693.

McLeod, J. G., and Penny, R. (1969). *J. Neurol. Neurosurg. Psychiatry* **32,** 297-304.

Mandelbaum-Shavit, F., Wolpert-DeFilippes, M. K., and Johns, D. G. (1976). *Biochem. Biophys. Res. Commun.* **72,** 47-54.

Mathé, G., Schneider, M., Band, P., Amiel, J. L., Schwarzenberg, L., Cattan, A., and Schlumberger, J. R. (1965). *Cancer Chemother. Rep.* **49,** 47-49.

Mathé, G., Misset, J. L., DeVassal, F., Gouveia, J., Hayat, M., Machover, D., Belpomme, D., Pico, J. L., Schwarzenberg, L., Riband, P., Musset, M., Jasmin, C., and DeLuca, L. (1978). *Cancer Treat. Rep.* **62,** 805-809.

Misra, N. C., and Roberts, D. (1975). *Cancer Res.* **35,** 99-105.

Ochs, S., and Worth, R. (1975). *Proc. Am. Assoc. Cancer Res.* **16,** 70.

Oldham, R. K., Greco, F., Richardson, R. L., and Stroup, S. L. (1978). *Proc. Am. Assoc. Cancer Res.* **19,** 361.

Owellen, R. J., Hartke, C. A., and Hains, F. O., (1977a). *Cancer Res.* **37,** 2597-2602.

Owellen, R. J., Root, M. A., and Hains, F. O. (1977b). *Cancer Res.* **37,** 2603-2607.

Pinkel, D. (1978). *In* "Cancer Chemotherapy III—The Forty-Sixth Hahnemann Symposium" (I. Brodsky, S. B. Kahn, and J. F. Conroy, eds.), pp. 429-436. Grune & Stratton, New York.

Remillard, S., Rebhun, L. I., Howie, G. A., and Kupchan, S. M. (1975). *Science* **189,** 1002-1005.

Robertson, J. H., and McCarthy, G. M. (1969). *Lancet* **ii,** 353-355.

Rozencweig, M., VonHoff, D. D., and Muggia, F. M. (1978). *In* "Cancer Chemotherapy III—the Forty-Sixth Hahnemann Symposium" (I. Brodsky, S. B. Kahn, and J. F. Conroy, eds.), pp. 75-85. Grune & Stratton, New York.

Samuels, M. L., Lanzotti, V. J., Holoye, P. Y., Boyle, L. E., Smith, T. L., and Johnson, D. E. (1976). *Cancer Treat. Rev.* **3,** 185-204.

Simone, J. V., Aur, R. J. A., Hustu, H. O., Verzosa, M., and Pinkel, D. (1975). *Cancer (Philadelphia)* **35,** 25-35.

Slater, L. M., Wainer, R. A., and Serpick, A. A. (1969). *Cancer (Philadelphia)* **23,** 122-125.

Svoboda, G. H., and Blake, D. A. (1975). *In* "The Catharanthus Alkaloids" (W. I. Taylor and N. R. Farnsworth, eds.), pp. 45-83. Dekker, New York.

Wilson, L. (1975). *Ann. N.Y. Acad. Sci.* **253,** 213-231.

Wolpert-DeFfilippes, M. K., Adamson, R. H., Cysyk, R. L., and Johns, D. G. (1975a).*Biochem. Pharmacol.* **24,** 751-754.

Wolpert-DeFfilippes, M. K., Bono, V. H., Jr., Dion, R. L., and Johns, D. G. (1975b). *Biochem. Pharmacol.* **24,** 1735-1738.

Wong, P. P., Yagoda, A., Currie, V. E., and Young, C. W. (1977). *Cancer Treat. Rep.* **61,** 1727-1729.

7

BLEOMYCIN—AN OVERVIEW
Stanley T. Crooke

I. INTRODUCTION

Bleomycin is an antitumor antibiotic initially isolated and characterized by Umezawa and colleagues (Umezawa *et al.*, 1966b). Subsequently, it was demonstrated to be active in a variety of animal tumor systems and to have significant clinical activity in the treatment of several malignancies. In addition to its antitumor activities, it is of interest because of its unique mechanism of action, toxicity profile, and its interesting clinical pharmacology.

II. CHEMISTRY

Bleomycin is produced by a strain of *Streptomyces verticillus* and is purified by ion exchange chromatography, which results in fractionation of the bleomycin complex into approximately 12 components (Umezawa *et al.*, 1966a,b).

CANCER AND CHEMOTHERAPY, VOL. III
97

Bleomycin A_2 accounts for 55–70% and bleomycin B_2, 25–32% of the material employed clinically. The other natural analogues account for less than 5% of the total. The clinically employed mixture is copper-free.

The proposed structure of bleomycin is shown in Fig. 1. It is composed of the bleomycinic acid nucleus shown in detail in Fig. 1 and a terminal amine structure (R). It has a molecular weight of approximately 1400, which varies, depending on the size of the terminal amine structure (Nakamura *et al.*, 1974; Umezawa, 1974).

Numerous analogues of bleomycin have been prepared as natural products, products of directed fermentations employing various amines as precursors, and semisynthesis (Takita *et al.*, 1972; Umezawa, 1973). These can be divided into three generations. First generation analogues can be thought of as the original analogues varying only in the terminal amine. Second generation analagues are the more than 250 analogues prepared subsequently which differ only in the terminal amine. Third generation analogues are those that differ significantly in the bleomycinic acid portion of the molecule. Although more than 300 second-generation analogues have been reported, only one third-generation analogue, Tallysomycin, has been reported (Konishi *et al.*, 1977).

Recently, a modification of the bleomycin structure has been proposed. The proposed modified bleomycin structure is shown in Fig. 2 and is essentially an equivalent structure in which the β-lactam ring system is opened (Umezawa,

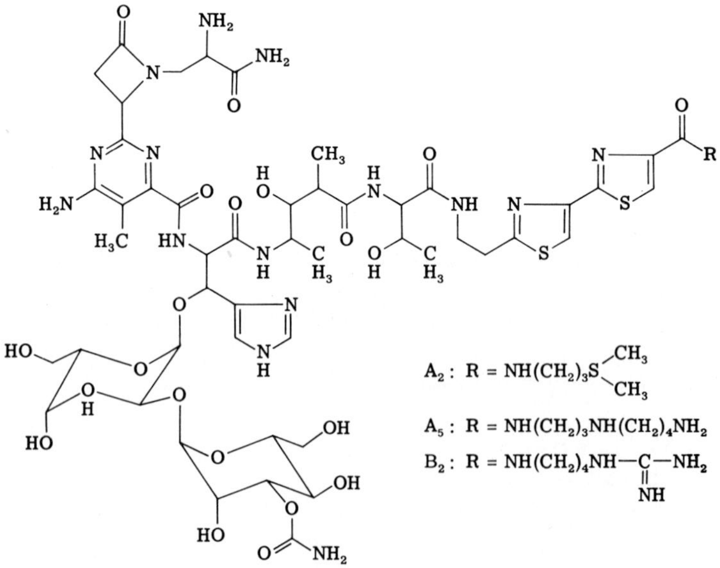

A_2 : R = $NH(CH_2)_3S\overset{\displaystyle CH_3}{\underset{\displaystyle CH_3}{<}}$

A_5 : R = $NH(CH_2)_3NH(CH_2)_4NH_2$

B_2 : R = $NH(CH_2)_4NH-\overset{\displaystyle O}{\underset{\displaystyle NH}{C}}-NH_2$

Fig. 1. Structure of bleomycin.

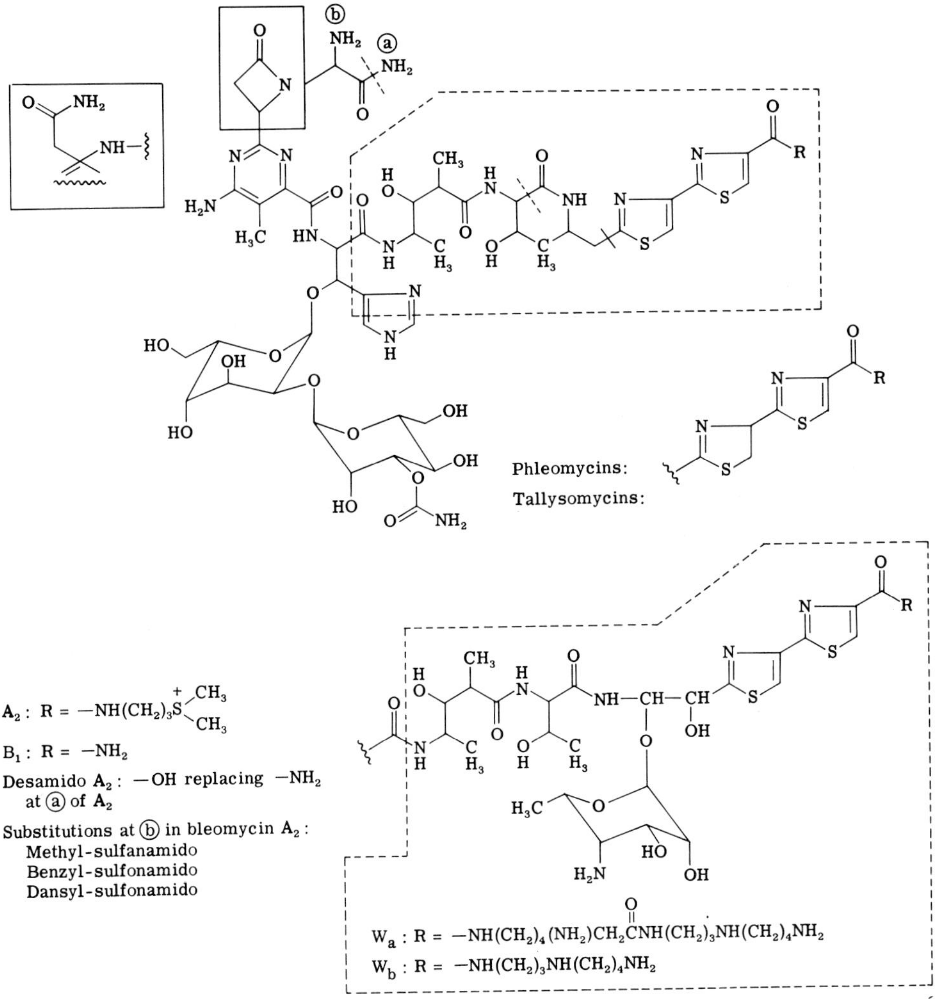

Fig. 2. Structure of tested bleomycin-related drug compounds.

1978). If the new structure is correct, this change would have no effect on the clinical activity but might alter certain structure activity relationship concepts, as well as concepts concerning metal binding.

III. MOLECULAR PHARMACOLOGY

That many of the effects of bleomycin may be related to its ability to degrade preformed DNA is now well established. Clearly, bleomycin binds to a variety of types of DNA and polydeoxynucleotides (Muller *et al.*, 1972; Umezawa, 1974). Subsequent to binding, the first effect observed is the release of free bases from DNA treated with bleomycin. At relatively low concentrations, thymine is selectively released, and at higher concentrations all four bases are released (Muller *et al.*, 1972; Muller and Zahn, 1976; Haidle *et al.*, 1972a,b).

After release of free bases, DNA degradation is observed. Bleomycin is specific for polydeoxyribonucleotides (Haidle, 1971; Haidle and Bearden, 1975; Muller *et al.*, 1972; Kuo and Haidle, 1973) and is more active against A-T-rich DNA molecules than G-C-rich DNA molecules (Muller *et al.*, 1972; Muller and Zahn, 1976; Crooke *et al.*, 1975). Bleomycin induces alkali labile sites and single- and double-strand breaks, and the rate of double-strand breaks is too great to be due to coincident single-strand breaks (Povirk *et al.*, 1977; Strong and Crooke, 1978). Bleomycin has been shown to induce intracellular DNA degradation at concentrations and times compatible with the concept that DNA degradation is a factor in its antitumor activity.

Bleomycin treatment of a variety of cells *in vitro* has been reported to produce a rapid and significant inhibition of DNA synthesis, but very little inhibition of RNA or protein synthesis (Muller *et al.*, 1972; Suzuki *et al.*, 1968; Watanabe *et al.*, 1973). In addition, marked nucleolar morphologic abnormalities have been reported (Daskal *et al.*, 1975). Bleomycin is most active in the G_2 and M phases of the cell cylce (Barranco and Humphrey, 1971; Nagatsu *et al.*, 1972; Tobey, 1972; Watanabe *et al.*, 1974).

IV. CLINICAL PHARMACOLOGY

The study of the clinical pharmacology of bleomycin has been facilitated by the development of a sensitive, specific radioimmunoassay. The most frequently employed radioimmunoassay uses ^{125}I-labeled bleomycin and either rabbit or goat antisera (Broughton and Strong, 1976). This assay was shown to be more than 20 times as sensitive as the microbiological assay and specific for bleomycin. Moreover, it was shown to cross-react with all the important naturally occurring analogues in the clinically employed mixture, Blenoxane (Strong *et al.*, 1977). Results obtained using the radioimmunoassay were comparable to results obtained with the microbiological assay within the range of sensitivity of the microbiological assay in serum, plasma, and urine (Crooke *et al.*, 1977b). Recently, another radioimmunoassay that employs [57]Co-labeled bleomycin has been developed and has been shown to give results comparable to the ^{125}I-radioimmunoassay and the microbiological assay (Elson *et al.*, 1977, 1978).

Bleomycin is absorbed when administered orally, subcutaneously, or intramuscularly. However, oral absorption is quite erratic. Bleomycin is also absorbed to a significant degree when administered either intrapleurally or intraperitoneally. In fact, the bioavailability of bleomycin administered intrapleurally or intraperitoneally has been estimated to be approximately 50% (Alberts *et al.*, 1978). It has been demonstrated that bleomycin is not absorbed to a significant degree after intravesical administration of doses as great as 120 units (Johnson *et al.*, 1976).

After intravenous administration, bleomycin is rapidly distributed. The distribution phase half-life is less than 10 min in man, and bleomycin pharmacokinetics are best described by a two-compartment model. The apparent volume of distribution is approximately 20 liters and is unaffected by variations in renal function (Crooke *et al.*, 1978). Elimination of bleomycin is effected primarily by renal excretion and is relatively rapid as the elimination half-life in patients with normal renal function has been reported to be approximately 120 min (Crooke *et al.*, 1977a; Prestayko and Crooke, 1978).

The rate of clearance of bleomycin from the blood is dependent on renal function. At creatinine clearances in excess of 25–35 ml/min, the elimination half-life of bleomycin was shown to be relatively constant, and approximately 120 min. At creatinine clearances below 25–35 ml/min, the elimination half-life observed after an intravenous bolus increased exponentially as the creatinine clearance decreased (Crooke *et al.*, 1978). This relationship is shown in Fig. 3.

The absorption of bleomycin after intramuscular administration was rapid, with peak serum concentrations observed within 30 min. The peak serum concentrations observed were approximately 50% of those observed after intravenous bolus administration (Elson *et al.*, 1978; Prestayko and Crooke, 1978). Elimination of bleomycin after intramuscular administration has been shown to be comparable to that observed after intravenous bolus administration (Prestayko and Crooke, 1978; Alberts *et al.*, 1978).

The pharmacokinetics of prolonged intravenous infusions have also been studied. As predicted on the basis of the two-compartment model, steady-state serum concentrations were obtained within approximately four half-lives, and the elimination half-life was comparable to that observed after an intravenous bolus. However, a third compartment was suggested by the observation of low concentrations of bleomycin in the serum several hours after discontinuation of the infusion. Unfortunately, since the concentrations were at the limit of sensitivity of the radioimmunoassay, the validity of these low concentrations is questionable. Table I summarizes these results.

In patients with normal renal function, approximately 50% of an intravenous bolus dose was excreted within 4 hr, and approximately 70% within 24 hr (Crooke *et al.*, 1977b). There are currently no data concerning other methods of clearance, and the bleomycin found in the urine was intact and active (Crooke *et al.*, 1977a). Nevertheless, in patients in frank renal failure, bleomycin was cleared within 48–72 hr after an intravenous bolus and was not dialyzable (Crooke *et al.*, 1977b).

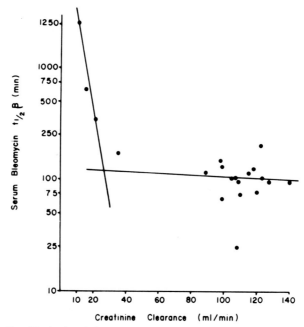

Fig. 3. Semilogarithmic plot of plasma and serum $t_{1/2}\beta$ of bleomycin versus creatinine clearance from values determined using the radioimmunoassay.

V. CLINICAL ACTIVITIES

Bleomycin has demonstrated activity as a single agent and in various combinations in the treatment of patients with testicular carcinomas, lymphomas, and squamous cell carcinomas (Blum *et al.*, 1973; Crooke and Bradner, 1976).

A. Testicular Cancer

In the treatment of metastatic testicular carcinomas of all histologic types, bleomycin is an important drug in first-line chemotherapeutic regimens. Most of the currently employed regimens are based on the combination of vinblastine and bleomycin (Samuels *et al.*, 1975). To this two-drug regimen is now added cisplatin, and in some combinations other agents such as actinomycin D. Perhaps the regimen that has generated the most enthusiasm is the Einhorn regimen. It consists of bleomycin 30 U/ week × 12 I.V., vinblastine 0.2 mg/kg daily for 2 days every 3 weeks, and cisplatin 20 mg/m² per day × 5 every 3 weeks given as a 15-min I.V. infusion with hydration (Einhorn and Donohue, 1977). In a study of 80 evaluable patients with stage III or IV testicular tumors, this regimen resulted in a complete remission rate of 54% and partial remission rate of 42%. More-

TABLE I

Comparison of $t_{\frac{1}{2}}\beta$ Bleomycin with Route of Administration[a]

Route	$t_{1/2}\beta$ RIA ^{125}I (min)	$t_{1/2}\beta$ RIA ^{57}Co (min)	$t_{1/2}\beta$ Micro-biological (min)
I.V. rapid injection	109	—	111
I.V. 10-min injection	122	—	—
I.V. continuous infusion	9.53 hr	—	—
	234 min	(<10 μU/ml values excluded)	
I.M. injection	158	144	175

[a] These values are for patients with creatinine clearance ≥ 60 ml/min.

over, the complete response rate was equivalent in all histologic types, and the regimen was as active in patients who had received prior chemotherapy as in those who had received no prior chemotherapy. The median survival time of all patients treated with this regimen has not been reached as yet, but more than 70% of all patients treated remain alive 20 months after initiation of therapy, and the survival of complete responders is significantly better than that of the partial responders.

Other regimens that employ bleomycin include the VAB regimens that in addition to vinblastine and bleomycin contain actinomycin D and, in the later VAB regimens, cisplatin. The VAB II regimen is the most extensively evaluated of the VAB regimens employing cisplatin, and it has resulted in a complete remission rate of 50% and a partial remission rate of 34%. The median survival time for all patients treated with VAB II was approximately 20 months (Wittes *et al.*, 1976). Also reported to be highly active is a regimen that involves a multimodality approach and employs a number of agents in addition to bleomycin, vinblastine, and cisplatin (Merrin *et al.*, 1977).

B. Lymphomas

Bleomycin is employed in a number of active combinations for patients with Hodgkin's disease. It has been added to the MOPP regimen and has proved of some value. Interestingly, low-dose bleomycin (2 U/m²/day × 2 during MOPP cycles 1 and 2) resulted in an improved complete remission rate ($P = .076$) and survival ($P = .06$) when compared to MOPP, but high-dose bleomycin did not. This may have been due to the increased toxicity due to high-dose bleomycin (Coltman *et al.*, 1978).

Alternatively, bleomycin has been employed in regimens that are thought to be non-cross-resistant to MOPP such as MABOP (bleomycin, adriamycin, nitrogen mustard, vincristine, and prednisone), (DeLena *et al.*, 1973). In general, these regimens are also active, but have not been clearly demonstrated to be superior to MOPP.

C. Squamous Cell Carcinoma

Bleomycin has demonstrated activity against squamous cell carcinomas of various sites and is currently employed in many active combinations (Crooke and Bradner, 1976). For the treatment of squamous cell carcinoma of the lung, bleomycin has been used in various combinations, but these combinations, and bleomycin in particular, have failed to demonstrate significant activity in this disease (Livingston, 1978). Bleomycin has been employed in combination with various other agents in the treatment of squamous cell carcinomas of other sites, but there are few data concerning the relative merits of the various combinations (Crooke and Bradner, 1976).

VI. CLINICAL TOXICITIES

A. Pulmonary Toxicity

1. Incidence

The most significant dose-limiting toxicity induced by bleomycin is pulmonary fibrosis. The reported incidence of pulmonary toxicities has varied from 0 to 40% (Crooke and Bradner, 1976). The variation in the incidence is a result of several factors. First, the method by which pulmonary toxicities were diagnosed has varied from accepting clinical findings to accepting only histopathologic evidence as adequate. Second, the patient population has varied significantly. Third, the total doses employed, and the concomitant and/or prior exposure to other potential pulmonary toxins, including radiotherapy to the chest, have varied. Thus an accurate figure for the incidence of pulmonary toxicities is difficult to provide. Perhaps the most reasonable estimates are an overall incidence of clinically significant pulmonary toxicities of approximately 10% and an incidence of fatal toxicities of approximately 1% of all patients treated with bleomycin (Comis, 1978; DeLena *et al.*, 1972).

Several factors are clearly related to the development of bleomycin-induced pulmonary toxicities. Although the relationship is not simple, the total dose of bleomycin to which a patient is exposed is an important factor. At total doses in excess of 400 U, the incidence of pulmonary toxicities increases significantly (Fig. 4) (Comis, 1978). Nevertheless, many patients have received very high doses and not experienced pulmonary toxicities (Samuels *et al.*, 1976). More-

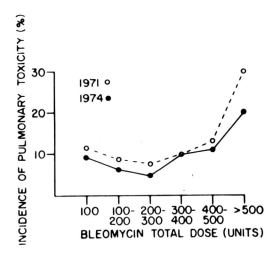

Fig. 4.   Incidence of all categories of bleomycin pulmonary toxicity related to total dose.

over fatal pulmonary toxicities have been reported at low total doses (Iacovino *et al.*, 1976).

Other important factors include the age of the patient but no clear increase in the incidence of the toxicities is observed until age 70 (Fig. 5). (Comis, 1978). Prior or concomitant exposure to radiotherapy to the chest is another important risk factor (Samuels *et al.*, 1975); Crooke *et al.*, 1978). In addition, exposure to other potential pulmonary toxins may contribute to the development of pulmonary toxicities.

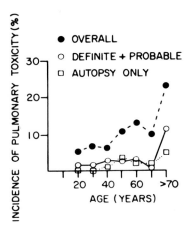

Fig. 5.   Incidence of bleomycin pulmonary toxicity related to age. (NDA Review, 1971, 808 patients.)

2. Clinicopathologic Characteristics

The clinical and pathologic characteristics of bleomycin are nonspecific. Physical findings, rales and rhonchi, may precede radiographic changes and may progress to signs and symptoms of respiratory failure. The radiographic presentation is typical of interstitial pneumonitis, which may progress to pulmonary fibrosis. It has been suggested that pulmonary toxicity may present either as a minimal or as a severe form. The severe form is associated with hypoxemia at rest and prominent radiographic findings; it is rapidly progressive. The minimal form is less severe and does not necessarily progress to fatality (Samuels *et al.*, 1976).

The histopathologic manifestations of bleomycin lung toxicity in humans are comparable to those noted in animals and do not differ significantly from interstitial pneumonitis and fibrosis associated with many other lung toxins. The lesions are found more frequently in the lower lobes and subpleural areas and consist of a fibrinous exudate, atypical proliferation of alveolar cells, hyaline membranes, interstitial and intra-alveolar fibrosis, and squamous metaplasia of the distal air spaces (DeLena *et al.*, 1972, 1973). Electronmicroscopic studies suggest type I alveolar cell destruction followed by type II cellular proliferation (Iacovino *et al.*, 1976). In addition, nucleolar fibrillar centers and granular nuclear bodies have been shown in type I and type II alveolar epithelial cells and fibroblasts.

3. Treatment

At present, no treatment has been demonstrated to be of value in ameliorating bleomycin-induced pulmonary toxicities. Thus prophylaxis is of heightened importance, and this can best be accomplished by limiting the total doses given and avoiding treating patients with bleomycin who have been exposed to radiotherapy to the chest. Unfortunately, pulmonary function tests have proven of little value in detecting early pulmonary toxicity (Pasqual *et al.*, 1973). However, recently, serial carbon monoxide difussion studies have been reported to be of use in patients with testicular carcinomas (Comis, 1978; Comis *et al.*, 1978).

B. Other Toxicities

Bleomycin induces hyperpyrexia in 20–50% of all patients treated (Blum *et al.*, 1973). In patients with lymphomas, the incidence of hyperpyrexia is greater than 50% and is occasionally associated with acute hypotensive responses that are rarely fatal. Hypotensive responses are usually noted within several hours of bleomycin administration, and treatment has included the administration of parenteral fluids, steroids, and antihistamines. There is no evidence that the administration of a test dose is of value in predicting hypotensive responses.

Mucocutaneous toxicities induced by bleomycin are frequent, occurring in approximately 47% of treated patients (Blum *et al.*, 1973; Crooke and Bradner, 1976), and occasionally are severe. Moreover, the severity of mucositis is enhanced when bleomycin is administered with radiotherapy to the head and neck.

VII. CONCLUSIONS

Bleomycin is a clinically useful antineoplastic agent. It has a unique structure, being a glycopeptide with a molecular weight of approximately 1400, and appears to be cytotoxic by degrading intracellular DNA. DNA degradation is thought to result from bleomycin binding to DNA, and facilitating the oxidation of Fe(II), producing free radicals that are the proximate DNA degradative compounds. Bleomycin is most active against nondividing cells. Of dividing cells, cells in M and G_2 are most sensitive.

Bleomycin is of value in the treatment of testicular carcinomas, lymphomas, and squamous cell carcinomas of various sites; however, it produces significant toxicities. The major dose-limiting toxicity is pulmonary fibrosis, which is thought to occur in approximately 10% of patients treated with bleomycin and to be fatal in 1% of the treated patients. It is total dose and age related and significantly exacerbated by prior or concomitant radiotherapy to the chest.

Bleomycin is well absorbed from all sites except the bladder, and after oral administration. It is cleared primarily by renal excretion and has an elimination half-life of approximately 120 min in patients with normal renal function. Essentially nothing is known about its distribution or metabolism in humans.

REFERENCES

Alberts, D., Chen, H.-S, Liu, R., Chen, J., Mayersohn, M., Perrier, D., Moon, T., Gross, J., Broughton, A., and Salmon, S. (1978). *In* "The Bleomycins: Current Status and New Developments" (S. K. Carter, S. T. Crooke, and H. Umezawa, eds.). Academic Press, New York.

Barranco, S. C., and Humphrey, R. M. (1971). *Cancer Res.* **31**, 1218–1223.

Blum, R. H., Carter, S. K., and Agre, K. A. (1973). *Cancer (Philadelphia)* **31**, 903–914.

Broughton, A., and Strong, J. (1976). *Cancer Res.* **36**, 1418–1421.

Coltman, C. A., Jones, S. E., Grozea, P. N., DePersio, E., and Moon, T. E. (1978). *In* "The Bleomycins: Current Status and New Developments" (S. K. Carter, S. T. Crooke, and H. Umezawa, eds.), pp. 227–242. Academic Press, New York.

Comis, R. L., (1978). *In* "The Bleomycins: Current Status and New Developments" (S. K. Carter, S. T. Crooke, and H. Umezawa, eds.), pp. 279–292. Academic Press, New York.

Comis, R. L., Ginsberg, S., Prestayko, A. W., Auchinclaus, J. H., and Crooke, S. T. (1978). *In* "Current Chemotherapy" (W. Siegenthaler and R. Luthy, eds.), Vol. 2, pp. 382–384. American Society for Microbiology, Washington, D.C.

Crooke, S. T., and Bradner, W. T. (1976). *J. Med. (Basel)* **7**, 333–428.

Crooke, S. T., Sitz, T. O., Bannon, M., and Busch, H. (1975). *Physiol. Chem. Phys.* **7**, 177–190.
Crooke, S. T., Comis, R. L., Einhorn, L. H., Strong, J. E., Broughton, A., and Prestayko, A. W. (1977a). *Cancer Treat. Rep.* **61**, 1631–1636.
Crooke, S. T., Luft, F., Broughton, A., Strong, J., Casson, K., and Einhorn, L. (1977b). *Cancer (Philadelphia)* **39**, 1430–1434.
Crooke, S. T., Einhorn, L., Comis, R. L., D'Aoust, J. C., and Prestayko, A. W. (1978). *Med. Pediatr. Oncol.* **5**, 93–98.
Daskal, Y., Crooke, S. T., Smetana, K., and Busch, H. (1975). *Cancer Res.* **35**, 374–381.
DeLana, M., Guzzon, A., Monfardini, S., and Bonadonna, G. (1972). *Cancer Chemother. Rep.* **56**, 343–356.
DeLana, M., Monfardini, S., Baretta, G., Fossati, F., and Bonadonna, G. (1973). *Natl. Cancer Inst. Monogr.* **36**, 403–422.
Einhorn, L. H., and Donohue, J. (1977). *Ann. Intern. Med.* **87**, 293–298.
Elson, M. K., Oken, M. M., and Shafer, R. B. (1977). *J. Nucl. Med.* **18**, 296–299.
Elson, M. K., Oken, M. M., Shafer, R. B., Broughton, A., Strong, J. E., Braun, C. T., and Crooke, S. T. (1978). *Med. Pediatr. Oncol.* **5**, 213–218.
Haidle, C. W. (1971). *Mol. Pharmacol.* **7**, 645–652.
Haidle, C. W., and Bearden, J. (1975). *Biochem. Biophys. Res. Commun.* **65**, 815–821.
Haidle, C. W., Kuo, M. T., and Weiss, K. K. (1972a). *Biochem. Pharmacol.* **21**, 3308–3312.
Haidle, C. W., Weiss, K. K., and Kuo, M. T. (1972b). *Mol. Pharmacol.* **8**, 531–537.
Iacovino, J. R., Leitner, J., Abbas, A. K., Lokich, J. L., and Snider, G. L. (1976). *J. Am. Med. Assoc.* **235**, 1253–1255.
Johnson, D. E., Bracken, B., Prestayko, A. W., Brown, T. E., and Crooke, S. T. (1976). *J. Am. Med. Assoc.* **236**, 1353–1354.
Konishi, M., Saito, K., Numata, K., Tsuno, T., Asama, K., Tsukiura, H., Naito, T., and Kawaguchi, H. (1977). *J. Antibiot.* **30**, 789–805.
Kuo, M. T., and Haidle, C. W. (1973). *Biochim. Biophys. Acta* **335**, 109–114.
Livingston, R. B. (1978). *In* "The Bleomycins: Current Status and New Developments" (S. K. Carter, S. T. Crooke, and H. Umezawa, eds.), pp. 165–172. Academic Press, New York.
Merrin, C., Takita, H., Beckley, S., and Kassis, J. (1977). *J. Urol.* **117**, 291–295.
Muller, W. E. G., and Zahn, R. K. (1976). *Gann Monogr.* **19**, 51–62.
Muller, W. E. G., Yamazaki, Z., Breter, H., and Zahn, R. K. (1972). *Eur. J. Biochem.* **31**, 518–525.
Nagatsu, M., Richart, R. M., and Lambert, A. (1972). *Cancer Res.* **32**, 1966–1970.
Nakamura, H., Takita, T., Umezawa, H., Muroaka, Y., and Iitaka Y. (1974). *J. Antibiot.* **27**, 352–355.
Pasqual, R. S., Mosher, M. B., Sikand, R. S., DeConti, R. C., and Bou Huys, A. (1973). *Am. Rev. Respir. Dis.* **108**, 211–217.
Povirk, L. F., Wubker, W., Kohnlein, W., and Hutchinson, F. (1977). *Nucleic Acids Res.* **4**, 3573–3580.
Prestayko, A. W., and Crooke, S. T. (1978). *In* "The Bleomycins: Current Status and New Developments" (S. K. Carter, S. T. Crooke, and H. Umezawa, eds.). Academic Press, New York.
Samuels, M. L., Holoye, P. Y., and Johnson, D. E. (1975). *In* "Cancer Chemotherapy: Fundamental Concepts and Recent Advances," pp. 483–492. Year Book Publ., Chicago, Illinois.
Samuels, M. L., Johnson, D. E., Holoye, P. Y., and Lanzotti, V. J. (1976). *J. Am. Med. Assoc.* **235**, 1117–1120.
Strong, J. E., and Crooke, S. T. (1978). *Cancer Res.* **38**, 3322–3326.
Strong, J. E., Broughton, A., and Crooke, S. T. (1977). *Cancer Treat. Rep.* **61**, 1509–1512.

Suzuki, H., Nagai, K., Yamaki, H., Tanaka, N., and Umezawa, H. (1968). *J. Antibiot.* **21**, 379–386.

Takita, T., Muraoka, Y., Yoshioka, T., Fuji, A., Maeda, K., and Umezawa, H. (1972). *J. Antibiot.* **25**, 755–759.

Tobey, R. A. (1972). *J. Cell. Physiol.* **79**, 259–266.

Umezawa, H. (1973). *Biomedicine* **18**, 459–475.

Umezawa, H. (1974). *Fred. Proc., Fed. Am. Soc. Exp. Biol.* **33**, 2296–2301.

Umezawa, H. (1978). *In* "The Bleomycins: Current Status and New Developments" (S. K. Carter, S. T. Crooke, and H. Umezawa, eds.). Academic Press, New York.

Umezawa, H., Surhara, Y., Takita, T., and Maeda, K. (1966a). *J. Antibiot., Ser. A* **19**, 210–219.

Umezawa, H., Maeda, K., Takeuchi, T., and Akami, Y. (1966b). *J. Antibiot., Ser. A* **19**, 200–209.

Watanabe, M., Takabe, Y., and Katsumata, T. (1973). *J. Antibiot.* **26**, 417–423.

Watanabe, M., Takabe, Y., Katsumata, T., and Terasima, T. (1974). *Cancer Res.* **34**, 878–881.

Wittes, R. E., Yagoda, A., Silven, O., Magill, G. B., Whitmore, W., Krakoff, I. H., and Golbey, R. B. (1976). *Cancer (Philadelphia)* **37**, 637–645.

8

THE ANTHRACYCLINES
Stanley T. Crooke

I. INTRODUCTION

The anthracyclines are a group of structurally related antibiotics that produce a wide variety of effects and have a rather broad spectrum of antineoplastic activity (Crooke and Reich, 1980). Adriamycin is prototypic and is the anthracycline that has been most extensively studied. Daunomycin, a closely related analogue, has also been evaluated clinically and has been shown to be active in the treatment of certain leukemias.

Because of the utility of adriamycin and daunomycin, substantial efforts to develop improved analogues have evolved and resulted in the preparation of several hundred anthracyclines. A number of these anthracyclines have been characterized, allowing partial definition of structure activity relationships relative to a number of aspects of drug action.

In this chapter the characteristics of adriamycin and daunomycin will be discussed and compared with a number of the anthracyclines currently being studied.

II. CHEMISTRY

In Figs. 1 and 2 are shown the general structural features of the anthracyclines. They are comprised of a tetracyclic aglycone and a glycosidic side chain of variable lengths. Figure 1 shows several analogues derived from or closely associated with adriamycin or daunomycin. In addition to adriamycin and daunomycin, carminomycin, rubidazone, and AD-32 are currently undergoing clinical evaluation. Figure 2 shows several analogues of the cinlrubin-aclacinomycin group of anthracyclines. These differ from the previous group in that a carbomethoxy group is present at C-10, the carbonyl function at C-13 is absent, and most of the members of this class are di- or trisaccharides (DuVernay et al., 1980b).

Because of the numerous analogues that have been studied, many structure activity relationships are understood. These will be discussed in more detail in a subsequent chapter, but will be discussed briefly here. The aglycones of both series of compounds are inactive. However, a number of modifications on the aglycone and the glycosidic side chain can be made without loss of activity, but more subtle molecular and clinical pharmacologic differences are induced by such modifications. The quinone also appears to be essential for the antitumor activity of compounds in both groups. Modifications at C-4, C-11, C-13, and C-14 of the compounds in the adriamycin–daunomycin group have been reported to result in active antitumor agents, but significant changes in activity, potency, and mechanism of action have also been reported (Arcamone et al., 1976;

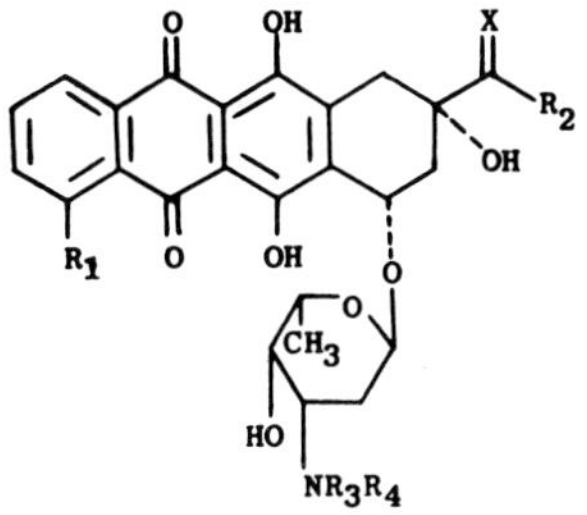

General Structure of the Adriamycin-
Daunomycin Class of Anthracyclines.

Compound	R_1	R_2	R_3	R_4	X-
ADRIAMYCIN	OCH_3	CH_2OH	H	H	O
DAUNOMYCIN	OCH_3	CH_3	H	H	O
CARMINOMYCIN	OH	CH_3	H	H	O
RUBIDAZONE	OCH_3	CH_3	H	H	$NNHCOC_6H_5$
AD-32	OCH_3	$CH_2OCOC_4H_9$	H	$COCF_3$	O
AD-41	OCH_3	CH_2OH	H	$COCF_3$	O

Fig. 1. Structural modifications in the adriamycin–daunomycin class of anthracyclines.

DiMarco *et al.*, 1977a; Brazhnikova *et al.*, 1974; Henry, 1975; DuVernay *et al.*, 1980b), Smith *et al.*, 1978).

III. MOLECULAR PHARMACOLOGY

A. Introduction

The anthracyclines produce a variety of effects that may contribute to their cytotoxicity, and the precise effects that are responsible for the cytotoxicity of any anthracycline are not fully delineated. Furthermore, recent studies have demonstrated that relatively minor structural modifications result in significant alterations in the molecular effects of anthracyclines, and that the anthracyclines can be divided into several mechanistic classes. Moreover, it is much simpler to define mechanisms of cytotoxicity and to compare the potency of various anthracyclines in various systems than to define those factors responsible for differential toxicities to malignant cells, i.e., antitumor efficacy. Thus a discussion of the molecular pharmacology of the anthracyclines must be relatively phenomenologic at present.

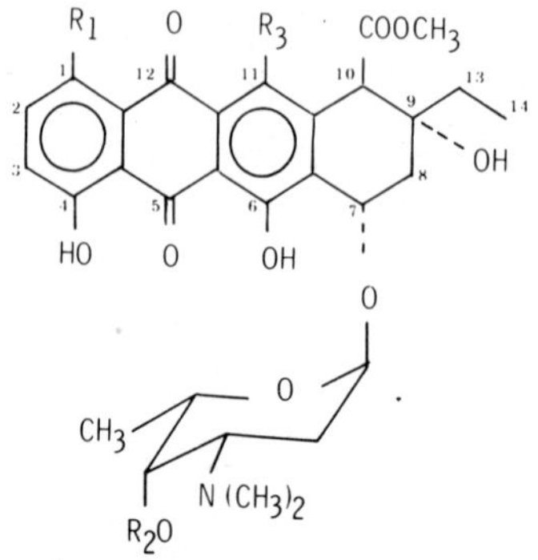

Structural Modifications in the cinerubin-
aclacinomycin class of anthracyclines

COMPOUND	R_1	R_2	R_3
PYRROMYCIN	OH	H	H
MUSETTAMYCIN	OH	DF	H
MARCELLOMYCIN	OH	DF-DF	H
CINERUBIN A	OH	DF-C	H
ACLACINOMYCIN	H	DF-C	H

Fig. 2. General structure of the cinerubin A–aclacinomycin class of anthracyclines.

B. Interactions with DNA

With a few exceptions the anthracyclines bind to DNA and depend on this interaction for at least one mechanism of cytotoxicity (Crooke and Reich, 1980). A variety of techniques has been employed to demonstrate that anthracyclines bind to DNA by partial intercalation of the aglycone and electrostatic interactions with the glycosidic side chain (Calendi et al., 1965; Waring, 1970; Zunino et al., 1972; DiMarco et al., 1977; DuVernay et al., 1979b,c). That modifications of the aglycone alter DNA interactions has been shown by variations in the apparent affinity constants and by alterations in the affinities of various anthracyclines for DNA species of different base compositions. Adriamycin, for example, has been shown to bind more avidly to DNA species with higher guanosine–cytosine content (Tsou and Yip, 1976; DuVernay et al., 1979b). However, several other anthracyclines that have been studied have been reported to prefer DNA species with higher adenosine–thymidine content (Du-Vernay et al., 1979b; Bhuyan and Smith, 1965; Ward et al., 1965; Reusser, 1975). A comparison of the apparent affinity constants for adriamycin and a number of anthracyclines of the aclacinomycin–cinerubin group demonstrates the base specificities for binding of these agents (see Fig. 10, DuVernay, Chap. 14; DuVernay et al., 1979b).

Removal or epimerization of the carbomethoxy group in marcellomycin has been shown to reduce the affinity for all DNA species studied (DuVernay *et al.*, 1979d). Modification of the hydroxyl group at position C-11 of carminomycin and the modifications present in the structure of AD-32 have been shown to reduce DNA binding (DuVernay *et al.*, 1980a; Sengupta *et al.*, 1976). Increasing the glycosidic side chain length of pyrromycinone-based anthracyclines has been shown to increase the binding affinities for various DNA species (DuVernay *et al.*, 1979b).

C. DNA Degradation

It has been reported that adriamycin induces degradation of isolated purified DNA (Lown *et al.*, 1977). However, the conditions employed included high concentrations of adriamycin, reducing agents, and harsh treatments. Another study (Mong *et al.*, 1980) reproduced the previously reported results but showed that the much more probable effects on DNA under physiologic conditions were those induced by intercalation, i.e., unwinding and rewinding phenomena.

Degradation of intracellular DNA after treatment of cells with anthracyclines *in vitro* has also been reported (Schwartz and Kanter, 1980). It has been suggested that intracellular DNA breakage may be correlated with cytotoxicity. However, it seems unlikely that DNA breakage induced by anthracyclines is a direct effect, and other studies have failed to demonstrate that DNA breakage can be observed at concentrations similar to those resulting in cytotoxicity (V. DuVernay, and S. T. Crooke unpublished results).

D. Effects on Macromolecular Syntheses

The effects of anthracyclines on DNA, RNA, and protein syntheses have been studied extensively, and it has been shown that most anthracyclines inhibit DNA and RNA syntheses but have little effect on protein synthesis (DuVernay *et al.*, 1980b). Studies in our laboratory have shown that anthracyclines can be divided into two groups, those that appear to inhibit nucleolar RNA synthesis selectively and those that do not demonstrate this property. Table I shows some of the compounds tested and the classification. The structure activity relationships responsible for nucleolar RNA synthesis inhibitory specificity include the presence and proper orientation of a carbomethoxy group at C-10 of the aglycone and the presence of a glycosidic side chain with at least two sugars (DuVernay *et al.*, 1979a,b,c, 1980b; Crooke *et al.*, 1978). Nogalomycin has also been reported to inhibit RNA synthesis selectively. Interestingly, all the nucleolar RNA synthesis selective agents appear to bind more effectively to adenosine–thymidine-rich DNA than guanosine–cytosine-rich DNA (Bhuyan *et al.*, 1980; DuVernay *et al.*, 1980b).

TABLE I

The Inhibition of Nucleolar RNA Synthesis Is Relative to Whole Cellular DNA and RNA Syntheses

Anthracycline	IC_{50} No-RNA[a] (μm)	IC_{50} DNA[c] IC_{50} WC-RNA[d]	IC_{50} DNA IC_{50} No-RNA	
Adriamycin	6.00[b]	1.89	1.02	
Carminomycin	13.10	1.64	1.12	Class I
Pyrromycin	6.15	1.26	0.93	
Marcellomycin	0.009	6.53	1256	
Musettamycin	0.014	6.66	714	Class II
Aclacinomycin	0.037	7.65	170	
Rudolfomycin	0.25	19.33	232	

[a] No-RNA = nucleolar RNA synthesis.
[b] IC_{50} values for nucleolar RNA synthesis were estimated by Probit analysis.
[c] DNA = DNA synthesis.
[d] WC-RNA = whole cellular RNA synthesis.

E. Generation of Free Radicals

It has been reported that anthracyclines may be reductively transformed intracellularly forming free radicals. It has been proposed that the free radicals may bind to DNA, labilizing the phosphodiester bonds and inducing DNA degradation (Handa and Sato, 1975; Bachur *et al.*, 1978).

F. Anthracyclines That May Not Depend on DNA Binding and/or Inhibition of Nucleic Acid Syntheses for Cytotoxicity

Studies on several compounds from several laboratories have suggested that some anthracyclines do not bind as effectively to DNA as others and do not inhibit nucleic acid syntheses at concentrations compatible with the concept that these effects are responsible for their cytotoxicity. AD32 (*N*-trifluoroacetyladriamycin-14-valerate) has been shown to bind poorly to DNA and to inhibit nucleic acid syntheses poorly (Israel *et al.*, 1980). Similar results have been reported for carminomycin, carminomycin 11-methyl ether, and 7-con-*o*-methylnogarol (DuVernay *et al.*, 1980b; Bhuyan *et al.*, 1980). At present the mechanisms of action of these compounds are not known. Effects on mitochondrial or membrane function may be important.

IV. CLINICAL PHARMACOLOGY

A. Adriamycin

The clinical pharmacology of adriamycin has been studied extensively by Bachur and co-workers and other groups. These studies have established the basic characteristics of adriamycin pharmacokinetics in man.

1. Absorption and Distribution

Adriamycin is inactive when administered orally, probably because of rapid inactivation in the gastrointestinal tract and liver. It is active when administered intravenously, and is rapidly and widely distributed (Bachur et al., 1974). Adriamycin binds to plasma proteins and cell membranes (Bachur, 1975).

2. Plasma Clearance

After adriamycin is administered as an intravenous bolus, it undergoes a rapid distribution phase followed by a more prolonged elimination phase. The elimination phase of adriamycin has been reported to be approximately 17 hr in patients with normal liver function (Benjamin et al., 1973). Metabolites have been shown to have a longer elimination half-life than the parent compound. The major metabolites are adriamycinol and adriamycin aglycone (Watson and Chan, 1976; Benjamin et al., 1973, 1974, 1977; Bachur et al., 1977; Bachur, 1975).

Clearance of Adriamycin and metabolites is primarily by biliary excretion (Riggs et al., 1977). Consequently, liver dysfunction results in substantially longer elimination half-lives and an increased incidence of toxicities (Benjamin et al., 1977). Treatment with phenobarbitol has been reported to enhance biliary excretion of adriamycin and metabolites (Harris, 1976; Riggs et al., 1977).

Urinary excretion accounts for significantly less of the clearance of adriamycin, accounting for less than 10% of the administered adriamycin in patients with normal hepatic and renal function (Benjamin et al., 1973).

3. Metabolism

Two enzymatic systems effect the significant metabolism of adriamycin. An aldo-keto reductase that requires NADPH as a cofactor and that is present in the cytosol is responsible for reducing adriamycin to adriamycinol, an active metabolite (Bachur, 1976). A reductive glycosidase that also requires NADPH and is localized to the microsomal fraction of cells cleaves the sugar moiety, resulting in the inactive aglycone (Bachur and Gee, 1976). Although all tissues were shown to have high levels of glycosidase activity that may be expressed when the oxygen tension is reduced, this is probably not a major metabolic pathway in normal clinical situations (Loveless et al., 1978).

In one patient biliary levels of adriamycin were studied and 41% of the administered dose was detected in 7 days. The major metabolite was adriamycinol, but other metabolites were detected (Riggs *et al.*, 1977).

4. Intra-Arterial Administration

Adriamycin has been administered by intrahepatic arterial infusion in two studies involving several patients. In both studies with continuous infusions, steady-state serum concentrations were obtained, and the steady-state concentration was proportionate to the dose, and the elimination of adriamycin was approximately equivalent to that observed with bolus administration after discontinuation of the infusion. Moreover, no significant differences in metabolism were detected (Garnick *et al.*, 1979; Bern *et al.*, 1978).

5. Dose Modification in the Presence of Hepatic Dysfunction

Clinical studies have shown that toxicity is increased in patients who have liver dysfunction. Consequently, dosage reductions in patients with liver dysfunction are recommended (Benjamin *et al.*, 1977).

B. Daunorubicin

Daunorubicin has also been studied extensively and has been shown to behave in a manner similar to adriamycin. However, it has been demonstrated that daunorubicin is converted to daunorubicinol at a more rapid rate than is adriamycin, and that this may be due to the fact that daunorubicin may be a better substrate for aldo-keto reductases (Benjamin *et al.*, 1973; Loveless *et al.*, 1978).

C. Other Anthracyclines

The pharmacokinetics of a number of other anthracyclines have been studied, and some interesting differences have been reported. The data relative to several of the more interesting agents will be discussed in this section.

1. Carminomycin

Following intravenous administration, the plasma disappearance of carminomycin was similar to that of adriamycin. However, the terminal half-life of the parent compound was only 10–12 hr (Bachur *et al.*, 1977; Crooke and Reich, 1980). On the other hand, carminomycin is rapidly and extensively converted to carminomycinol, which has an elimination half-life of 30–50 hr. Figure 3 shows a typical plasma clearance curve for carminomycin and carminomycinol. Inasmuch as carminomycinol is as active and toxic as carminomycin, it is possible

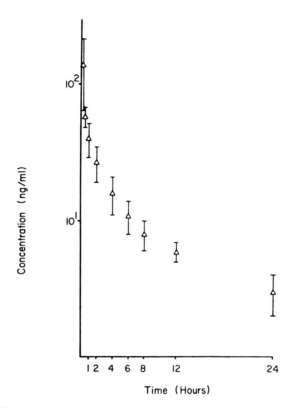

Fig. 3.   Serum pharmacokinetics of carminomycin. Composite phase I data.

that a portion of the activity of carminomycin is due to its primary metabolite (Fandrich *et al.*, 1980). Preliminary observations also suggest that the toxicities of carminomycin may be exacerbated in patients with liver dysfunction.

2. N-Trifluoroacetyladriamycin-14-valerate (AD-32)

The pharmacokinetic characteristics of AD-32 have been determined in mice and monkeys. Table II shows several pharmacokinetic parameters of adriamycin and AD-32 in the monkey. It demonstrates that AD-32 was found to have a biphasic plasma elimination curve and that it had a shorter elimination half-life ($t_{\frac{1}{2}}\beta$) and smaller peripheral compartment than adriamycin (Israel *et al.*, 1980). Approximately 30% and 11% of the administered AD-32 dose were detected in the bile and urine, respectively. Studies currently in progress should determine its characteristics in man.

TABLE II

Characteristics of the Two Exponential Components of the Plasma Concentration versus Time Curve (Total Fluorescence) in Monkey (*M. fasicularis*) Following the Single I.V. Administration of Adriamycin (35 mg/m^2) and AD-32 (350 mg/m^2)

	Adriamycin	AD-32
$t_{1/2}\alpha$ (min)	2.70	7.00
$t_{1/2}\beta$ (hr)	12.15	3.80
Elimination clearance (ml/min)	17.90	12.80
Central compartment volume (liters)	0.83	1.13
Peripheral compartment volume (liters)	18.11	3.00

V. CLINICAL ACTIVITIES OF ADRIAMYCIN AND DAUNORUBICIN

A. Adriamycin

1. Leukemias

Adriamycin is rarely used in the initial treatment of standard risk children with acute lymphocytic leukemia but may be useful in the treatment of acute lymphocytic leukemia in relapse and has been reported to extend the duration of remissions if administered intermittently during remission (Minow *et al.*, 1975) (Wiernik, 1980; Sallon *et al.*, 1978). Adriamycin has little if any role in the management of chronic leukemias.

2. Lymphomas

Adriamycin is an important drug in the treatment of patients with advanced Hodgkin's disease refractory to treatment with nitrogen mustard, vincristine, procarbazine, and prednisone (MOPP) (Wiernik, 1980). Combinations such as bleomycin, vinblastine, adriamycin, and streptozotocin (Santoro and Bonadonna, 1979) have been reported to result in significant complete remission rates in patients who are refractory to MOPP. In addition, in some studies adriamycin-containing combinations have been employed in an alternating fashion with MOPP (Bonadonna *et al.*, 1978). The precise role of adriamycin in this regard remains to be defined.

A large number of adriamycin-containing regimens have also been developed to treat patients with non-Hodgkin's lymphomas. In studies performed by the Southwest Oncology Group, addition of adriamycin to treatment regimens for nodular lymphomas appeared to be of no benefit. However, a better complete remission rate and a statistically significantly longer duration of remission were observed in patients with diffuse lymphomas (Jones *et al.*, 1979). Adriamycin is also a useful agent in the management of patients with advanced mycoses fungoides (Levi *et al.*, 1977).

3. Breast Cancer

Significant activity for adriamycin against metastatic breast cancer was identified in phase II studies (O'Bryan *et al.*, 1973; Tan *et al.*, 1973). Moreover, as a single agent adriamycin was reported to be equally active in patients who had or had not received prior chemotherapy, with approximately one-third of the patients in each group achieving a partial remission (Hoogstraten *et al.*, 1976).

The addition of adriamycin to various combinations has also been studied, and adriamycin has proved to be a valuable drug in combination chemotherapy of advanced breast cancer. However, relative few randomized comparative trials have been reported. In one study, for example, the combination of cyclophosphamide, 5-fluorouracil, and methotrexate was compared to the same combination to which adriamycin was added. In this study the four-drug combination resulted in a 62% response rate, whereas the three-drug regimen resulted in a 49% response rate, which is not a statistically significant difference. However, the response rate to the four-drug regimen for poorer-risk patients was significantly better than that of the three-drug regimen (Creech *et al.*, 1979). In both patient groups the toxicities due to the adriamycin-containing regimen were greater. Thus, although adriamycin is of value in the treatment of breast cancer, its precise role and a "best regimen" are not defined.

4. Gastrointestinal Malignancies

Adriamycin has been demonstrated clearly to be active against gastric and liver cnacers (Wiernik, 1980; Vogel *et al.*, 1977; Falkson *et al.*, 1976). As a single agent it induces approximately a 20–30% response rate in patients with gastric cancer, and in combination with 5-fluorouracil and mitomycin C, a 50% response rate has been reported (MacDonald *et al.*, 1979). As a single agent adriamycin has been reported to induce a 19–25% response rate in patients with hepatocellular carcinomas (Vogel *et al.*, 1977; Falkson *et al.*, 1976). Addition of 5-fluorouracil to adriamycin did not improve the activity (Baker and Vaitkevicius, 1976).

Adriamycin has failed to demonstrate significant activity against colorectal cancer and has had limited activity and limited trials against carcinomas of other sites in the gastrointestinal tract (Wiernik, 1980).

5. Lung Cancer

Adriamycin has demonstrated activity in the treatment of small-cell carcinoma of the lung and adriamycin-containing regimens have resulted in responses in nearly three-fourths of patients with small-cell carcinoma of the lung (Einhorn *et al.*, 1976). However, the overall contribution of adriamycin to the therapy of small-cell carcinoma of the lung is difficult to assess (Wiernik, 1980). Although adriamycin has shown activity in non-small-cell carcinoma of the lung, none of the combinations studied have resulted in demonstrable improvement in survival characteristics (Wiernik, 1980).

6. Genitourinary Cancer

Adriamycin is an active agent in the treatment of ovarian carcinomas, resulting, as a single agent, in a response in approximately one-third of the women treated (DeVita *et al.*, 1976; Fisher and Young, 1978). Moreover, trials of adriamycin and cyclophosphamide suggest that this combination may produce responses in 50% of the treated patients (Bruckner *et al.*, 1978). Adriamycin is also an active agent in the treatment of endometrial cancer (Horton *et al.*, 1978). It has also demonstrated activity against metastatic prostate cancer (DeWys *et al.*, 1977), refractory metastatic testicular cancer (Blum and Carter, 1974), and bladder cancer. However, in each of these diseases much must be learned before its role is understood.

7. Sarcomas

Adriamycin is highly effective in the treatment of metastatic sarcomas and in an adjuvant setting (Benjamin *et al.*, 1975). A combination of cyclophosphamide, dacarbazine, adriamycin, and vincristine was reported to induce a response rate of 60% in patients with metastatic sarcomas (Benjamin *et al.*, 1976). However, in other studies employing less intensive regimens, the response rates were much lower (Douglas and Karakovsis, 1975; Creagan *et al.*, 1978). It is also known that different histologies of sarcomas may respond differently to adriamycin-containing regimens (Levine *et al.*, 1978).

Inasmuch as adriamycin proved to be active against metastatic sarcomas, it and combinations using adriamycin have been studied as adjuvants to surgical therapy of osteogenic sarcomas. The use of adriamycin alone has been reported to result in a 5-year disease-free period in 39% of treated patients, an improvement over historical controls. Combinations have been studied but it is not yet clear that they are superior to adriamycin alone (Pratt *et al.*, 1977; Sutow *et al.*, 1978). In other sarcomas such as childhood rhabdomyosarcoma and Ewing's sarcoma, adriamycin-containing regimens have been reported to be effective adjuvant therapy (Ransom *et al.*, 1977; Bellani *et al.*, 1977).

8. Head and Neck Cancer

Adriamycin had demonstrated activity in the range of 30–50% response rates in patients with head and neck cancer (Tan *et al.*, 1973). However, the precise role of adriamycin-containing combinations in the treatment of this disease is not yet defined.

B. Daunorubicin

Daunorubicin has been evaluated much less extensively than adriamycin. Nonetheless, it has clear utility in the treatment of acute nonlymphocytic leukemias (Wiernik and Serpick, 1972) and in acute lymphocytic leukemias (Aur *et al.*, 1971). The combination of cytosine arabinoside and daunorubicin has proved very effective in the treatment of acute nonlymphocytic leukemia.

VI. TOXICITIES OF ADRIAMYCIN

The acute dose-limiting toxicity of adriamycin is myelosuppression. Other acute toxicities include mucositis, alopecia, nausea and vomiting, and cardiac rhythm disturbances. The subacute or chronic administration of adriamycin is associated with the development of myocardial fiber degeneration, which ultimately may result in intractable congestive heart failure. This toxicity is total dose limiting.

A. Myelosuppression

Myelosuppression is the acute dose-limiting toxicity and is clearly dose related. At doses lower than 60 mg/m^2, only modest myelosuppression has been observed. At doses greater than 60 mg/m^2, pancytopenia develops, which usually becomes most pronounced 10–16 days after a dose. However, the myelosuppression is not cumulative if schedules employing doses no more frequently than every 3 weeks are administered (Skovsgaard and Nissen, 1975; Blum and Carter, 1974). When employed in myelosuppressive combinations the dose of adriamycin should be reduced. Other factors that may require dose reduction include extensive prior myelosuppressive therapy, radiotherapy to a large area of bone marrow, or liver dysfunction (Wiernik, 1980).

B. Cardiotoxicity

1. Incidence and Clinical Manifestations

Adriamycin induces acute and chronic cardiac toxicities, and the chronic congestive heart failure reported due to adriamycin is apparently not related to the acute toxicities. The acute manifestations are electrocardiographic changes that are transient. These include supraventricular tachyarrhythmias, premature ventricular and supraventricular contractions, conduction abnormalities, and a variety of nonspecific S-T wave abnormalities. None of these abnormalities has been shown to be associated with long-term toxicities. The incidence of transient electrocardiographic disturbances reported in the literature has varied from 0 to 41.2% of treated patients and is approximately 11% if all published patients are included (Lenaz and Page, 1976).

Congestive heart failure is a toxicity associated with long-term therapy with adriamycin. The clinical manifestations are those of congestive failure induced by any cause. Antecedent symptoms are rare and congestive heart failure may occur as much as 6 months after the last dose of the drug (Minow et al., 1975). After development of congestive heart, survival is short, usually 1–10 days (Lenaz and Page, 1976).

Cardiomyopathy has been observed in approximately 2% of treated patients and was fatal in approximately 1%. Congestive heart failure is clearly total dose related as the incidence of cardiomyopathy is 0 at doses less than 450 mg/m² and increases to 41% in patients receiving more than 600 mg/m².

2. Methods of Clinical Evaluation

In addition to physical examination a variety of noninvasive and invasive methods have been evaluated as potential methods of early diagnosis of adriamycin cardiomyopathy. A reduction of 30% in the QRS voltage has been reported to predict for the development of cardiomyopathy. Serial estimates of systolic time interval has also been reported to be of value (Rinehart et al., 1974). However, other studies have failed to confirm these results (Bristow et al., 1978). Serial cardiac catheterizations and right ventricular biopsies have been reported to be predictive, but these results have not been widely reported.

3. Risk Factors

In addition to the increased risk associated with higher total doses of adriamycin, several other risk factors have been identified. Radiotherapy to the mediastinum clearly reduces the dose of adriamycin necessary to induce cardiomyotherapy. Biopsies have been reported to be of value (Bristow et al., 1978). However, this remains to be confirmed, and its precise utility is difficult to determine. Other factors that may increase the risk of cardiac toxicicty include concomitant cyclophosphamide therapy, uncontrolled hypertension, and liver dysfunction (Minow et al., 1977). Other compounds that may exacerbate the problem include actinomycin D and mithramycin (Lenaz and Page, 1976).

4. Pathology

The morphologic effects of adriamycin on the heart include nucleolar damage (Daskal and Crooke, 1980) and myocardial fiber dropout (Bristow, 1980). The cellular damage is focal but often widespread and appears to increase with increasing dose. Mitochondrial swelling and intramitochondrial dense bodies are also observed (LeFrak *et al.*, 1973).

5. *Methods of Amelioration*

Several techniques or compounds have been reported to ameliorate the cardiotoxicity of adriamycin. However, none of the proposed methods has as yet been shown to be effective in well-designed randomized comparative clinical trials. Administration of adriamycin on a weekly schedule has been reported to reduce the incidence of cardiotoxicity while not affecting the activity or incidence of myelotoxicity of the drug (Weiss *et al.*, 1976). This remains to be demonstrated in a randomized comparative trial. In animals, the coadministration of α-tocopherol has been reported to reduce the toxicity of adriamycin, and this has been extrapolated to the concept that it may inhibit the cardiotoxicity of adriamycin (Myers *et al.*, 1976). However, other laboratories have had difficulty reproducing the earlier data, and there is the suggestion that α-tocopherol may enhance the myelotoxicity of adriamycin (Alberts *et al.*, 1978). The coadministration of coenzyme Q10 with adriamycin has been reported to reduce the cardiotoxicity of adriamycin in cultured cardiac cells in animals (Bertazzoli and Ghione, 1977; Kishi *et al.*, 1976). In rats, the coadministration of acetyl-daunomycin has been reported to inhibit the development of adriamycin cardiotoxicity (Zbinden, 1975). Based on a very small series of patients, one report has suggested that digoxin may prevent the development of adriamycin-induced cardiotoxicity (Guthrie and Gibson, 1977). In hamsters, ICRF-187 has also been suggested to reduce the lethality and cardiotoxicity of adriamycin (Herman *et al.*, 1979). Obviously none of the reported methods of amelioration are proved, and much research is necessary to determine if any technique will reduce the clinical cardiotoxicity of adriamycin.

VII. ANTHRACYCLINES IN DEVELOPMENT

The very significant clinical activities of adriamycin and the obvious deficiencies of the drug have resulted in several extensive analogue programs that have, in general, focused on the toxicities of adriamycin. Thus the major goals of anthracycline development are to develop new analogues with equivalent clinical activity but reduced cardiotoxicity and/or myelosuppression. Secondary objectives include the development of compounds that induce less alopecia, or compounds that are orally active, active against adriamycin-resistant tumors, or potentially less costly (Crooke, 1980; Muggia and Rozencweig, 1980). As a consequence of the various programs, a number of anthracyclines have been developed. In this section several of these compounds are reviewed.

A. *N*-Trifluoroacetyladriamycin (AD-32)

AD-32 is a semisynthetic adriamycin analogue synthesized by Israel and colleagues (1975). Its molecular and clinical pharmacologic characteristics have been discussed in previous sections. It is currently in clinical trials primarily as a result of three significant differences from adriamycin. It has been shown to have activity superior to adriamycin in a variety of experimental animal tumor systems (Israel *et al.*, 1975; Parker *et al.*, 1978; Vecchi *et al.*, 1978). Second, several studies have suggested that AD-32 has less cardiotoxicity (Israel *et al.*, 1975; Henderson *et al.*, 1978; Parker *et al.*, 1978). Third, the molecular and clinical pharmacologic differences are of interest. The major difficulty with the drug, however, is its lack of water solubility, which necessitates the use of specialized vehicles for administration (e.g., emulphor).

AD-32 has undergone phase I clinical investigation. The maximal tolerated dose has been shown to be 600 mg/m² in patients with normal liver function. The dose-limiting clinical toxicity in this study was myelosuppression, and clinical antitumor activity against breast and bladder cancer was reported. No evidence of cardiotoxicity was observed (Blum *et al.*, 1979).

B. Carminomycin

Carminomycin is a close structural analogue of adriamycin that was discovered by Gauze and colleagues (Gauze *et al.*, 1974) and developed initially in the Soviet Union. Studies in the Soviet Union suggested that it has a broad spectrum of antitumor activity and reduced cardiotoxicity (Crooke, 1977). Moreover, studies in the United States have suggested that carminomycin differs from adriamycin molecular and clinical pharmacologically and has lower cardiotoxicity in animals than adriamycin (Crooke and Reich, 1980). Its principal toxicity appears to be myelosuppression.

Phase I trials of intravenously administered carminomycin have been completed. The maximal tolerated dose in patients with normal liver function was shown to be approximately 20 mg/m² every 3 weeks, and the dose-limiting toxicity was myelosuppression. No evidence of cardiotoxicity was detected, and the incidence and extent of alopecia observed were significantly less than those induced by adriamycin. Substantial differences in clinical pharmacologic characteristics were also observed (described in detail in previous section). An oral phase I study is in progress, and at doses of 36 mg/m² every 3 weeks evidence of activity and the presence of carminomycin and carminomycinol were detected (Crooke and Reich, 1980).

C. Aclacinomycin

Aclacinomycin A is an anthracycline discovered and developed in Japan by Umezawa and colleagues (Oki *et al.*, 1975; Oki, 1980). It is a triassacharide anthracycline that has been shown to be a class II anthracycline, i.e., it inhibits nucleolar RNA synthesis at much lower concentrations than those necessary to inhibit DNA synthesis (DuVernay *et al.*, 1980b).

Although studies in various animal tumor systems showed aclacinomycin was less potent than adriamycin, it was highly active against a variety of animal tumors (Oki, 1980). It was also shown to have oral activity and has been demonstrated to be nonmutagenic in the Ames test. Its cardiotoxicity has been evaluated in several species, including hamsters, rats, rabbits, and dogs; and the studies have suggested that it is less cardiotoxic than adriamycin (Hori *et al.*, 1977; Oki, 1980).

Phase I and II clinical trials have been completed in Japan. The cumulative maximal tolerated dose in phase I studies was 4 mg/kg. The dose-limiting toxicity was myelosuppression, but that alopecia and cardiotoxicity were reported to be less apparent. Phase II trials demonstrated acute electrocardiographic changes, but no evidence of congestive failure. The trials were reported to have demonstrated antitumor activity. Phase I trials are beginning in the United States (Oki, 1980).

D. Marcellomycin

Marcellomycin is a trissacharide anthracycline that is approaching phase I clinical trials in the United States (Nettleton *et al.*, 1977). Molecular pharmacologic studies have demonstrated that it is a class II anthracycline and has a mechanism of action different from adriamycin (Reich *et al.*, 1980). Marcellomycin has been shown to have activity against several animal tumors, albeit less activity than adriamycin.

Studies in several species have shown that marcellomycin is markedly less myelotoxic than adriamycin. Interestingly, musettamycin, which differs from marcellomycin only by the loss of the terminal sugar, deoxyfucose, is myelotoxic, as is rudolphomycin, which has a different terminal sugar. Marcellomycin has also been reported to be less cardiotoxic. The dose-limiting toxicity appears to be gastrointestinal (Reich *et al.*, 1980).

E. Quelamycin

Quelamycin is a triferric chelate of adriamycin prepared and studied by Gosalvez *et al.* (1978). It has been shown to bind to DNA more avidly than adriamycin, but little else is known about its mechanism of action. It is active against a variety of animal tumor systems, and little is known about its toxicities.

F. 4′-Epiadriamycin

A number of analogues at position 4 in the anthracycline ring system and at position 4′ of amino sugar have been developed in Italy (Casazza *et al.*, 1979).

4'-Epiadriamycin is one of these analogues and has undergone extensive studies. *In vitro* studies demonstrated that 4-epiadriamycin was as active as adriamycin in nucleic acid synthesis inhibition but that it was taken up more extensively by cultured L1210 cells (DiMarco *et al.*, 1977). Against L1210 and P388 leukemias *in vivo* it was as active or more active than adriamycin. Toxicologic studies in several species suggested that 4-epiadriamycin may be slightly less cardiotoxic than adriamycin (Casazza *et al.*, 1980).

A phase I clinical trial has been completed in Italy. In that study, at doses comparable to those used for adriamycin, 4-epiadriamycin was reported to produce less vomiting and alopecia than adriamycin. It also demonstrated activity against several tumors, and no evidence of significant differences in cardiotoxicity was found (Bonfante *et al.*, 1979). Phase II studies are in progress.

G. 7-con-*o*-Methylnogarol (7-con-Omen)

7-con-Omen is an analogue of nogalomycin developed in the United States. It is an monosaccharide that apparently prefermentally inhibits RNA synthesis, and intercalates preferentially in adenine–thymine-rich DNA species. It is active against a wide variety of experimental tumors, and it has been suggested that it may be relatively less cardiotoxic than adriamycin. It is currently under advanced preclinical investigation (Bhuyan *et al.*, 1980).

H. Rubidazone

Rubidazone can be considered a prodrug for adriamycin, being metabolized to adriamycin and other metabolites. Initial clinical trials suggested that it might be more active than adriamycin and less cardiotoxic. More recent trials have failed to confirm this (Jacquillat *et al.*, 1976).

REFERENCES

Alberts, D. S., Peng, Y. M., and Moon, T. E. (1978). *Biomedicine* **29,** 189–191.
Arcamone, F., Bernardi, L., Giardino, P., Patelli, B., DiMarco, A., Casazza, A. M., Pratesi, G., and Reggiani, P. (1976). *Cancer Treat. Rep.* **60,** 829–834.
Aur, R. J. A., Simon, J. V., and Pratt, C. B. (1971). *Cancer (Philadelphia)* **27,** 1332–1336.
Bachur, N. R. (1975). *Cancer Chemother. Rep., Part 3* **6,** 103–108.
Bachur, N. R. (1976). *Science* **193,** 595–597.
Bachur, N. R., and Gee, M. (1976). *J. Pharmacol. Exp. Ther.* **197,** 681–686.
Bachur, N. R., Hildebrand, R. C., and Jaenke, R. S. (1974). *J. Pharmacol. Exp. Ther.* **191,** 331–340.
Bachur, N. R., Riggs, C. E., Green, M. R., Langone, J. J., VanVanaris, H., and Levine, L. (1977). *Clin. Pharmacol. Ther.* **21,** 70–77.
Bachur, N. R., Gordon, S. L., and Gee, M. V. (1978). *Cancer Res.* **38,** 1745–1750.

Baker, L. H., and Vaitkevicius, V. K. (1976). *Proc. Am. Assoc. Cancer Res.* **17,** 215.

Bellani, R. F., Barni, S., Gaspauni, M., Lombardi, F., Lattuada, A., and Bonadanna, G. (1977). *In* "Adjuvant Therapy of Cancer" (S. E. Salman and S. K. Jones, eds.), pp. 373–380. Elsevier/ North-Holland, Amsterdam.

Benjamin, R. S., Riggs, C. R., Jr., and Bachur, N. R. (1973). *Clin. Pharmacol. Ther.* **14,** 592–600.

Benjamin, R. S., Wiernik, P. H., and Bachur, N. R. (1974). *Cancer (Philadelphia)* **33,** 19–27.

Benjamin, R. S., Wiernik, P. H., and Bachur, N. R. (1975). *Med. Pediatr. Oncol.* **1,** 63–76.

Benjamin, R. S., Gottlieb, J. A., and Baker, L. H. (1976). *Proc. Am. Assoc. Cancer Res.* **17,** 256.

Benjamin, R. S., Riggs, C. E., and Bachur, N. R. (1977). *Cancer Res.* **37,** 1416–1420.

Bern, M. M., McDermott, W., Cady, B., Oberfield, R. A., Trey, C., Clouse, M. E., Tullis, J. L., and Parker, L. M. (1978). *Cancer (Philadelphia)* **42,** 399–405.

Bertazzoli, C., and Ghione, M. (1977). *Pharmacol. Res. Commun.* **9,** 235–250.

Bhuyan, B. K., and Smith, C. G. (1965). *Proc. Natl. Acad. Sci. U.S.A.* **54,** 566–572.

Bhuyan, B. K., Neil, G. L., Li, L. H., McGovern, J. P., and Wiley, P. F. (1980). *In* "Anthracyclines: Current Status and New Developments" (S. T. Crooke and S. D. Reich, eds.). Academic Press, New York. pp.365–396·

Blum, R. M., and Carter, S. K. (1974). *Ann. Intern. Med.* **80,** 249–259.

Blum, R. H., Henderson, I. C., Mayer, R. J., Skarin, A., Parker, L. M., Canellos, G. P., Israel, M., and Frei, E., III (1979). *Proc. Am. Assoc. Cancer Res.* **20,** 327.

Bonadonna, G., Fossati, V., and DeLena, M. (1978). *Proc. Am. Assoc. Cancer Res.* **19,** 363.

Bonfante, V., Villani, F., Bonadonna, G., and Veronesi, U. (1979). *Proc. Am. Assoc. Cancer Res.* **20,** 372.

Brazhnikova, M. G., Zbarsky, V. B., Ponomarenko, V. T., and Potapova, N. P. (1974). *J. Antibiot.* **27,** 254–259.

Bristow, M. R. (1980). *In* "Anthracyclines: Current Status and New Developments" (S. T. Crooke and S. D. Reich, eds.). Academic Press, New York. pp.255–272·

Bristow, M. R., Mason, J. W., Billingham, M. E., and Daniels, J. E. (1978). *Ann. Intern. Med.* **88,** 168–175.

Bruckner, H. W., Ratner, L. H., Cohen, C. J., Wallach, R., Kabakow, B., Greenspan, E. M., and Holland, J. F. (1978). *Cancer Treat. Rep.* **62,** 1021–1023.

Calendi, E., DiMarco, H., Reggiani, M., Scarpinato, B., and Valentini, L. (1965). *Biochim. Biophys. Acta* **103,** 25–49.

Casazza, A. M., Bertazzoli, C., Pratesi, G., Bellini, O., and DiMarco, A. (1979). *Proc. Am. Assoc. Cancer Res.* **20,** 16.

Casazza, A. M., DiMarco, A., Bonadonna, G., Bonfante, V., Bertazzoli, C., Bellini, O., Pratesi, G., Sala, L., and Ballerini, L. (1980). *In* "Anthracyclines: Current Status and New Developments" (S. T. Crooke and S. D. Reich, eds.). Academic Press, New York. pp.403–430·

Creagan, E. T., Edmonson, J. H., Hahn, R. G., Ohman, D. L., Bisel, H. F., and Eagan, R. T. (1978). *Med. Pediatr. Oncol.* **4,** 85–86.

Creech, R. H., Catalano, R. B., Harris, D. T., Engstrom, P. K., and Grotzinger, P. J. (1979). *Cancer (Philadelphia)* **43,** 51–59.

Crooke, S. T. (1977). *J. Med.* **8:**295–316.

Crooke, S. T. (1980). *In* "Anthracyclines: Current Status and New Developments" (S. T. Crooke and S. D. Reich, eds.). Academic Press, New York. pp. 11–15·

Crooke, S. T., and Reich, S. D., eds. (1980). *In* "Anthracyclines: Current Status and New Developments." Academic Press, New York.

Crooke, S. T.,DuVernay, V. H., Galvan, L., and Prestayko, A. W. (1978). *Mol. Pharmacol.* **14,** 290–298.

Daskal, Y., and Crooke, S. T. (1980). *In* "Anthracyclines: Current Status and New Developments" (S. T. Crooke and S. D. Reich, eds.). Academic Press, New York. Pp. 193–220.

DeVita, V. T., Jr., Wasserman, T. H., Young, R. C., and Carter, S. K. (1976). *Cancer (Philadelphia)* **38**, 509–525.

DeWys, W. D., Bauer, M., Colsky, J., Cooper, R. A., Creech, R., and Carbone, P.P. (1977). *Cancer Treat. Rep.* **61**, 325–328.

DiMarco, A., Casazza, A. M., and Pratesi, G. (1977a). *Cancer Treat. Rep.* **61**, 893–894.

DiMarco, A., Casazza, A. M., Dasdia, T., Necco, A., Pratesi, G., Rivolta, P., Velcich, A., Zaccara, A., and Zunino, F. (1977b). *Chem.-Biol. Interact.* **19**, 291–302.

Douglas, H. O., Jr., and Karakovsis, C. (1975). *Cancer Chemother. Rep.* **59**, 1035–1037.

DuVernay, V. H., Pachter, J. A., and Crooke, S. T. (1979a). *Proc. Am. Assoc. Cancer Res.* **20**, 35.

DuVernay, V. H., Pachter, J. A., and Crooke, S. T. (1979b). *Biochemistry* **18**, 4024–4030.

DuVernay, V. H., Pachter, J. A., and Crooke, S. T. (1979c). *Mol. Pharmacol.* **16**, 623–632.

DuVernay, V. H., Essery, J. M., Doyle, T. W., Bradner, W. T., and Crooke, S. T. (1979d). *Mol. Pharmacol.* **15**, 341–356.

DuVernay, V. H., Pachter, J. A., and Crooke, S. T. (1980a). *Cancer Res.* **40**, 387–394.

DuVernay, V. H., Mong, S., and Crooke, S. T. (1980b). *In* "Anthracyclines: Current Status and New Developments" (S. T. Crooke and S. D. Reich, eds.). Academic Press, New York. In press.

Einhorn, L. H., Fee, W. H., Farber, M. O., Livingston, R. B., and Gottlieb, J. A. (1976). *J. Am. Med. Assoc.* **235**, 1225–1229.

Falkson, G., Moertel, C. G., and Lavin, P. T. (1976). *Proc. Am. Assoc. Cancer Res.* **17**, 21.

Fandrich, S., Pittman, K. A., Rozencweig, M., Lenaz, L., and Crooke, S. T. (1980). *Fed. Proc.* **39,**2528, 1980.

Fisher, R. I., and Young, R. C. (1978). *Surg. Clin. North Am.* **58**, 143–150.

Garnick, M. C., Fensminger, W. D., and Israel, M. (1979). *Cancer Res.* **39**, 4105–4110.

Gauze, G. F., Brazhnikova, M. G., and Shorin, V. A. (1974). *Cancer Chemotherp. Rep., Part 2* **58**, 255–256.

Gosalvez, M., Blanco, M. F., Vivero, F. , and Valles, F. (1978). *Eur. J. Cancer* **14**, 1185–1190.

Guthrie, D., and Gibson, R. L. (1977). *Br. Med. J.* **ii**, 1447–1449.

Handa, K., and Sato, S. (1975). *Gann* **66**, 43–47.

Harris, D. A. (1976). *Proc. Am. Assoc. Cancer Res.* **17**, 131.

Henderson, I. C., Billingham, M., Israel, M., Krisham, A., and Frei, E., III (1978). *Proc. Am. Assoc. Cancer Res.* **19**, 158.

Henry, D. W. (1975). *Cancer Chemother., Meet. Am. Chem. Soc., 169th, Div. Med. Chem. Symp., Philadelphia, Pa.* pp. 15–57.

Herman, E., Ardalan, B., Bier, C., Waravdekor, V., and Krop, S. (1979). *Cancer Treat. Rep.* **63**, 89–92.

Hoogstraten, B., George, S. L., Samal, B., Rivkin, S. E., Costanzi, J. J., Bonnet, J. D., Thigpen, T., and Braine, H. (1976). *Cancer (Philadelphia)* **38**, 13–20.

Hori, S., Shirai, M., Hirano, S., Oki, T., Inui, T., Tsukagoshi, S., Ishizuka, M., Takeuchi, T., and Umezawa, H. (1977). *Gann* **68**, 685–690.

Horton, J., Begg, C. B., Arseneault, J., Bruckner, H., Creech, R., and Hahn, R. G. (1978). *Cancer Treat. Rep.* **61**, 1385–1387.

Israel, M., Modest, E. J., and Frei, E., III (1975). *Cancer Res.* **35**, 1365–1368.

Israel, M., Wilkinson, P. M., and Osteen, R. T. (1980). *In* "Anthracyclines: Current Status and New Developments" (S. T. Crooke and S. D. Reich, eds.). Academic Press, New York. pp. 431–444 .

Jacquillat, C. L., Weil, M., Germon-Auclerc, G., Izrael, V., Bussel, A., Boirdon, M., and Bernard, J. (1976). *Cancer (Philadelphia)* **37**, 653–659.

Jones, S. E., Grozea, P. N., Metz, E. N., Hant, A., Stephens, R. L., Morrison, F. S., Butler, J. J., Byrne, G. E., Jr., Moon, T. E., Fisher, R., Haskins, C. L., and Coltman, C. A., Jr. (1979). *Cancer (Philadelphia)* **43**, 417–425.

Kishi, T., Watanabe, T., and Folkers, K. (1976). *Proc. Natl. Acad. Sci. U.S.A.* **73**, 4653–4656.

LeFrak, E. A., Pitha, J., Rosenheim, S., and Gottlieb, J. A. (1973). *Cancer (Philadelphia)* **32**, 302–314.

Lenaz, L., and Page, J. A. (1976). *Cancer Treat. Rev.* **3**, 111–120.

Levi, J. A., Diggs, C. H., and Wiernik, P. H. (1977). *Cancer (Philadelphia)* **39**, 1967–1970.

Levine, A. S., Appelbaum, F. R., Graw, R. C., Jr., Magrath, I. T., Pizzo, P. A., Poplack, D. G., and Ziegler, J. L. (1978). *Cancer Treat. Rep.* **62**, 247–250.

Loveless, H., Arena, E., Felsted, R. L., and Bachur, N. R. (1978). *Cancer Res.* **38**, 593–598.

Lown, J. W., Sim, S. K., Majunder, K. C., and Chang, R. Y. (1977). *Biochem. Biophys. Res. Commun.* **76**, 705–710.

MacDonald, J. S., Woolley, P. V., Smythe, T., Yend, O., Hoth, D., and Schein, P. S. (1979). *Cancer (Philadelphia)* **44**, 42–47.

Minow, R. A., Benjamin, R. S., and Gottlieb, J. A. (1975). *Cancer Chemother. Rep.* **6**, 195–199.

Minow, R. A., Benjamin, R. S., Lee, E. T., and Gottlieb, J. A. (1977). *Cancer (Philadelphia)* **39**, 1397–1402.

Mong, S., Strong, J. E., DuVernay, V. H., and Crooke, S. T. (1980). *Mol. Pharmacol.* **17**, 100–104.

Muggia, F. M., and Rozencweig, M. (1980). *In* "Anthracyclines: Current Status and New Development" (S. T. Crooke and S. D. Reich, eds.). Academic Press, New York. pp. 1–10, 1980.

Myers, C. E., McGuire, W., and Young, R. (1976). *Cancer Treat. Rep.* **7**, 961–962.

Nettleton, D. E., Bradner, W. T., Busch, J. A., Coon, A. B., Moseley, J. E., Myelymafi, R. W., O'Herron, F. A., Schreiber, R. H., and Vulcano, A. L. (1977). *J. Antibiot.* **30**, 525–529.

O'Bryan, R. M., Luce, J. K., Talley, R. W., Gottlieb, J. A., Baker, L. H., and Bonadonna, G. (1973). *Cancer (Philadelphia)* **32**, 1–8.

Oki, T. (1980). *In* "Anthracyclines: Current Status and New Developments" (S. T. Crooke and S. D. Reich, eds.). Academic Press, New York. pp 373–342.

Oki, T., Matsuzawa, Y., Yoshimoto, A., Numata, K., Kitamura, I., Hosi, G., Takamatsu, A., Umezawa, H., Ishizuka, M., Naganawa, H., Suda, H., Hamada, M., and Takeuchi, T. (1975). *J. Antibiot.* **28**, 830–834.

Parker, L. M., Hirst, M., and Israel, M. (1978). *Cancer Treat. Rep.* **61**, 119–127.

Pratt, C., Shanks, E., Husta, O., Rivera, G., Smith, J., and Kumar, A. P. M. (1977). *Cancer (Philadelphia)* **39**, 51–57.

Ransom, J. L., Pratt, C. B., and Shanks, E. (1977). *Cancer (Philadelphia)* **40**, 2810–2816.

Reich, S. D., Bradner, W. T., Rose, W. C., Schurig, J. E., Madissoo, H., Johnson, D. F., DuVernay, V. H., and Crooke, S. T. (1980). *In* "Anthracyclines: Current Status and New Developments" (S. T. Crooke and S. D. Reich, eds.). Academic Press, New York. pp. 343–364.

Reusser, R. (1975). *Biochim. Biophys. Acta* **383**, 266–273.

Riggs, C. E., Benjamin, R. S., Serpich, A. A., and Bachur, N. R. (1977). *Clin. Pharmacol. Ther.* **22**, 234–241.

Rinehart, J. J., Lewis, R. P., and Balcerzak, S. P. (1974). *Ann. Intern. Med.* **81**, 475–478.

Sallon, S. E., Camitta, B. M., Cassady, J. R., Nathan, D. G., and Frei, E., III (1978). *Blood* **51**, 425–433.

Santoro, A., and Bonadonna, G. (1979). *Cancer Chemother. Pharmacol.* **2**, 101–105.

Schwartz, H. S., and Kanter, P. M. (1980). *In* "Anthracyclines: Current Status and New Developments" (S. T. Crooke and S. D. Reich, eds.). Academic Press, New York. pp. 43–62.

Sengupta, S. K., Seshadir, R., Modest, E. J., and Israel, M. (1976). *Proc. Am. Assoc. Cancer Res.* **17**, 109.

Skovsgaard, T., and Nissen, N. J. (1975). *Dan. Med. Bull.* **22**, 62–73.

Smith, T. H., Fujiwara, A. N., and Henry, D. W. (1978). *J. Med. Chem.* **21**, 280–283.

Sutow, W. W., Gehan, E. A., Dyment, P. G., Vietti, T., and Miale, T. (1978). *Cancer Treat. Rep.* **62**, 265–269.

Tan, C., Etcubanes, E., Wollner, N., Rosen, G., Gilladoga, A., Showel, J., Murphy, M. L., and Kradoff, I. H. (1973). *Cancer (Philadelphia)* **32**, 9–17.

Tsou, K. C., and Yip, K. F. (1976). *Cancer Res.* **36**, 3367–3373.

Vecchi, A., Cairo, M., Mantovani, A., Sironi, M., and Speafico, F. (1978). *Cancer Treat. Rep.* **61**, 111–116.

Vogel, C. L., Bayley, A. C., Brooker, R. J., Anthony, P. P., and Ziegler, J. L. (1977). *Cancer (Philadelphia)* **39**, 1923–1929.

Ward, D. C., Reich, E., and Goldberg, I. H. (1965). *Science* **149**, 1259–1263.

Waring, M. (1970). *J. Mol. Biol.* **54**, 247–279.

Watson, E., and Chan, K. K. (1976). *Cancer Treat. Rep.* **60**:1611–1618. (1976).

Weiss, A. J., Mether, G. E., Fletcher, W. S., Wilson, W. L., Grage, T. B., and Ramirez, G. (1976). *Cancer Treat. Rep.* **60**, 813–822.

Wiernik, P. H. (1980). *In* "Anthracyclines: Current Status and New Developments" (S. T. Crooke and S. D. Reich, eds.). Academic Press, New York. pp. 273–294.

Wiernik, P. H., and Serpick, A. A. (1972). *Cancer Res.* **37**, 2023–2026.

Zbinden, G. (1975). *Experientia* **31**, 1058–1060.

Zunino, F., Gambetta, R., DiMarco, A., and Zaccara, A. (1972). *Biochim. Biophys. Acta* **277**, 489–498.

9

CISPLATIN AND ANALOGUES: A NEW CLASS OF ANTICANCER DRUGS

Archie W. Prestayko

I. INTRODUCTION

Cisplatin (*cis*-diamminedichloroplatinum II,) is an anticancer drug that is indicated for the treatment of metastatic testicular and ovarian carcinomas. It has also

CANCER AND CHEMOTHERAPY, VOL. III

demonstrated significant activity in carcinomas of the urinary bladder, prostate, and head and neck and in osteogenic sarcomas in children. This chapter will deal with the antitumor activity and toxicity of cisplatin in animal and human studies. A brief discussion of studies with analogues of cisplatin will also be included. For a discussion of the mechanism of action and clinical pharmacology of cisplatin, the reader is referred to separate chapters in this volume.

II. ANTITUMOR ACTIVITY IN ANIMAL TUMORS

Cisplatin has demonstrated antitumor activity in a number of experimental systems, including B-16 melanoma and Walker 256 carcinosarcoma (Kociba *et al.*, 1970), sarcoma 180 and leukemia L1210 (Rosenberg *et al.*, 1969), and DMBA-induced mammary tumors in rats (Welsch, 1971).

Mice bearing the L1210 leukemia and treated with cisplatin appeared normal and healthy and remained in remission for 10 months. Sixty-three to 100% of the animals bearing the sarcoma 180 tumors had complete regression of tumor with no apparent irreversible damage to the host. Cisplatin was more effective in this tumor than mercaptopurine, which to date had been the most effective therapy for the sarcoma 180 tumor.

In a study of DMBA-induced mammary tumor (Welsch, 1971), cisplatin produced complete remission in 14 animals, with 3 of them being "cured" of tumor. When tested against the Rous sarcoma-induced tumor, cisplatin produced tumor regression in 95% of the chickens bearing the tumor.

Cisplatin has been combined with cyclophosphamide, iphosphamide, thioguanine, 5-thiouracil, methotrexate, and daunomycin in the treatment of L1210 leukemia in mice (Woodman *et al.*, 1973; Woodman, 1974; Gale *et al.*, 1974; Walker and Gale, 1973; Hill *et al.*, 1972). Enhanced therapeutic effects were observed with combination chemotherapy compared with either drug used alone. In combination with 2,2'-anhydro-1-β-D-arabinofuranosyl-5fluorocytosine, cisplatin showed synergism in L1210 and P-388 leukemia, which were resistant to 5-fluorouracil or methotrexate (Burchenal *et al.*, 1977).

III. ANIMAL TOXICOLOGY

Table I shows doses of cisplatin that induced various degrees of toxicity in beagle dogs and Rhesus monkeys (Madias and Harrington, 1978; Schaeppi *et al.*, 1973). The toxicities observed in the treated animals included the toxicities described in the following sections.

A. Kidney

The toxicologic studies in beagle dogs and Rhesus monkeys have identified nephrotoxicity as the principal dose-limiting toxicity of cisplatin. Dogs de-

TABLE I

Toxicity of Cisplatin in Animals

	Dog				Monkey	
	Single dose		qd × 5 days		qd × 5 days	
	mg/kg	(mg/m^2)	mg/kg	(mg/m^2)	mg/kg	(mg/m^2)
Highest nontoxic dose (HNTD)	0.625	(13.2)	0.187	(3.75)	0.156 (or less)	(1.94)
Toxic dose low (TDL)	1.25	(22.5)	0.375	(7.75)	.0313	(8.0)
Toxic dose high (TDH)	2.5	(47.3)	0.75	(14.9)	1.25	(15.9)
Lethal dose (LD)			1.5	(31.1)	2.5	(33.6)

veloped azotemia and hypochloremia. Histologically, cisplatin induced acute tubular necrosis in dogs, whereas monkeys developed focal subacute interstitial nephritis. In some animals return of the BUN to normal values suggested reversibility of cisplatin renal toxicity.

B. Gastrointestinal Tract

Doses of ≥2.5 mg/kg cisplatin produced prompt and severe emesis, anorexia, abdominal tenderness, and diarrhea in both dogs and monkeys.

C. Lymphatic System

In both dogs and monkeys doses of ≥2.5 mg/kg cisplatin rapidly destroyed circulating lymphocytes and induced striking lymphoid atrophy. This action was not detected at lower doses.

D. Liver

Although elevation of liver transaminases and slight changes in fatty acid levels were noted, no significant histopathologic alterations were observed after cisplatin administration.

E. Bone Marrow

Severe bone marrow hypoplasia was produced by ≥2.5 mg/kg cisplatin in dogs and monkeys, but peripheral blood elements were not severely decreased in some animals.

F. Ototoxicity

Transient loss of hearing was noted in some monkeys, rats, and guinea pigs after cisplatin doses. In addition, animals experienced a loss of outer and inner hair cells in the inner ear, but no apparent vestibular toxicity was detected.

G. Other Toxicities

Additional occasional toxicities included atrophy of the testes, prostate, and salivary glands as well as pancreatitis and myocarditis. The induction of an allergic reaction by cisplatin was studied in rats (Khan *et al.*, 1977; Mota, 1963). Cutaneous reactions were observed in two of the 12 rats after two injections of cisplatin and pertussis vaccine. When repeated weekly injections were given, a higher percentage of animals developed allergic manifestations, suggesting that frequently repeated injections of cisplatin in rats may have been allergenic.

In studies using the Ames test (Monti-Bragadin *et al.*, 1975) and induction of auxotrophic mutants in *E. coli* (Beck and Brubaker, 1975), cisplatin was shown to possess mild to moderate mutagenic activity. Cisplatin has also been shown to be teratogenic in Swiss mice (Lazar *et al.*, 1979).

IV. EFFICACY

Cisplatin is an active anticancer agent in malignancies of the testes and ovaries and is recommended as treatment in these metastatic tumors. Cisplatin has also shown activity in cancers of the urinary bladder. head and neck, cervix, prostate, osteogenic sarcoma, and neuroblastoma and to a limited extent in lung cancer. Most of the treatments include combination chemotherapy, which will be discussed in this chapter.

A. Testicular Cancer

During the past 15 years many new agents have been developed that have substantial activity in testicular tumors, notably vinblastine, bleomycin, actinomycin D, adriamycin, mithramycin, and cisplatin. Table II summarizes the response rate and duration of response in patients treated with single drugs. In general, complete responses (CR) were few and durations of remission were short.

Seven studies evaluated the efficacy of cisplatin as a single agent in germ cell tumors of the testes (Cavalli *et al.*, 1976; Chary *et al.*, 1977; Corder *et al.*, 1977; Higby *et al.*, 1974a; Merrin, 1976; Piel *et al.*, 1974; Rossof, 1976). Tumor types when specified included teratocarcinomas, seminomas, and embryonal cell carcinomas. All patients had advanced, disseminated disease refractory to previous chemotherapy. The overall response rate in 74 patients was 55%,

TABLE II

Activity of Single Agents in Testicular Cancer

		Remission[a]			
Agent	Evaluable patients	CR (%)	PR (%)	Response rate	Duration of remission (months)
Cyclophosphamide	14	4 (28.5)	7 (50)	79%	4–24
Bleomycin	54	6 (11)	17 (31)	43%	9–28
Vinblastine	41	5 (12)	10 (24)	37%	4–5
Actinomycin D	61	11 (18)	9 (15)	33%	9–63
Adriamycin	29	0	5 (17)	17%	5–12 (PR)
Cisplatin	74	15 (20)	26 (35)	55%	
Mithramycin	74	5 (6)	14 (19)	26%	6–77

[a] CR = complete response; PR = partial response.

including 15 complete responders and 26 partial responders. The most frequently employed regimen was 20 mg/m² given as a rapid intravenous infusion daily for 5 days and repeated at 4-week intervals. Moderate myelosuppression and transient increases in serum creatinine were reported.

While active as a single agent, the major role of cisplatin in the treatment of testicular cancer is in combination with other agents (Table III). Most combination induction regimens contained cisplatin, vinblastine, and bleomycin with or without other agents. Cisplatin-containing therapy has been shown to be active in patients with prior chemotherapy and/or radiotherapy and in tumors of all histologic types, resulting in greater response rates and longer survival than other regimens.

A series of 86 patients were treated by the Einhorn regimen utilizing a combination of cisplatin (20 mg/m² daily for 5 days every 3 weeks), vinblastine (0.3 or 0.4 mg/kg every 3 weeks), and bleomycin (30 units per week). Of 80 evaluable patients, 64% achieved CR and 32.5% achieved PR. Six partial responders had subsequent surgical resection of residual tumor and were rendered free of disease. Response rate and survival were not significantly affected by site of metastasis, tumor histology, or prior therapy. The addition of adriamycin (30–40 mg/m² every 3 weeks) to the regimen (eight patients) likewise did not significantly affect response rate or survival.

Kaplan-Meier survival curves were generated for all 86 patients (Fig. 1). The difference in survival of CR and PR patients was highly significant ($P = .0001$). Median survival was not reached in an observation period of 51 months. Sixty patients were alive, 53 of whom were free of disease from 17+ to 51+ months at the latest time of analysis.

To determine whether survival was influenced by the addition of cisplatin,

TABLE III

Cisplatin Combination Therapy of Metastatic Germ Cell Tumors of the Testes

Reference	Regimen	No. evaluable patients	CR[a]	PR	% Response (CR + PR)
Einhorn (1978)	Bleomycin, vinblastine, cisplatin	47	33	14	100%
D'Aoust et al. (1979)	Bleomycin, vinblastine, cisplatin	80	51	26	96%
Wittes et al. (1976)	VAB (vinblastine, actinomycin D, bleomycin)	68	15	17	47%
Cheng et al. (1978)	VAB-II (VAB + cisplatin)	50	25	17	84%
Golbey (personal communication)	VAB-III (VAB + cyclophosphamide)	90	54	23	86%
Golbey (personal communication)	VAB-IV (VAB-III—increase bleomycin)	49	29	13	86%
Merrin et al. (1977); Merrin (1978a,b)	A-bleomycin, vinblastine, cisplatin, adriamycin, cyclophosphamide	30	17	5	73%
Merrin et al. (1977); Merrin (1978a,b)	B-bleomycin, vinblastine, cisplatin, prednisone, actinomycin D, vincristine	40	32	8	100%
Samson and Stephens (1978)	Bleomycin, vinblastine, cisplatin	57	32	17	86%
Einhorn and Williams (1978)	Adriamycin, cisplatin	10	1	9	100%
Vogl et al. (1976)	Adriamycin, cisplatin	5	0	1	20%
Kwong and Kennedy (1977)	Adriamycin, cisplatin	3	1	1	67%
Wallace et al. (1975)	Adriamycin, cisplatin	3	2	1	100%

[a] CR = complete remission; PR = partial response.

survival characteristics of 78 patients (eight patients who received adriamycin were excluded) were compared to those of a series of 70 patients who received bleomycin and vinblastine (VB-1) combination therapy of testicular cancer (Samuels, 1976).

In addition to receiving similar doses of vinblastine and bleomycin, the two series of patients were comparable with respect to tumor histologies, prior therapy, extent of disease, and duration of follow-up. The difference between the survival of patients treated by VB-1 and by the Einhorn regimen was highly significant ($P = .001$). The median survival time was 60 weeks for the patients treated with VB-1. The median survival time was not reached for patients receiving the cisplatin-containing regimen. Seventy-seven percent of these patients were alive 60 weeks after beginning therapy (D'Aoust et al., 1979). The survival characteristics reflect the differences in CR rates in the two studies. Sixty-two percent of patients treated with the Einhorn regimen achieved CR, compared to 31% of VB-1 patients.

Two hundred and fifty-seven patients with testicular cancer have been treated at the Memorial Sloan-Kettering Cancer Center in a series of studies employing successive versions of the VAB regimens (Cheng *et al.*, 1978; Golbey, personal communication; Wittes *et al.*, 1976). VAB-I consisted of vinblastine, actinomycin, and bleomycin (Wittes *et al.*, 1977). VAB-II consisted of VAB-I plus cisplatin 120 mg/m², and the bleomycin was changed from an intermittent schedule to a 7-day infusion. Cyclophosphamide was added in VAB-III and VAB-IV. Cisplatin was administered by intravenous infusion with hydration and diuresis. Response rates for the VAB studies are summarized in Table III. The data suggest that the addition of cisplatin to the VAB-I regimen resulted in increased response and survival. Relatively few data have been reported for VAB-III, -IV, but the difference in response rate (CR + PR) to VAB-I (47%) and VAB-II (84%) regimens is highly significant (*P* = .0001) (Golbey, 1978). As in the results noted with the Einborn regimen, a major difference between the efficacy of VAB-I and VAB-II is the response rate of patients who received prior chemotherapy. Nine percent of VAB-I patients with prior chemotherapy achieved complete remission, whereas 40% of pretreated VAB-II patients achieved complete remission. The median survival time was 12 and 20 months for VAB-I and VAB-II patients, respectively. The toxicities observed for VAB-I and VAB-II-IV were comparable except for cisplatin-related nausea and vomiting.

Seventy patients were treated with combined multisequential chemotherapy and radical reductive surgery by Merrin at Roswell Park Memorial Hospital (Cisplatin, 1978; Merrin, 1978a,b). Cisplatin was administered by a 6–8-hr infusion with saline hydration plus mannitol diuresis. This administration

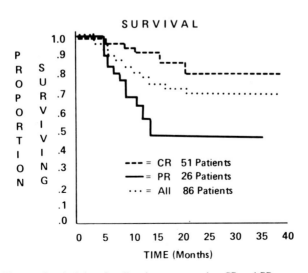

Fig. 1. Survival time for all patients compared to CR and PR groups.

schedule appears to be less toxic than other cisplatin administration schedules currently employed.

Thus the combination of cisplatin, vinblastine, and bleomycin with or without other agents is currently the most effective first-line therapy for testicular cancer. Given the natural history of testicular cancer, long-term survivors (>24 months) may represent clinical cures.

B. Ovarian Tumors

Cisplatin is active both as a single agent and in combined therapy of advanced or recurrent ovarian tumors (Table IV). Although the dose commonly administered in single-agent studies was 50 mg/m², it appears likely that the optimum dose and schedule have not been defined. Fifty-two patients received cisplatin 30–50 mg/m² every 3–4 weeks and 29 patients received 100 mg/m² every 4 weeks with hydration and mannitol diuresis (Wiltshaw, 1977). The CR rate was 15.4% and 31% for the low- and high-dose regimen, respectively. The overall response rate was 31% and 52%, respectively. In another study (Bruckner et al., 1978), in which 19 patients received cisplatin 50 mg/m² as a I.V. bolus injection every 3 weeks, only six patients achieved objective response and four patients experienced subjective improvement.

Cisplatin combination therapy of ovarian cancer appears to be more effective than single-agent therapy in both patients with or without previous chemotherapy. The most widely used combination consisted of cisplatin and adriamycin with or without cyclophosphamide. In a comparative study (Holland, personal communication), 52 previously untreated patients were randomized to receive either cisplatin, cisplatin plus adriamycin, or thio-TEPA plus methotrexate. Overall response to single-agent cisplatin was 41%, with three (18%) complete remissions. There were six complete remissions (33%) and an overall response rate of 67% to the cisplatin and adriamycin combination. Thio-TEPA and methotrexate therapy resulted in a 12% complete remission and a 35% overall response rate. Fifty percent of the patients receiving cisplatin and adriamycin were alive 18 months after beginning therapy. The survival time of this group was significantly longer ($P = .04$) than that of the thio-TEPA and methotrexate group. Survival of the cisplatin single-agent group was not significantly longer than that of the thio-TEPA and methotrexate group ($P = .14$). Ehrlich et al. (1978) reported a 45% CR rate in 29 patients when cyclophosphamide was added to the adriamycin and cisplatin combination. In another study of 24 patients treated with 60 mg/m² cisplatin and 60 mg/m² adriamycin (Briscoe et al., 1978), 20 patients had received prior chemotherapy. Complete remissions were observed in four patients (two previously untreated), with an overall response rate of 38%. Toxicities were predictable and manageable. The lower overall response rate observed in this study compared to that observed in

TABLE IV

Cisplatin Therapy of Metastatic Ovarian Tumors

Reference	Regimen	No. evaluable patients	CR[a]	PR	Response (CR + PR) (%)	Patients with prior chemo. (%)
Wiltshaw (1977)	Cisplatin (low)	52	8	8	31	100
Wiltshaw (1977)	Cisplatin (high)	29	9	6	52	100
Bruckner et al. (1978)	Cisplatin	19	0	6	31.5	100
Holland (personal communication)	Cisplatin	17	3	4	41	0
Holland (personal communication)	Cisplatin, adriamycin	18	6	6	67	0
Briscoe et al. (1978)	Cisplatin, adriamycin	24	4	5	38	83
Ehrlich et al. (1978)	Cisplatin, adriamycin cyclophosphamide	29	13	8	72	0
Wiltshaw (1977)	Cisplatin, chlorambucil	35	0	19	54	0
Wiltshaw (1977)	Cisplatin, chlorambucil, adriamycin	22	0	13	59	0
Greenwald et al. (1978)	Cisplatin, adriamycin, hexamethylmelamine	12	3	3	50	100
Greenwald et al. (1978)	Cisplatin, hexamethyl-malamine	5	0	4	80	100
Kane et al. (1978)	Cisplatin, adriamycin, cyclophosphamide, hexamethylmelamine	22	4	7	50	100

[a] CR = complete remission; PR = partial remission.

others suggests that cisplatin and adriamycin are not as effective in second-line therapy as in first-line therapy.

It is not yet clear whether the addition of an alkylating agent other than cyclophosphamide increases the efficacy of the cisplatin and adriamycin combination (see Table IV). The response rate to the combination of cisplatin and adriamycin with or without other agents (50-72%) approximates those obtained with another active combination, Hexa-CAF (76%) (Young *et al.*, 1978). In most studies survival data are unavailable or preliminary. Randomized studies comparing the response and survival data for these combination regimens and melphalan are needed to define the exact role of cisplatin in first-line combination therapy of advanced ovarian cancer.

C. Head and Neck Cancer

Cisplatin is active as a single agent in squamous cell cancer of the head and neck (Hill *et al.*, 1975; Wittes *et al.*, 1977; Panettiere *et al.*, 1978; Jacobs *et al.*, 1978).

Wittes *et al.* (1977) treated 26 patients with high-dose cisplatin, 120 mg/m² as a rapid intravenous infusion every 3 weeks. All 26 patients had received prior radiotherapy to local disease, 14 had had major ablative surgery, and all but 5 had been previously treated with chemotherapy. Responses included 2 CR, 6 PR, 10 less than PR, and 8 who had no change in their disease. This study demonstrated that cisplatin was definitely active in this group of patients with a poor prognosis.

Eighteen patients were treated with cisplatin by Jacobs *et al.* (1978) for advanced squamous cell carcinoma of the head and neck. Twelve of the 18 patients had recurrent disease following treatment with surgery and radiation. Cisplatin was given intravenously as a 24-hr infusion in a dose of 80 mg/m². The overall response rate was 72%, with one complete remission. Six patients experienced a partial remission of tumor and six patients experienced less than a partial response.

Standard therapy for early stages of head and neck cancer includes surgery and radiotherapy. Patients with early stages of disease can often be cured by this treatment, but patients with more advanced disease have a poor prognosis. Cisplatin has been utilized in combination with bleomycin, methotrexate, and vincristine in treatment of advanced head and neck cancer (Table V). The best response rates have been obtained with cisplatin and bleomycin. Methotrexate has been added to these two drugs, and although toxicities are generally greater, this three-drug regimen has been utilized in an outpatient clinic (Vogl and Kaplan, 1979).

Forty patients with advanced head and neck cancer unamenable to surgery were treated with cisplatin and bleomycin as induction therapy to decrease the tumor mass (Hong *et al.*, 1979). Patients were then treated with surgery and/or

TABLE V

Cisplatin Combination Therapy in Head and Neck Cancer

Reference	Therapy	No. evaluable patients	CR[a]	PR	CR + PR (%)
Wittes et al. (1975)	Cisplatin 2 mg/kg, bleomycin	24	0	3	13
Wittes et al. (1977)	Cisplatin 3 mg/kg, bleomycin	21	2	6	38
Randolf et al. (1978)	Cisplatin 3 mg/kg, bleomycin	21	4	11	71
Hong et al. (1979)	Cisplatin 120 mg/m², bleomycin	39	8	22	76
Amer et al. (1978)	Cisplatin, 100–120 mg/m², bleomycin, vincristine	16	0	6	38
Caradonna et al. (1978)	Cisplatin 120 mg/m², bleomycin, methotrexate	14	2	9	79
Elias et al. (1978)	Cisplatin 100 mg/m², bleomycin, methotrexate, Leucovorin Rescue	23	0	14	61

[a] CR = complete remission; PR = partial remission.

radiotherapy. Cisplatin was administered in a dose of 120 mg/m². Of 39 patients evaluable for response to induction chemotherapy, 8 achieved CR (20%) and 22 achieved PR (56%), for an overall response rate of 76%. This drug combination appears to be effective in reducing tumor bulk in previously untreated patients. Twenty of these patients are alive with no evidence of recurrent disease, for a median follow-up time of 9.5 months (range 5.5–21 months).

The early results of cisplatin plus bleomycin chemotherapy in conjunction with surgery and radiation therapy suggest that this combined modality may significantly improve the survival of patients with head and neck cancer. Randomized comparative studies comparing surgery and radiation therapy to this same therapy with the addition of chemotherapy are currently under way.

D. Bladder and Other Genitourinary Tumors

Recent phase II clinical trials have defined the therapeutic efficacy of cisplatin in metastatic transitional cell carcinoma. Cisplatin was first considered for treatment of this disease after bladder tumors in animal models showed response to this agent (Soloway et al., 1973). Table VI summarizes clinical results of three studies using single-agent cisplatin. Although the duration of response was relatively short, cisplatin produced a higher response rate than any other single chemotherapeutic agent in bladder cancer.

Higher response rates utilizing cisplatin in combination with other drugs have been reported (Yagoda et al., 1978); Sternberg et al., 1977; Williams et al., 1978). However, since duration of remission is also relatively short after combination drug therapy, it is questionable whether combination chemotherapy should be used when the greater toxicity is considered compared to single-agent cisplatin. New agents with which to combine cisplatin in the treatment of bladder cancer await further new drug screening studies.

TABLE VI

Cisplatin Therapy of Metastatic Bladder Cancer

Reference	No. Evaluable Patients	CR[a]	PR	Response CR + PR (%)
Soloway (1977)	13	0	6	46
Yagoda (1979)	28	0	10	36
Merrin (1978)	19	1	8	47

[a] CR = complete remission; PR = partial remission.

Cisplatin has shown activity in prostate cancer (Merrin, 1978a); however, objective responses are difficult to measure in this disease and meaningful objective responses were not observed in another study (Yagoda, 1979). Although cisplatin has affinity for kidney tissue, no meaningful antitumor activity has been observed in renal cell carcinoma.

E. Lung Cancer

When used as a single agent in lung cancer patients, cisplatin has shown only slight activity in a small number of studies. Rossof (1976), using cisplatin at a dose of 75 mg/m^2 every 3 weeks, found that only 1 of 17 patients with lung cancer achieved a partial response. This response was seen in a patient with adenocarcinoma. Only one other response had been reported previously by Hill et al. (1972) in a broad phase II study that included seven patients with lung cancer. A later study in adenocarcinoma of the lung compared cisplatin alone with a cisplatin-containing regimen and showed that cisplatin monotherapy resulted in a 9% response rate in 22 patients (Kvols et al., 1978).

Despite evidence for the low activity of displatin as a single agent, the reported synergy of cisplatin with adriamycin and cyclophosphamide in animal models (Ohnuma et al., 1975; Woodman et al., 1973) encouraged investigators to evaluate cisplatin in combination with other chemotherapy in lung cancer patients. Table VII summarizes the major studies reported. The median survival times of patients in three studies was 6 months. Cisplatin-containing regimens appear to have equivalent activities for squamous cell carcinoma, adenocarcinoma, and large-cell anaplastic carcinoma of the lung (Bjornsson et al., 1978; Eagan et al., 1977; Gralla et al., 1978; Issell et al., 1978a; Kvols et al., 1978). However, the role of cisplatin in small-cell lung cancer, the most chemotherapeutically sensitive lung cancer, is more difficult to evaluate from the limited number of studies reported. No activity was demonstrated in four patients with small-cell lung cancer who received cisplatin alone (Rossof, 1976). Eagan et al. (1977), using cisplatin combined with cyclophosphamide and adriamycin, reported four partial remissions in eight small-cell lung cancer patients after one course of therapy, but this response rate might be expected for cyclophosphamide and adriamycin without cisplatin. Sierocki *et al.* (1978) have recently reported that three of six patients with small-cell lung cancer responsed to cisplatin and VP16-213. However, VP16-213 is probably the most effective single compound in this disease, and the small number of patients do not allow an assessment of the contribution of cisplatin in this study.

Cisplatin-containing chemotherapy is active in lung cancer patients, but it is not possible to evaluate its role in extending survival on the basis of available data. Median survivals of 6 months are not uncommonly reported with other non-cisplatin-containing regimens in non-small-cell lung cancer (Hansen *et al.*, 1976; Issell *et al.*, 1978b; Lanzotti *et al.*, 1976; Livingston *et al.*, 1976). Clearly, further studies comparing survival times of patients treated with cisplatin-containing combination chemotherapy to those treated with noncisplatin chemotherapy are indicated.

F. Other Malignancies

Other malignancies in which cisplatin has been reported to be active either as a single agent or in combination regimens include osteogenic sarcoma, pediatric neuroblastoma, and esophageal carcinoma. One complete response and four partial responses were reported in eight patients with advanced metastatic osteogenic sarcoma who had received prior chemotherapy (Ochs *et al.*, 1978). Baum *et al.* (1978) reported complete response in one of eight patients with extensive osteogenic sarcoma who had failed high-dose methotrexate and adriamycin chemotherapy. Ettinger *et al.* (1978) reported on an adjuvant study using cisplatin combined with adriamycin in surgically treated osteogenic sarcoma. All eight patients have remained disease-free at intervals varying from 3 to 21 months following study entry.

Cisplatin, as single agent, has demonstrated activity in children with neuroblastoma. Six of 22 patients (Nitschke *et al.*, 1978) and one of three patients (Kamalakar *et al.*, 1977) were reported to experience remission of disease after cisplatin therapy.

A 21% complete plus partial remission rate was reported in 28 patients with squamous cell esophageal carcinoma when cisplatin was combined with bleomycin (Kelsen *et al.*, 1978). Survival data from this study were not reported and it is difficult to evaluate the contribution of cisplatin to the regimen.

Malignancies in which cisplatin has reported activity but where insufficient numbers of patients have been studied include cloacogenic carcinoma of the anus (Fisher *et al.*, 1978) and medullary carcinoma of the thyroid (Kamalakar *et al.*, 1977).

Cisplatin appears to have little activity in breast and colorectal tumors. Only

TABLE VII

Cisplatin Combination Therapy in Lung Cancer

References	Histology	Therapy	Evaluable patients (number)	CR[a]	PR	CR + PR (%)	Median survival (months)
Bjornsson et al. (1978)	All types	Cisplatin, adriamycin, cyclo-phosphamide, vincristine	64	0	14	22	6
Issell et al. (1978)	Adenocarcinoma, large cell	Cisplatin, adriamycin, ftorafur	43	2	9	26	6
Eagan et al. (1977)	Non-small cell	Cisplatin, adriamycin, cyclophosphamide	41	1	7	20	6
Gralla et al. (1978)	Non-small cell	Cisplatin, adriamycin, cyclophosphamide	36	0	11	31	Not reported
Kvols et al. (1978)	Adenocarcinoma	Cisplatin, adriamycin, cyclophosphamide	19	1	3	21	Not reported

[a] CR = Complete recovery; PR = partial recovery.

two partial responses were observed in 65 patients with metastatic breast cancer who received cisplatin therapy (Bull *et al.*, 1978; Samal *et al.*, 1978; Yap *et al.*, 1978). In colorectal adenocarcinoma only one partial response was observed in 19 patients treated with cisplatin (Samal *et al.*, 1978).

V. TOXICITY

The major toxicities induced by cisplatin include nephrotoxicity, nausea and vomiting, myelosuppression, and ototoxicity. Other toxicities include anaphylactic-like reactions; neurotoxicity characterized primarily by peripheral neuropathies, hypocalcemia secondary to renal damage, and occasionally cardiac abnormalities; elevation of liver enzymes; and allergic reactions. All toxicities appear to be dose related (with the exception of anaphylactic-like reactions), and nephrotoxicity, ototoxicity, and neurotoxicity appear to be cumulative also. Each of these toxicities will be discussed in some detail.

A. Renal Toxicity

Renal toxicity is one of the major dose-limiting toxicities of cisplatin and appears to be cumulative. In early studies in which cisplatin was administered in a variety of doses and dose schedules without hydration and diuresis, the incidence of nephrotoxicity in 396 patients, as measured by increase in BUN and/or serum creatinine to above-normal limits, ranged from 26 to 36% (De Conti *et al.*, 1973; Higby *et al.*, 1973, 1974a,b; Hill *et al.*, 1974, 1975; Kovach *et al.*, 1973; Krakoff and Lippman, 1974; Lippman *et al.*, 1973; Rossof *et al.*, 1972; Talley *et al.*, 1973; Wallace and Higby, 1974; Wiltshaw and Carr, 1974; Wiltshaw and Kroner, 1976; Yagoda *et al.*, 1976). These manifestations of renal toxicity were first noted during the second week after cisplatin therapy. In most cases the renal toxicity was reversible.

Subsequently, various methods were used to alleviate cisplatin-induced nephrotoxicity, including slow intravenous infusion of the drug and intravenous saline hydration with/without furosemide and/or mannitol diuresis (Chary *et al.*, 1977; Cheng *et al.*, 1978; Corder *et al.*, 1977; Einhorn and Donohue, 1977; Hayes *et al.*, 1977; Merrin, 1976, 1978a,b,c; Merrin *et al.*, 1977; Stark *et al.*, 1977; Stark and Howell, 1978). Patients received subsequent hydration to replace fluids lost as a result of emesis and diuresis. Even at doses of 20 mg/m^2 hydration is necessary to decrease renal toxicity (Table VIII).

Renal pathology has been reported in patients who received cisplatin therapy (Dentino *et al.*, 1977; Gonzalez-Vitale, 1977; Higby *et al.*, 1973, 1974a; Hill *et al.*, 1972). In patients receiving cisplatin (low dose and high dose) with hydration and diuresis (Gonzalez-Vitale, 1977) pathologic changes in the kidneys were

TABLE VIII

Severity of Nephrotoxicity versus Hydration

	No. patients	Degree of nephrotoxicity[a]			
		None	Mild	Moderate	Severe
Patients receiving hydration	51	45 (88%)	2 (4%)	2 (4%)	2 (4%)
Patients not receiving hydration	31	19 (61%)	6 (19%)	3 (9.6%)	3 (9.6%)

[a] Mild = serum creatinine 1.5–2.0 mg/100 ml or BUN 25–35 mg/100 ml; moderate = serum creatinine 2.1–2.5 mg/100 ml or BUN 36–50 mg/100 ml; severe = serum creatinine >2.5 mg/100 ml or BUN >50 mg/100 ml.

essentially the same in both groups and consisted of focal acute necrosis of the distal convoluted tubules and collection ducts, dilatation of convoluted tubules, and formation of casts. Similar results were reported in patients 5–6 months after the last course of cisplatin therapy, suggesting that permanent subclinical renal injury may be induced by cisplatin (Dentino et al., 1977).

Major studies of animal and human nephrotoxicity have been reviewed recently by Madias and Harrington (1978).

B. Nausea and Vomiting

The incidence of moderate to severe nausea and vomiting after cisplatin administration is significant and probably dose related. In phase II studies (Higby et al., 1974b; Kovach et al., 1973; Wiltshaw and Carr, 1974; Wiltshaw and Kroner, 1976; Yagoda et al., 1978) the incidence of gastrointestinal toxicity was 100% in 102 patients treated with cisplatin at doses of 30–100 mg/m².

Nausea and vomiting usually began within 1–2 hr after administration and lasted 24–48 hr. However, some patients experienced variable degrees of gastrointestinal toxicity for up to 1 week after treatment. In most instances antiemetics have been ineffective in controlling emesis.

C. Myelosuppression

Although hydration and diuresis were effective in reducing nephrotoxicity, the incidence and severity of myelosuppression was not altered by this treatment and occurred in 20–30% of patients (Chary et al., 1977; Cheng et al., 1978; Einhorn and Donohue, 1977; Hill et al., 1975; Merrin, 1976, 1978a,b,c; Merrin et al., 1977; Monti-Bragadin et al., 1975; Stark et al., 1977; Stark and Howell, 1978).

At intermittent doses of 50–60 mg/m^2, leukopenia below 2000 cells/mm^3 or thrombocytopenia below 50,000 cells/mm^3 rarely occurred. Anemia, reported as a decrease of > 2.0 g/100 ml hemoglobin was observed in 11% of the patients.

D. Other Toxicities

Ototoxicity, manifested as tinnitus and loss of hearing in the high-frequency range (4000–8000 Hz), occurred in approximately 11% of patients treated with cisplatin in phase I trials (De Conti *et al.*, 1973; Higby *et al.*, 1973, 1974b; Krakoff and Lippman, 1974; Lippman *et al.*, 1973; Piel *et al.*, 1974; Rossof *et al.*, 1972; Talley *et al.*, 1973). Ototoxicity appeared to be dose related and cumulative and occurred both unilaterally and bilaterally. Speech discrimination threshold showed no consistent change with cisplatin dosage. The incidence of hearing loss in the 4000–8000 Hz range did not appear to be lessened by administration of cisplatin with hydration and diuresis (Hayes *et al.*, 1977). No vestibular symptoms appeared to be associated with the audiologic toxicities.

Neurotoxicity has been reported to occur in patients treated with cisplatin (Von Hoff *et al.*, 1979) and was characterized by peripheral neuropathies, including paresthesia in both upper and lower extremities, tremor, leg weakness, loss of taste, and light-headedness. Seizures were also reported to occur in some patients. These neurologic symptoms generally occurred in patients who were treated with cisplatin from 4 to 7 months and received cisplatin at doses of 2.5 mg/kg and 15 mg/m^2 daily $\times$ 5 at 3–4-week intervals with total doses ranging from 500 to 1470 mg. However, neurotoxicity occurred in two patients receiving only one dose of cisplatin 50 mg/m^2.

Cases of anaphylacticlike reactions possibly secondary to cisplatin were reported to have occurred (Rozencweig *et al.*, 1977). The reactions consisted of facial edema, wheezing, tachycardia, and hypotension within a few minutes after intravenous drug administration. All reactions were controlled with intravenous adrenaline, corticosteroids, or antihistamines.

Hyperuricemia has been reported to occur in patients treated with cisplatin at approximately the same frequency as the increase in BUN and serum creatinine. It is more pronounced after doses greater than 50 mg/m^2 cisplatin, and peak levels of uric acid generally occur between 3 and 5 days after dose administration. Allopurinol was reported to reduce uric acid levels effectively (Hill *et al.*, 1974; Rossof *et al.*, 1972).

E. Serum Electrolyte Decrease

A decrease in serum electrolyte has been correlated with renal toxicity in patients receiving cisplatin (Schilsky and Anderson, 1979). Hypomagnesemia developed in 23 of 44 evaluable patients. Symptomatic patients demonstrated muscular irritability, twitching, and tetany. Other reports have indicated hypokalemia and hyponatremia occurring secondary to hypomagnesemia. Serum magnesium must be carefully monitored in patients receiving cisplatin, and signs of hypomagnesemia can be treated with supplemental magnesium gluconate or magnesium sulfate.

VI. CISPLATIN ANALOGUES

Many analogues of cisplatin have been synthesized, including substitution of ligands for both the ammonia and chloride groups of the molecule. A number of these compounds have been reported to possess antitumor activity in experimental animal tumors (Cleare *et al.*, 1978; Prestayko *et al.*, 1979). In addition, many of these analogues have demonstrated significantly lower nephrotoxicity compared to cisplatin (Guarino *et al.*, 1979; Prestayko *et al.*, 1979).

A class of analogues that contains a 1,2-diaminocyclohexyl moiety was shown to be active in a line of L1210 leukemia cells that had developed resistance to cisplatin (Burchenal *et al.*, 1977). One of these compounds, 1,2-diaminocyclohexyl platinum II malonate, has demonstrated antitumor activity in human tumors (Hill *et al.*, 1977; Ribaud *et al.*, 1979), some of which may have been resistant to cisplatin.

Another group of analogues in which platinum has a 4^+ valence state (platinum IV) may possess additional activity on DNA that is different from that of the platinum II compounds. One such compound, bis(isopropyl)-*trans*-dihydroxy-dichloro platinum IV, is scheduled for clinical trials in the very near future.

VII. CONCLUSION

Cisplatin and analogues show considerable promise in the chemotherapy of human neoplasms. The lack of cross-resistance with alkylating agents and the relative lack of myelosuppression make cisplatin a useful drug to include in combination chemotherapy. Approximate dosing schedules must still be worked out to utilize cisplatin most efficaciously and to minimize the associated toxicities.

REFERENCES

Amer, M. H., Izbicki, R., and Al-Sarraf, M. (1978). *Proc. Am. Soc. Clin. Oncol.* **19**, 312.
Baum, E., Greenberg, L., Gaynon, P., Krivit, W., and Hammond D. (1978). *Proc. Am. Soc. Clin. Oncol.* **19**, 385.

Beck, D. J., and Brubaker, R. R. (1975). *Mutat. Res.* **27**, 181–189.

Bjornsson, S., Takita, H., Kuberka, N., Priesler, H., Cantane, H., Higby, D., and Henderson, E. (1978). *Cancer Treat. Rep.* **62**, 505–510.

Briscoe, K., Pasmantier, M., Brown, J., and Kennedy, B. J. (1978). *Proc. Am. Soc. Clin. Oncol.* **19**, 378.

Bruckner, H. W., Cohen, C. J., Wallach, R. C., Kabakow, B., Deppe, G., Greenspan, E. M., Gusberg, S. B., and Holland, J. F. (1978). *Cancer Treat. Rep.* **62**, 555–558.

Bull, J. M., Anderson, T., Lippman, M. E., Cassidy, J. G., Gormley, P. E., and Young, R. C. (1978). *Proc. Am. Assoc. Cancer Res.* **19**, 87.

Burchenal, J. H., Kalaher, K., O'Toole, T., and Chisholm, J. (1977). *Cancer Res.* **37**, 3455–3457.

Caradonna, R., Paladine, W., Goldstein, J., Ruckdeschel, J., Hillinger, S., and Horton, J. (1978). *Proc. Am. Soc. Clin. Oncol.* **19**, 401.

Cavalli, F., Sonntag, R. W., Ryssel, H. J., Tschopp, L., and Brunner, K. W. (1976). *Schweiz. Med. Wochenschr.* **106**, 754–757.

Chary, K. K., Higby, D. J., and Henderson, E. S. (1977). *J. Clin. Hematol. Oncol.* **7**, 633–644.

Cheng, E., Cvitkovic, E., Wittes, R. E., and Golbey, R. B. (1978). *Cancer (Philadelphia)* **42**, 2162–2168.

Cisplatin (1978). NDA No. 18–057 Amendment, Vol. 2.1, pp. 100104–100124. Bristol Lab., Syracuse, New York.

Cleare, M., Hydesm, P. C., Malerbi, B. W., and Watkins, D. M. (1978). *Biochimie* **60**, 835–850.

Corder, M. P., Elliott, T. E., and Bell, S. J. (1977). *J. Clin. Hematol. Oncol.* **7**, 645–651.

D'Aoust, J. C., Prestayko, A. W., Archambault, W. A. T., Einhorn, L. H., Comis, R. L., and Crooke, S. T. (1979). *Med. Pediatr. Oncol.* **6**, 195–205.

De Conti, R. C., Toftness, B. R., Lange, R. C., and Creasey, W. A. (1973). *Cancer Res.* **33**, 1310–1361.

Dentino, M. E., Luft, F. C., Yum, M. N., Williams, S. D., and Einhorn, L. H. (1977). *Cancer (Philadelphia)* **41**, 1274–1281.

Eagan, R. T., Carr, D. T., Lee, R. E., Frytak, S., Rubin, J., and Coles, D. T. (1977). *Cancer Treat. Rep.* **6**, 93–95.

Ehrlich, C. E., Einhorn, L. H., and Morgan, J. L. (1978). *Proc. Am. Soc. Clin. Oncol.* **19**, 379.

Einhorn, L. H. (1978). *Proc. Am. Soc. Clin. Oncol.* **19**, 308.

Einhorn, L. H., and Donohue, J. (1977). *Ann. Intern. Med.* **87**, 293–298.

Einhorn, J. H., and Williams, S. D. (1978). *Cancer Treat. Rep.* **62**, 1351–1353.

Elias, E. G., Chretein, P. B., Monnard, E., and Wiernik, P. H. (1978). *Proc. Am. Soc. Clin. Oncol.* **19**, 376.

Ettinger, L. J., Douglass, H. O., Higby, D. J., Bjornsson, S., Mindell, E. R., and Freeman, A. I. (1978). *Proc. Am. Assoc. Cancer Res.* **19**, 323.

Fisher, W. B., Herbst, K. D., Sims, J. E., and Critchfield, C. F. (1978). *Cancer Treat. Rep.* **62**, 91–97.

Gale, G. E., Walker, E. M., Jr., Atkins, L., Smith, A. B., and Meischen, S. J. (1974). *Res. Commun. Chem. Pathol. Pharmacol.* **7**, 529–538.

Goldbey, R. B. (1978) Personal Communication. Cited in: *Cisplatin New Drug Application Amendment*, V. **2.1**, p 90.

Gonzalez-Vitale, J. C., Hayes, D. M., Cvitkovic, E., and Sternberg, S. S. (1977). *Cancer (Philadelphia)* **39**, 1362–1371.

Gralla, R. J., Cvitkovic, E., and Boldbey, R. B. (1978). *Proc. Am. Soc. Clin. Oncol.* **19**, 353.

Greenwald, E., Vogl, S. E., Kaplan, B. H., and Wallner, D. (1978). *Proc. Am. Soc. Clin. Oncol.* **19**, 327.

Guarino, A., Miller, D. S., Arnold, S. T., Pritchard, J. B., Davis, R. D., Urbanek, M. A., Miller, T. J., and Litterst, C. L. (1979). *Cancer Treat. Rep.* **63**, 1475–1483.

Hansen, H. H., Selawry, O. S., Simon, R., Carr, D. T., Van Wyk, C. E., Tucker, R. D., and Sealy, R. (1976). *Cancer (Philadelphia)* **38**, 2201–2207.

Hayes, D. M., Cvitkovic, E., Golbey, R. B., Scheiner, E., Helson, L., and Krakoff, I. H. (1977). *Cancer (Philadelphia)* **39**, 1372–1381.

Higby, D. J., Wallace, H. J., and Holland, J. F. (1973). *Cancer Chemother. Rep., Part 1* **57**, 459–463.

Higby, D. J., Wallace, H. J., Albert, D. J., and Holland, J. F. (1974a). *Cancer (Philadelphia)* **33**, 1219–1225.

Higby, D. J., Wallace, H. J., Albert, D., and Holland, J. F. (1974b). *J. Urol.* **112**, 100–104.

Hill, J. M., Cardona, F. A., Loeb, E., MacLellan, A. S., Hill, N. O., and Khan, A. (1972). *Wadley Med. Bull.* **2**(3), 45.

Hill, J. M., Loeb, E., MacLellan, A. S., Hill, N. O., Khan, A., and Kogler, J. (1974). *In* "Platinum Coordination Complexes in Cancer Chemotherapy,": Springer-Verlag, New York and Berlin, pp 145–152.

Hill, J. M., Loeb, E., MacLellan, A., Hill, N., Khan, A., and King, J. J. (1975). *Cancer Chemother, Rep.* **59**, 647–659.

Hill, J. M., Loeb, E., Pardue, A. S., Hill, N. O., and Khan, J. J. (1977). *J. Clin. Hematol. Oncol.* **7**, 681–700.

Hong, W. K., Shapshay, S. M., Bhutani, R., Craft, M. L., Alptekin, U., Yamaguchi, K. T., Vaughan, C. W., and Strong, M. S. (1979). *Cancer Res.* **44**, 26–31.

Issell, B. F., Valdivieso, M., and Bodey, G. P. (1978a). *Cancer Treat. Rep.* **62**, 1089–1091.

Issell, B. F., Valdivieso, M., Hersh, E. M., Richman, S., Gutterman, J. U., and Bodey, G. P. (1978b). *Cancer Treat. Rep.* **62**, 1059–1063.

Jacobs, C., Bertino, J. R., Goffinet, D. R., Fee, W. E., and Goode, R. L. (1978). *Cancer (Philadelphia)* **42**, 2135–2140.

Kamalakar, P., Freeman, A. I., Higby, D. I., Wallace, H. I., and Sinks, L. F. (1977). *Cancer Treat. Rep.* **61**, 835–840.

Kane, R., Andrews, T., Bernath, A., Curry, S., Dixon, R., Gottlieb, R., Harvey, H., Kukrika, M., Lipton, A., Mortel, R., Ricci, J., and White, D. (1978). *Proc. Am. Soc. Clin. Oncol.* **19**, 320.

Kelsen, D. P., Cvitkovic, E., Bains, M., Shils, M., Howard, J., Hopfan, S., and Golbey, R. (1978). *Cancer Treat. Rep.* **62**, 1041–1046.

Khan, A., Wakasugi, K., Hill, B., Richardson, D., Disabato, J., and Hill, J. M. (1977). *J. Clin. Hematol. Oncol.* **7**, 797–816.

Kociba, R. J., Sleight, S. D., and Rosenberg, B. (1970). *Cancer Chemother. Rep.* **54**, 325–328.

Kovach, J. S., Moertel, C. G., Schutt, A. J., Reitemeier, R. G., and Hahn, R. G. (1973). *Cancer Chemother. Rep.* **57**, 357–359.

Krakoff, I. H., and Lippman, A. J. (1974). *In* "Platinum Coordination Complexes in Cancer Chemotherapy" (T. A. Connors and J. J. Roberts, eds.), pp. 183–190. Springer-Verlag, Berlin and New York.

Kvols, L. K., Eagan, R. T., Creagan, E. T., and Dalton, R. J. (1978). *Proc. Am. Assoc. Cancer Res.* **19**, 82.

Kwong, R. W., and Kennedy, B. J. (1977). *Proc. Am. Soc. Clin. Oncol.* **18**, 317.

Lanzotti, V. J., Thomas, D. R., Holoye, P. Y., Boyle, L. E., Smith, T. L., and Samuels, M. L. (1976). *Cancer Treat. Rep.* **60**, 61–68.

Lazar, R., Conran, P. B., and Damjanov, I. (1979). *Experientia* **114**, 1082.

Lippman, A. J., Helson, C., Helson, L., and Krakoff, I. H. (1973). *Cancer Chemother. Rep.* **57**, 191–200.

Livingston, R. B., Fee, W. H., Einhorn, L. H., Burgess, M. A., Freireich, R. J., Gottlieb, J. A. M., and Farber, M. O. (1976). *Cancer (Philadelphia)* **37**, 1237–1242.

Madias, N. E., and Harrington, J. T. (1978). *Am. J. Med.* **65**, 307–314.

Merrin, C. (1976). *Proc. Am. Soc. Clin. Oncol.* **17,** 243.

Merrin, C. (1978a). *J. Urol.* **119,** 493–495.

Merrin, C. (1978b). *J. Urol.* **119,** 522–524.

Merrin, C. E. (1978c). *Proc. Int. Workshop Pulm. Metastases.*

Merrin, C. E., Takita, H., Beckley, S., and Kassis, J. (1977). *J. Urol.* **117,** 291–295.

Monti-Bragadin, C., Tamaro, M., and Banji, E. (1975). *Chem.-Biol. Interact.* **11,** 469–472.

Mota, I. (1963). *Life Sci.* **2,** 917–927.

Nitschke, R., Starling, K. A., Vats, T., and Bryan, H. (1978). *Med. Pediatr. Oncol.* **4,** 127–132.

Ochs, J. J., Freeman, A. I., Douglass, H. O., Jr., Higby, D. S., Mindell, E. R., and Sinks, L. F. (1978). *Cancer Treat. Rep.* **62,** 239–245.

Ohnuma, T., Holland, J. F., and Vogl. S. (1975). *Proc. Am. Assoc. Cancer Res.* **16,** 272.

Panettiere, F. J., Lane, M., and Lehane, D. (1978). *Proc. Am. Soc. Clin. Oncol.* **19,** 410.

Piel, I. J., Meyer, D., Perlia, C. P., and Wolf, V. I. (1974). *Cancer Chemother. Rep. Part 1* **58,** 871–875.

Prestayko, A. W., Bradner, W. T., Huftalen, J. B., Rose, W. C., Schurig, J. E., Cleare, M. J., Hydes, P. A., and Crooke, S. T. (1979). *Cancer Treat. Rep.* **63,** 1503–1507.

Randolf, V. J., Vallejo, A., Sprio, R. H., Shah, J., Strong, E., Huvos, A. G., and Wittes, R. E. (1978). *Cancer (Philadelphia)* **41,** 460–467.

Ribaud, P., Alcock, N., Burchenal, J. H., Young, C., Muggia, F., and Mathé, G. (1979). *Proc. Am. Assoc. Clin. Oncol.* **20,** 336.

Rosenberg, B., Van Camp, L., Trosko, J., and Mansour, V. H. (1969). *Nature (London)* **222,** 385–386.

Rossof, A. H. (1976). SWOG Rep., Cisplatin NDA No. 18–057, Vol. 1.6, pp. 1200531–1200540. Bristol Laborarories Syracuse, N.Y.

Rossof, A. H., Slayton, R. E., and Perlia, C. P. (1972). *Cancer (Philadelphia)* **30,** 1451–1456.

Rozenscweig, M., Von Hoff, D. D., Slavik, M., and Muggia, F. (1977). *Ann. Intern. Med.* **86,** 803–812.

Samal, B., Vaitkevicius, V., Singhakowinta, A., O'Bryan, R., Buroker, T., Samson, M., and Baker, L. (1978). *Proc. Am. Soc. Clin. Oncol.* **19,** 347.

Samson, M. K., and Stephens, R. L. (1978). *Proc. Am. Assoc. Cancer Res.* **19,** 12.

Samuels, M. L. (1976). In "Testicular Tumors" (D. E. Johnson, ed.), 2nd ed., pp. 204–219. Med. Exam. Publ. Co., Flushing, New York.

Schaeppi, U., Heyman, I. A., Fleischman, R. W., Rosenkrantz, H., Ilievski, V., Phelan, R. A., Cooney, D. A., and Davis, R. D. (1973). *Toxicol. Appl. Pharmacol.* **25,** 230–241.

Schilsky, R. L., and Anderson, T. (1979). *Ann. Intern. Med.* **90,** 929–931.

Sierocki, J. S., Golbey, R. B., and Wittes, R. E. (1978). *Proc. Am. Soc. Clin. Oncol.* **19,** 352.

Soloway, M. S. (1977). *J. Urol.* **120,** 716–719.

Soloway, M. S., deKernion, J. G., Rose, D., and Persky, L. (1973). *Surg. Forum* **13,** 542–544.

Stark, J. J., and Howell, S. B. (1978). *Clin. Pharmacol. Ther.* **23,** 461–466.

Stark, J. J., Howell, S. B., and Carmody, J. (1977). *Clin. Res.* **25,** 412.

Sternberg, J. J., Bracken, R. B., Handel, P. B., and Johnson, D. E. (1977). *J. Am. Med. Assoc.* **238,** 2282–2287.

Talley, R. W., O'Bryan, R. M., Gutterman, J. U., Brounlee, R. W., and McCredie, K. B. (1973). *Cancer Chemother. Rep. Part 1* **57,** 465–471.

Vogl, S. E., and Kaplan, B. H. (1979). *Cancer (Philadelphia)* **44,** 26–31.

Vogl, S., Ohnuma, T., Perloff, M., and Holland, J. F. (1976). *Cancer (Philadelphia)* **38,** 21–26.

Von Hoff, D. D., Schilsky, R., Reichert, C. M., Reddick, R. L., Rozencweig, M., Young, R. C., and Muggia, F. M. (1979). *Cancer Treat. Rep.* **63,** 1527–1531.

Walker, E. M., Jr., and Gale, G. R. (1973). *Res. Commun. Chem. Pathol. Pharmacol.* **6,** 419–425.

Wallace, H. J., and Higby, D. J. (1974). In "Platinum Coordination Complexes in Cancer

Chemotherapy'' (T. A. Connors and J. J. Roberts, eds.), pp. 167–177. Springer-Verlag, Berlin and New York.

Wallace, H. J., Higby, D. J., Wilbur, D. W., and Cortes, E. P. (1975). *Proc. Am. Soc. Clin. Oncol.* **16,** 1092.

Welsch, C. W. (1971). *Proc. Am. Assoc. Cancer Res.* **12,** 25.

Williams, S. D., Rohn, R. J., Donohue, J. P., and Einhorn, L. H. (1978). *Proc. Am. Soc. Clin. Oncol.* **19,** 316.

Wiltshaw, E. (1977). Cisplatin NDA Amendment, Vol. 4.2, pp. 00163–00165.

Wiltshaw, E., and Carr, B. (1974). *In* ''Platinum Coordination Complexes in Cancer Chemotherapy'' (T. A. Connors and J. J. Roberts, eds.), pp. 178–182. Springer-Verlag, Berlin and New York.

Wiltshaw, E., and Kroner, T. (1976). *Cancer Treat. Rep.* **60,** 55–60.

Wittes, R. E., Brescia, F., Young, C. W., Magil, G. B., Golbey, R. B., and Krakoff, I. H. (1975). *Oncology* **32,** 202–207.

Wittes, R. E., Yagoda, A., Silvag, O., Magil, G. B., Whitmore, W., Krakoff, I. H., and Golbey, R. B. (1976). *Cancer (Philadelphia)* **37,** 637–645.

Wittes, R. E., Cvitkovic, E., Shah, J., Gerold, P. F., and Strong, E. W. (1977). *Cancer Treat. Rep.* **61,** 359–366.

Woodman, R. J. (1974). *Cancer Chemother. Rep., Part 1,* **4,** 45–52.

Woodman, R. J., Sirica, A. E., Gang, M., Kling, I., and Vendetti, J. M. (1973). *Chemotherapy (Basel)* **18,** 169–283.

Yagoda, A. (1979). *Cancer Treat. Rep.* **63,** 1565–1572.

Yagoda, A., Watson, R. C., Gonzalez-Vitale, J. C., Grabstald, H., and Whitmore, W. F. (1976). *Cancer Treat. Rep.* **60,** 917–923.

Yagoda, A., Watson, R. C., Kemeny, M., Barzell, W. E., Grabstald, H., and Whitmore, W. F. (1978). *Cancer (Philadelphia)* **41,** 2121–2130.

Yap, H. Y., Salem, P., Hortobagyi, G. N., Bodey, G. P., Sr., Buzdar, A. U., Tashima, C. K., and Blumenschein, G. R. (1978). *Cancer Treat. Rep.* **62,** 404–408.

Young, R. C., Chabner, B. A., Hubbard, S. P., Fisher, R. I., Bender, R. A., Anderson, T., and DeVita, V. T. (1978). *Proc. Am. Soc. Clin. Oncol.* **19,** 393.

10

INVESTIGATIONAL CANCER DRUGS
Manuel L. Gutierrez

I. INTRODUCTION

In the past few years, rapid advances have been made in research and development of compounds with potential tumor-inhibitory properties. As a result of this activity, therapeutic breakthroughs in several types of human cancer have occurred. The development of a comprehensive screening program involving a large number of compounds has increased the number of available effective antineoplastic agents.

The identification and acquisition of agents for antitumor studies have been accomplished by various means. They include screening of natural products and synthetic compounds, structural modification of known, active agents, and the use of a rational approach based on available biological information.

From the thousands of compounds that are available, only a few are chosen for clinical trial. The steps involved in developing antitumor agents have become increasingly complex and tedious. They include

1. Selection of materials to be tested
2. Screening of the selected materials in appropriate experimental tumor systems
3. Preclinical evaluation (formulation, toxicology, and pharmacology)
4. Clinical evaluation in man
5. Introduction into clinical practice

Relatively few of all the anticancer agents still considered investigational both here and abroad are mentioned in this section. It was not feasible to include more agents. Those selected are among many that were deemed promising. The more commonly used criteria for classifying antineoplastic agents has been used— alkylating, anthracycline analogues, antitumor antibiotics, tubulin binding agents, nitrosoureas, antimetabolites, and miscellaneous agents. Such classifications are based on origin or mechanisms of action.

II. ALKYLATING AGENTS

A. Isophosphamide

An analogue of cyclophosphamide, isophosphamide has been extensively evaluated, primarily by German investigators. It has characteristics comparable to cyclophosphamide. In experimental tumor systems isophosphamide has superior activity in L1210 leukemia. It is also active in Lewis lung carcinoma, Ehrlich ascites tumor, and Yoshida sarcoma. In early studies, responses to isophosphamide have been reported in oat cell tumor of the lung, ovarian cancer, breast cancer, and lymphomas (Carter, 1978; EORTC, 1975). Myelosuppression and genitourinary side effects are the dose-limiting toxicities, similar to those of cyclophosphamide. However, isophosphamide-induced myelosuppression and hemorrhagic cystitis are reported to be less frequent and less severe than those produced by cyclophosphamide (Posey *et al.*, 1978). The administration of isophosphamide in fractional doses has significantly reduced its renal toxicity while retaining its desired antitumor effects (Rodriquez *et al.*, 1976b).

Clinical studies of isophosphamide have also been conducted in the United States. Phase II studies have shown favorable responses in the following tumor types: acute lymphocytic leukemia, acute undifferentiated leukemia, malignant lymphomas, bronchogenic carcinoma, and epidermoid carcinoma of the lung (Rodriquez *et al.*, 1978; Posey *et al.*, 1978; Costanzi *et al.*, 1978).

B. Dianhydrogalactitol

Dianhydrogalactitol (DAG) belongs to the group of compounds referred to as the hexitols, which have been evaluated as anticancer agents since the 1950s (Eckhardt *et al.*, 1963, 1964; Eckhardt, 1978). Hexitol derivatives studied earlier for possible antitumor activity include dibromomannitol, dibromodulcitol, and dianhydromannitol. DAG is the diepoxide of dibromodulcitol, sharing the same biological and biochemical properties but appearing to possess greater antitumor activity. It inhibits DNA and RNA protein synthesis (Institoris *et al.*, 1967a,b). Inhibition is greater than that seen with dibromomannitol and dibromodulcitol. Like the dihalogenated hexitols, it is presumed that DAG exhibits cross resistance to alkylating agents.

Studies in various tumor systems show DAG has produced growth inhibition in L1210 leukemia, S180 sarcoma, Ehrlich ascites tumor, Walker carcinosarcoma 256, Yoshida sarcoma, NK/Ly ascites tumor, and ependymoblastoma (Nemeth *et al.*, 1972; Keller, 1976).

Based on the phase I clinical trials conducted in several institutions in the United States, the following dose range has been recommended for phase II studies: 20–30 mg/m^2 daily for 5 days or 55–70 mg/m^2 administered weekly (Haas *et al.*, 1976). Eagan and co-workers (1976) at the Mayo Clinic treated patients with lung cancer with DAG at doses of 30 mg/m^2/day × 5 days every 5 weeks. Responses were observed in 4/7 squamous cell, 1/3 large cell, and 0/12 adenocarcinoma patients.

The Southwest Oncology Group has evaluated DAG in patients with advanced breast cancer. One partial response was observed in 26 evaluable cases (Hoogstraten *et al.*, 1978).

C. Peptichemio

Peptichemio is a multipeptide complex composed of six synthetic peptides of *m*-L-phenylalanine mustard (DeBarbieri, 1968; DeBarbieri *et al.*, 1970). It pos-

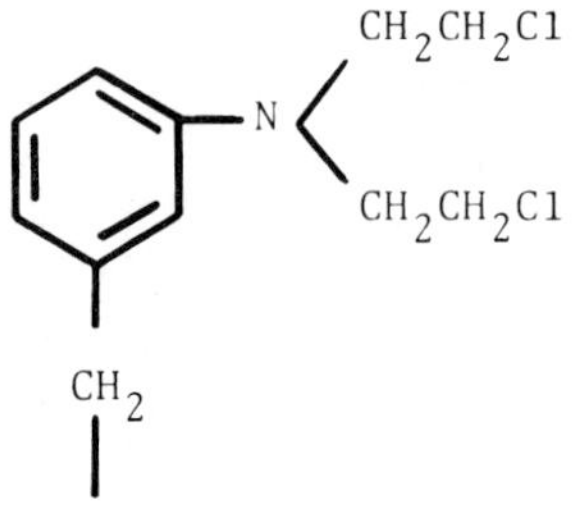

$$
\begin{array}{c}
\text{CH}_2\text{CH}_2\text{Cl} \\
\diagup \\
\text{N} \\
\diagdown \\
\text{CH}_2\text{CH}_2\text{Cl}
\end{array}
$$

$$
\text{CH}_2
$$

$$
\text{R}_1\text{-NH-CH-CO-R}_2
$$

$\downarrow$	$\downarrow$
H-	-(NO$_2$)Arg.Nval
Ser.pFPhe-	-OH
Pro-	-pFPhe
pFPhe-	-Asn
m-SL.Arg.Lys-	-His
pFPhe.Gly-	-Nval

Fig. 1. Peptichemio structural formula.

sesses both alkylating and antimetabolic properties. The alkylating activity of this compound is due to the dichlorodiethyl-amino group whereas the peptidic moiety accounts for its antimetabolic effect. The structural formula is shown in Fig. 1.

Clinical evaluation of peptichemio has been conducted since 1970 in Italy and other European countries. It is now available commercially in Italy. Data from the European studies have shown peptichemio to be effective in tumors affecting the lungs, ovary, breast, and the head and neck (Astaldi, 1975; Ruzicka and Nowotny, 1973; Battelli *et al.*, 1975; Gingold *et al.*, 1974). Activity in non-Hodgkin's lymphoma, multiple myeloma, and chronic leukemia has likewise been reported (Pittermann *et al.*, 1974; Astaldi *et al.*, 1973; Bruckner *et al.*, 1972; Carella *et al.*, 1975; Luporini, 1973; Marmont *et al.*, 1973). DeBernardi *et al.* (1978) treated 12 patients with advanced neuroblastoma with peptichemio alone. Although the duration of remission was relatively short, a 92% response rate was obtained. Toxicities include myelosuppression, nausea and vomiting, alopecia, and phlebosclerosis.

D. Prednimustine

Prednimustine is a steroidal alkylating agent formed by a combination of prednisolone and chlorambucil through an ester bond linkage (Konyves *et al.*, 1974; Konyves and Liljekvist, 1976). It is one in the group of new antineoplastic agents in which the early and initial clinical studies were conducted in Europe.

In a series of multiinstitutional phase II trials in Europe, prednimustine has demonstrated promising results in chronic lymphocytic leukemia, non-Hodgkin's lymphoma, acute myelogenous leukemia, breast carcinoma, and melanoma (Moller *et al.*, 1978; Konyves *et al.*, 1975; Hakansson *et al.*, 1978; Harrap *et al.*, 1977). The only clinical trials to date in the United States were reported by the group from Roswell Park Memorial Institute. The responses obtained in chronic lymphocytic leukemia, non-Hodgkin's lymphoma, prostatic adenocarcinoma, and some gynecologic tumors were comparable to those obtained in the European studies (Catane *et al.*, 1978; Kaufman *et al.*, 1976; LeLe *et al.*, 1978).

III. ANTHRACYCLINE ANALOGUES

A. Rubidazone

Rubidazone is a semisynthetic benzoylhydrazone derivative of daunorubicin. The compound is reported to be rapidly converted to daunorubicin; hence the mechanism of action is thought to be similar to the latter. Antitumor activity of rubidazone against Ehrlich ascites tumor, sarcoma 180, and L1210 leukemia is similar to that of daunorubicin and adriamycin (Maral *et al.*, 1972; Skovsgaard, 1975). In B16 melanoma, rubidazone has superior activity compared to daunorubicin (Goldin and Johnson, 1975).

Experimental animal studies have shown that rubidazone has milder cardiotoxic and myelosuppressive effects (Maral *et al.*, 1972). Cardiac toxicity as shown in the Zbinden model is delayed (Zbinden and Brandle, 1975). The clinical data on the cardiotoxicity of rubidazone are, however, too preliminary to draw a definite conclusion.

Promising results have been obtained with rubidazone in acute leukemias (Jacquillat *et al.*, 1972, 1976; Benjamin *et al.*, 1976), although early studies have demonstrated modest antitumor activity against solid tumors (Skovsgaard *et al.*, 1978).

B. Carminomycin

Isolated in the Soviet Union from the mycelium of *Actinomadura carminata*, carminomycin is an anthracycline antitumor antibiotic (Gause *et al.*, 1975). Biochemically, carminomycin is closely related to adriamycin; i.e., it binds to DNA, inhibits DNA synthesis to a greater extent than RNA synthesis, and has little effect on protein synthesis (Dudnik *et al.*, 1974). It has demonstrated significant antitumor activity against a number of animal tumors including L1210 and sarcoma 180.

The principal acute and subacute toxicity in animals is myelosuppression (Vertogradova *et al.*, 1974). Significant myocardial toxicity was not noted in

dogs. Minimal EKG changes did not correlate with other m
cardiac toxicity. Studies employing the Zbinden rat model s
minomycin administered at doses equipotent to adriamycin result
icant EKG changes (Zbinden and Brandle, 1975). Electron mid
failed to demonstrate focal necrosis characteristic of adriamyci
1976).

Phase II studies in the Soviet Union have shown that carminomycin is effective
in leukemia, soft tissue sarcomas, and other types of malignant neoplasms involving lungs, stomach, ovary, and breast (Lichinitser et al., 1977; Perevodchikova et al., 1977; Crooke, 1977). It appears that carminomycin has a spectrum of activity similar to that of adriamycin. In a small number of patients
treated chronically (3-9 months) with total doses ranging from 126-135 mg/m^2,
serial EKGs did not demonstrate any permanent abnormalities (Perevodchikova
et al., 1975).

C. Aclacinomycin A

Aclacinomycin A is an anthracycline antibiotic isolated in Japan from a culture
broth of *Streptomyces galilaeus*. It is related to doxorubicin, with each molecule
having three deoxysugars linked by glycosidic bonds and bound to the ring at the
C-7 position (Oki et al., 1975).

Aclacinomycin inhibits DNA and RNA synthesis, with inhibition of the latter
occurring at concentrations as low as one-tenth of that required for DNA synthesis inhibition [Sanraku-Ocean Co., Ltd., Aclacinomycin A, NCI Meeting,
1978]. The antitumor activity of aclacinomycin A in L1210 leukemia, CD8F,
mammary carcinoma, and sarcoma 180 were comparable to that of doxorubicin
[Sanraku-Ocean Co., Ltd., Aclacinomycin A, Section VIII, June 1978] (Kubota
et al., 1978a,b).

Clinical studies have been ongoing in Japan since 1976. Aclacinomycin has
been found to be active in lymphomas, breast cancer, lung carcinoma, and
gastric and ovarian tumors (Konno et al., 1978; Furue et al., 1978; Ishibiki et
al., 1978). Gastrointestinal side effects as manifested by nausea, vomiting, and
anorexia were the most frequent toxicities encountered while the dose-limiting
toxicity was myelosuppression. Stomatitis, alopecia, EKG changes, and liver
function abnormalities were the only other observed toxic effects (Furue et al.,
1978; Sakano et al., 1978).

IV. TUBULIN BINDING AGENTS

A. Maytansine

Maytansine was the first of the ansa macrolides to have shown significant
antitumor activity. Kupchan and associates first isolated maytansine in 1971

from the alcoholic extracts of the East African shrub *Maytenus serrata* (Kupchan, 1974; Kupchan *et al.*, 1974). The structural formula is shown in Fig. 2.

Maytansine has been found to be highly active against mouse P388 lymphocytic leukemia and, to a lesser degree, against the L1210 mouse leukemia, Lewis lung carcinoma, and B16 melanoma solid tumors (Kupchan, 1974; Kupchan *et al.*, 1974).

Maytansine shares the same mechanism of action as the vinca alkaloids vincristine and vinblastine. However, preclinical studies have suggested that it is more potent than the preceding two compounds. Dose-limiting toxicities are mainly gastrointestinal and neural (Cabanillas *et al.*, 1978a,b; Eagan *et al.*, 1978; Chabner *et al.*, 1978; Blum and Kahlert, 1978). Maytansine does produce peripheral neuropathy like vincristine (Blum and Kahlert, 1978). The development of central nervous system toxic symptoms would seem to indicate that maytansine crosses the blood–brain barrier (Chabner *et al.*, 1978; Blum and Kahlert, 1978). The maximum tolerated dose ranged from 1.8 to 2.25 mg/m^2, either administered as a bolus or in divided dose (Cabanillas *et al.*, 1978a,b; Eagan *et al.*, 1978; Chabner *et al.*, 1978).

Early phase II studies have suggested activity in lymphoblastic leukemia and malignant lymphoma (Cabanillas *et al.*, 1978a,b; Eagan *et al.*, 1978; Chabner *et al.*, 1978; Blum and Kahlert, 1978).

B. Epipodophyllotoxin Analogues

Podophyllotoxin, a crystalline derivative of podophyllin derived from the root of May apple or American mandrake (*Podophyllum peltatum*) plant has demonstrated distinct antimitotic properties (Kelly and Hartwell, 1954). In 1963, Sandoz Laboratories synthesized two podophyllin derivatives, SPI-77 (podophyllic acid, 2-ethyl hydrozide) and SPG-827 (podophyllotoxin, 4,6-0-benzylidine-β-D-glucoside). Both drugs exhibited minimal antitumor activity and severe tox-

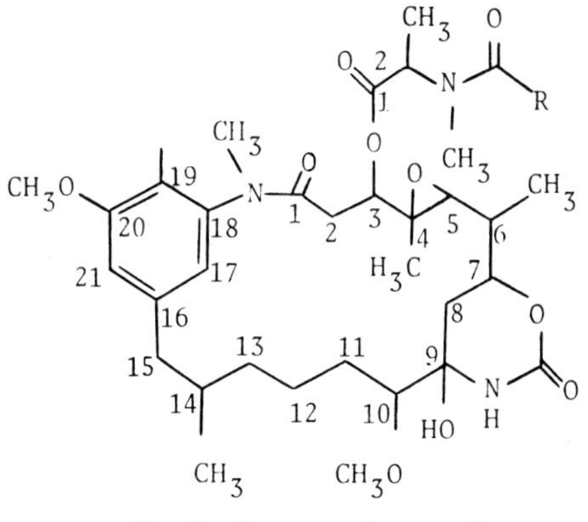

Fig. 2. Structure of maytansine.

icities, thereby eliminating possible use in the clinic (Chakravorty *et al.*, 1967; Vaitkevicius and Reed, 1966).

Recently, two semisynthetic derivatives of podophyllotoxin were synthesized, VM-26 (teniposide) and VP-16 (etoposide). These two compounds have shown antineoplastic activity against experimental animal tumors including L1210 leukemia, Walker 256 carcinosarcoma, and sarcoma 180 (Avery *et al.*, 1973; Dombernowsky and Nissen, 1973; Stahelin, 1970, 1973; Venditti, 1971). VP-16 and VM-26 are both known to damage the spindle apparatus of cells, resulting in mitotic arrest of cells with chromosomes in metaphase (Cornman and Cornman, 1951; Krishan *et al.*, 1975). Cell cultures exposed to these two compounds have also shown mitotic arrest in metaphase (Krishan *et al.*, 1975; Stahelin, 1970) as well as inhibition of the incorporation of tritiated thymidine (Clinical Brochure, VP-16, NCI).

Clinical trials in adults have demonstrated etoposide to be active against advanced neoplasms, especially acute myelocytic leukemia, malignant lymphomas, lung cancer, and ovarian and thyroid carcinoma (Nissen *et al.*, 1972; Falkson *et al.*, 1975). Teniposide's spectrum of clinical antitumor activities includes Hodgkin's disease, non-Hodgkin's lymphomas, brain tumors, and bladder carcinoma (EORTC, 1972; Sonntag *et al.*, 1974; Sklansky *et al.*, 1974).

Both teniposide and etoposide have likewise been investigated in childhood tumors. In a limited number of early phase I and phase II clinical trials, teniposide has shown activity against neuroblastoma and acute lymphocytic leukemia (Bleyer and Chard, 1978; Rivera *et al.*, 1975), whereas VP-16 has been shown to be active against acute nonlymphocytic leukemia (Bleyer and Chard, 1978; Rivera *et al.*, 1975). A number of NCI-sponsored studies are currently in progress using both compounds in various combination regimens.

C. Vindesine

Vindesine is an analogue of vinblastine and vincristine differing only in two functional groups. The structural formulas of vindesine, vinblastine, and vincristine are shown in Fig. 3.

Studies in experimental animals have shown that vindesine is more toxic than vinblastine but less toxic than vincristine (Todd *et al.*, 1976). Comparative studies on the antitumor activities of vindesine, vinblastine, and vincristine have been reported. The activity of all these agents was more or less similar against P388 leukemia, B16 melanoma, and ascites tumors. Vindesine, however, demonstrated better activity than vinblastine against some other tumor types such as Gardner lymphosarcoma, Ridgway osteogenic sarcoma, and mammary carcinoma (Dyke and Nelson, 1977).

Vindesine has been extensively investigated in phase I and phase II studies. Responses in the following tumors have been reported: acute lymphocytic

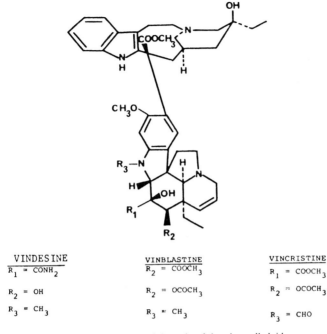

VINDESINE	VINBLASTINE	VINCRISTINE
$R_1 = \overline{CONH_2}$	$R_2 = COOCH_3$	$R_1 = COOCH_3$
$R_2 = OH$	$R_2 = OCOCH_3$	$R_2 = OCOCH_3$
$R_3 = CH_3$	$R_3 = CH_3$	$R_3 = CHO$

Fig. 3.   General structural formula of the vinca alkaloids.

leukemia (40%), Hodgkin's disease (35%), non-Hodgkin's lymphoma (30%), malignant melanoma (13%), breast cancer (20%), and non-oat-cell lung cancer (10%) (Dyke, 1978). It has been suggested that there is no cross resistance between vincristine and vindesine in patients with acute lymphocytic leukemia (Mathe *et al.*, 1978).

The most toxic effects of vindesine are neutropenia and thrombocytopenia. Neurotoxic effects were considered minimal. Alopecia, vomiting, fever, jaw pain, skin rash, and phlebitis are the other reported side effects (Dyke and Nelson, 1977; Mathe *et al.*, 1978).

V. ANTITUMOR ANTIBIOTICS

A. Zinostatin

Zinostatin is a protein antibiotic isolated and purified from *Streptomyces carzinostaticus* var. F47 in Japan in 1965 (Ishida *et al.*, 1965). It has been shown to selectively inhibit DNA synthesis in *Sarcina lutea*, HeLa cells, and Burkett lymphoma cells (Ono *et al.*, 1968; Kumagai *et al.*, 1970; Kawai and Katoh,

1972). Instead of being degraded into an acid-soluble form, DNA strand scission by zinostatin results in relatively larger acid-precipitable fragments (Beerman and Goldberg, 1974). Zinostatin has also been found to block the growth of Chinese hamster ovary cells at phase G_2 of the cell cycle. The G_2 block has been found in synchronized cells independent of when the drug was added during the cell cycle (Tobey, 1972).

Animal antitumor studies have shown zinostatin to be active against L1210 leukemia, Ehrlich ascites carcinoma, ascites sarcoma 180, and mouse leukemia SN-36 (Bradner and Hutchinson, 1966; Nishikawa et al., 1965; Kumagai and Miyazaki, 1963). Synergistic effects have been found when used in combination with cytosine arabinoside, 6-mercaptopurine, and methotrexate (Bradner and Hutchinson, 1966; Bradner and Rossomano, 1968).

In clinical trials conducted in Japan, antitumor activity was reported in acute leukemia, gastric and pancreatic carcinoma, and malignant melanoma (Legha et al., 1976). Phase I clinical trials in the United States have been completed and the results indicate that zinostatin has a wide dose toxicity range. In solid tumor patients the Maximum Tolerated Doses (MTD) of zinostatin given daily for 5 days ranges from 2250 to 3600 U/m^2 when given by intermittent infusion and from 3000 to 4500 U/m^2 when given by continuous infusion (Issell et al., 1979). A wider dose range schedule has been reported for patients with leukemia. Phase II evaluation of this compound is in progress.

B. Piperazinedione

Piperazinedione is a crystalline antibiotic isolated from the fermented broth of the actinomycete *Streptomyces griseoluteus*. The compound probably acts as an alkylating agent. Piperazinedione is highly active in the L1210 system.

Phase II evaluation of piperazinedione against squamous cell carcinoma of the cervix, renal cell carcinoma, metastatic breast carcinoma, lymphomas, and multiple myeloma have been reported (Thigpen et al., 1978; Palmer et al., 1977; Jones et al., 1977; Koons et al., 1977; Pasmantier et al., 1977; Pratt et al., 1975). The dose schedule used in most of these studies was 9–12 mg/m^2 intravenously given every 3 weeks. Table I summarizes the results obtained from these studies.

Clinical evaluation of piperazinedione in children with leukemia and solid tumor was conducted by Pratt and associates at St. Jude Children's Research Hospital (Pratt et al., 1975). Doses of 5 mg/m^2 I.V. daily $\times$ 5 for leukemic children and 3 mg/m^2 I.V. daily $\times$ 5 for solid tumors have been suggested. One patient each with neuroblastoma and rhabdomyosarcoma showed reduction in the size of metastases. Two patients with ALL and two patients with AML had reduction in the blast counts and organomegaly.

TABLE I

Phase II Studies with Piperazinedione

Investigator	Tumor types	No. of Evaluable Patients	Responses
Thigpen *et al.* (1978)	Advanced squamous cell carcinoma, cervix	33	1 CR 1 PR 13 Stable disease
Palmer *et al.* (1977)	Metastatic breast carcinoma	42	3 PR
Jones *et al.* (1977)	Hodgkin's disease	7	5 PR
	Non-Hodgkin's lymphoma	16	3 PR
	Multiple myeloma	13	0
Koons *et al.* (1977)	Advanced squamous cell carcinoma, lung	28	0
Pasmantier *et al.* (1977)	Metastatic renal carcinoma	12	0

C. Anguidine

Anguidine is a sesquiterpenoid isolated from the parasitic fungi *Fusarium equiseti* (Brian *et al.*, 1961; Dawkins *et al.*, 1965; Flury *et al.*, 1965). It is closely related structurally to nivalenol, fusarenon-X, and T-2 toxin, compounds produced from fungi that damage wheat (Ohtsubo *et al.*, 1972; Rauen and Norpoth, 1966).

The biochemical mechanism of action of anguidine is not known. Grollman has shown that anguidine inhibits synthesis of protein in HeLa cells and in intact rabbit reticulocytes by 50% at a concentration of 5×10^{-8} M. This effect is irreversible after incubation of HeLa cells with 10^{-7} M anguidine for 30 min. The primary effect of this drug in HeLa cells appears to be on the biosynthesis of protein (Helman *et al.*, 1976).

Experimental antitumor studies have demonstrated activity against P388 leukemia, L1210 leukemia, and B16 melanocarcinoma. No activity was seen against implanted Lewis lung carcinoma.

Murphy *et al.* (1978) reported a phase I study of anguidine in a relatively small number of patients. The drug was administered by rapid I.V. infusion daily for 5 days at 2-week intervals starting at a dose of 0.1 mg/m$^2 \cdot$ day. Significant toxicity was observed at doses of ≥ 3 mg/m^2 and consisted mainly of nausea and vomiting, myelosuppression, hypotension, central nervous system symptoms, and diarrhea.

It has been observed that the severity of side effects correlates with the presence or absence of liver metastases. Based on this study, a dose of 5 mg/m^2 daily for 5 days is recommended for patients with normal liver function in phase II clinical trials. For patients with liver abnormalities, an initial dose of 3 mg/m^2 for 5 days is suggested.

D. Pepleomycin

Pepleomycin is one of several semisynthetic analogues of bleomycin that has undergone extensive clinical evaluation in Japan. Chemically, pepleomycin is a basic glycopeptide of the bleomycin group and is a sulfate of 3-[(S)-1-phenylethyl amino]propylamino bleomycin.

The selection of pepleomycin for drug development in Japan has been brought about by its superiority over bleomycin in preclinical studies (Matsuda *et al.*, 1978). Pepleomycin has a spectrum of antitumor activity comparable to that of bleomycin; however, it possesses greater antineoplastic activity against cultured cancer cells (HeLa S$_3$) and transplanted tumors (Ehrlich solid carcinoma). Pepleomycin also exhibits an antitumor effect against some strains of ascites hepatoma not included in the antitumor spectrum of bleomycin. The incidence of pepleomycin-induced pulmonary fibrosis is approximately one-third as high as bleomycin whereas the severity is about one-fourth that of bleomycin. Pepleomycin achieves a tissue concentration in both normal and tumor-bearing tissues 1.5 times as high as that of bleomycin.

Early clinical trials of pepleomycin in Japan have shown encouraging results in malignant lymphomas, head and neck cancer, and squamous cell carcinoma of the lungs and skin (Ikeda *et al.*, 1978; Inuyama *et al.*, 1978; Tojo *et al.*, 1978).

VI. NITROSOUREAS

A. Chlorozotocin (NSC-178248) (DCNU)

Chlorozotocin is the 2-chloroethyl analogue of the nitrosourea streptozotocin. The structure is illustrated in Fig. 4. For a nitrosourea derivative, chlorozotocin is relatively cell cycle specific with a much higher killing action of G$_1$ arrest cells than for cells in exponential growth phase (Tobey *et al.*, 1975). Chlorozotocin has the highest alkylating and the lowest carbamylating activity of the nitrosoureas.

In experimental tumor systems, chlorozotocin has somewhat better activity than streptozotocin but a narrower spectrum of action than BCNU, CCNU, or MeCCNU [Chlorozotocin (NSC-178248) Clinical Brochure, 1976]. DCNU is active against L1210 leukemia, P388 leukemia, and B16 melanocarcinoma.

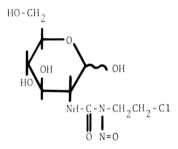

Fig. 4. Structure of chlorozotocin.

Marginal activity against Lewis lung carcinoma implanted subcutaneously has also been shown.

Phase I clinical trials have been conducted utilizing both the single dose and daily × 5 dosage schedules. Single doses of ≤120 mg/m² produced no dose-limiting toxicity (Hoth *et al.*, 1977) although dosages of 150 and 200 mg/m² administered singly were associated with higher incidences of thrombocytopenia and leukopenia than the same total dosages given over a 5 day period (Kovach *et al.*, 1978). Tan and co-workers (1978) of Memorial Sloan-Kettering Cancer Center have recommended a dose of 30–40 mg/m² per day × 5 days. This regimen has been associated with predictable and reversible hematologic toxicity.

Preliminary reports on early phase II trials have shown responses in patients with melanoma, colon cancer, lymphomas, and lung cancer (Hoth *et al.*, 1978) [Chlorozotocin (NSC-178748) Annual Report to the FDA-NCI, 1977 and Minutes of the Phase I Working Group Meeting, May 15, 1978]. The number of cases reported is still relatively few and more studies are in progress.

B. Streptozotocin

Streptozotocin is another member of the nitrosourea group that has been in clinical trials for several years. The compound was originally isolated and purified from *Streptomyces acromogenes* fermentation broth (Vavra *et al.*, 1960). Structurally, streptozotocin is composed of a nitrosourea moiety with a methyl group attached on one end and a glucosamine on the other. It primarily inhibits DNA synthesis and interferes with enzymes involved in gluconeogenesis and NADH metabolism (Rosenkranz and Carr, 1970; Bhuyan, 1970).

The drug is active in the L1210 systems (Handelsman *et al.*, 1974). Toxic side effects are mainly referrable to the renal and hepatic systems, although another major toxicity is the development of diabetes mellitus (Rakieten *et al.*, 1963; Brosky and Logothetopoulos, 1969; Schein *et al.*, 1971). In contrast to the other nitrosoureas, streptozotocin is nonmyelosuppressive. Streptozotocin has shown distinct activity in malignant tumors of neural crest origin like islet cell carcinoma of the pancreas and carcinoid tumors.

VII. ANTIMETABOLITES

A. Baker's Antifol

Baker's Antifol, also called triazinate (TZI), is a triazine folic acid metabolite that causes inhibition of DNA synthesis by blocking the enzyme dihydrofolate reductase [Baker's Antifol (NSC-139105) Clinical Brochure, 1975] (Frei *et al.*, 1975).

Animal antitumor studies have shown Walker 256 carcinoma to be most sensitive to Baker's Antifol [Baker's Antifol (NSC-139105) Clinical Brochure, 1975]. Comparable activity is seen when the drug is given either subcutaneously or intraperitoneally. In addition, significant activity was seen against Dunning leukemia in rats and AK leukemia in mice. The drug was, however, ineffective against L1210 leukemia.

Dose-finding studies in adults have shown clinical responses to occur at doses greater than 100 mg/m² per day for 3–5 days (Rodriguez *et al.*, 1976a). Manageable toxicity has been reported at doses ranging from 200 to 300 mg/m². Phase II clinical trials have utilized either one of the following dosage regimens: 250 mg/m² per day × 3 days or 100–150 mg/m² per day × 5 days. Rodriquez *et al.* (1977) reported the result of a phase II study of Baker's Antifol in 138 patients with various types of solid tumors. Responses were observed in lung adenocarcinoma, colorectal cancer, and renal cell carcinoma. Padilla and co-workers (1978), however, have shown no superiority of Baker's Antifol over methotrexate in patients with colorectal carcinoma. The drug has also been shown to be of very little therapeutic value in metastatic sarcoma (Thigpen *et al.*, 1977).

B. Diglycoaldehyde

Diglycoaldehyde is the periodate-oxidation product of the purine nucleoside inosine in which carbons 2 and 3 of the riboside ring have been oxidized to formyl groups with resistant cleavage of the ring. The structure of diglycoaldehyde is illustrated in Fig. 5.

Early studies have indicated that the earliest effect of diglycoaldehyde in L1210 cultures is the inhibition of the incorporation of [³H]uridine-5 into RNA followed shortly by inhibition of protein and DNA synthesis [Diglycoaldehyde Clinical Brochure, 1976]. Diglycoaldehyde also causes inhibition of the incorporation of C^{14} formate into nucleic acids [Diglycoaldehyde Clinical Brochure,

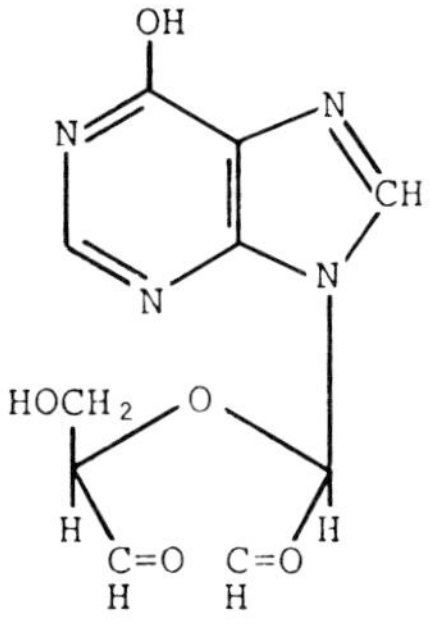

Fig. 5. Structure of diglycoaldehyde.

1976]. Activity is maximal against cells in early S or late G phase (Bhuyan and Fraser, 1974).

Diglycoaldehyde has been selected for clinical trials because of its activity against L1210, P388, and AKR murine leukemias. Marginal activity has been shown against Lewis lung carcinoma while no activity was demonstrated against B16 melanoma, Walker 256 carcinosarcoma, and rodent ependymoblastoma [Diglycoaldehyde Clinical Brochure, 1976].

Diglycoaldehyde was evaluated by the Children's Cancer Study Group (CCSG) using an induction dose of 1.5 g/m² per day × 5 given every 14 days and a maintenance dose of 1.5 g/m² per day × 5 every 28 days. No significant antitumor activity was seen in leukemia and solid tumor patients [Diglycoaldehyde, CCSG Minutes of the February 1977 Meeting].

Kaufman and Mittelman reported the results of a phase I clinical trial in 40 patients with various types of tumor refractory to standard chemotherapeutic regimens. Objective tumor responses were observed in 3 out of 20 patients (seminoma, sarcoma, oat cell carcinoma) who received doses of ≥2 g/m² (Kaufman and Mittelman, 1975a,b).

Preliminary data on the ECOG study on diglycoaldehyde against colorectal cancer showed three responses in 32 evaluable patients [Diglycoaldehyde, Minutes of the New Drug Liaison Meeting, March 1978].

C. Ftorafur

Structurally similar to 5-fluorodeoxyuridine (FUDR), Ftorafur is a pyrimidine antimetabolite first synthesized in the Soviet Union in 1966. The compound acts as a weak inhibitor of DNA thymine and RNA pyrimidine synthesis and is neither a substrate nor an inhibitor of pyrimidine nucleoside phosphorylases (Meiren and Belousova, 1972).

Experimental and clinical studies have shown that Ftorafur exhibits the same activity as 5-FU. It has been reported that the metabolism of Ftorafur releases small amounts of 5-FU and that the effect of the former is comparable to a continuous low-dose infusion of the latter [Ftorafur (FT-209) (NSC-148958) Clinical Brochure, 1974].

In the Soviet Union the dose of Ftorafur used in clinical trials was 30 mg/kg I.V. given every 12 hr with a total dose of 30–40 g. (First All-Union Conference, 1968). When the dose was given orally, the Japanese investigators obtained results similar to that of the I.V. infusion (Hattori *et al.*, 1973). Phase I studies in the United States have recommended an optimal dose of between 1.0 and 2.5 g/m^2 per day × 5.

Ftorafur has been extensively studied clinically and has shown activity against a variety of gastrointestinal tumors, breast carcinoma and possibly adenocarcinoma of the lung [Ftorafur (FT-209) (NSC-148958) Clinical Brochure, 1974] (Blokhina *et al.*, 1972; Karev *et al.*, 1972; Toguchi *et al.*, 1972; Konda *et al.*, 1974; Saito and Yokoyama, 1974; Valdivieso *et al.*, 1976; Smart *et al.*, 1975).

The minimal myelosuppression produced by ftorafur relative to 5-FU has generated studies aimed at replacing 5-FU infusion with ftorafur. Buroker *et al.* (1978) reported that the results of a combination of ftorafur with either mitomycin C or methyl-CCNU in untreated colorectal cancer were not superior to those produced by 5-FU alone or in combination with either of the two agents mentioned earlier. Similarly, Woolley *et al.* (1977) have obtained similar response rates using a combination of 5-FU or ftorafur plus adriamycin and mitomycin C in advanced gastric cancer patients. The ftorafur-containing regimen, however, was associated with a lower marrow toxicity.

D. 5-Azacytidine

5-Azacytidine (4-amino-1-β-D-ribofuranosyl-1,3,5-triazine-2-one or 1-β-D-ribofuranosyl-5-azacytosine) is a ring analogue of the pyrimidine nucleoside cytidine. It was isolated from a fermentation of *Streptoverticillium ladakanus* (Hanka *et al.*, 1966) and has been in clinical trials in the United States since 1970. 5-Azacytidine interferes with nucleic acid metabolism and four mechanisms have been postulated:

1. Incorporation of 5-azacytidine into DNA (Zadrazil *et al.*, 1965)
2. Incorporation into RNA, thereby interfering with protein synthesis (Cihak *et al.*, 1966)
3. Competition for uridine kinase (Vadlamudi *et al.*, 1970)
4. Inhibition of orotidylic and decarboxylase (Vesely *et al.*, 1968; Raska *et al.*, 1965)

In animal tumors, 5-azacytidine appears to be most active against the L1210 system (Sorm and Vesely, 1964). It is ineffective in Walker 256 tumor, murine myeloma tumor, and transplants of slow-growing experimental solid tumors (Von Hoff *et al.*, 1975).

Maximally tolerated doses of 150–200 mg/m^2 per day × 5 and 150–300 mg/m^2 per day × 5 have been established for childhood and adult leukemia, respectively (Von Hoff *et al.*, 1975).

5-Azacytidine has demonstrated definite antitumor activity in acute myelogenous leukemia with a reported response rate of approximately 40% (Karon *et al.*, 1973; McCredie *et al.*, 1973; Vogler *et al.*, 1975). Dose-limiting toxicities were mainly gastrointestinal and hematologic (Leukopenia). Liver toxicity has also been reported.

E. PALA

PALA [*N*-(phosphonacetyl)-L-aspartate] is an analogue of the transition state for the aspartate transcarbamylase reaction and is reported to be a potent and specific inhibitor of *de novo* pyrimidine nucleotide biosynthesis (Collins and Stark, 1971).

A unique antitumor activity against various animal tumors has been reported (Johnson *et al.*, 1976). Growth inhibition was observed in Lewis lung carcinoma, B16 melanoma, and glioma 26. The effect of PALA in the Lewis lung system is evident at doses well below the maximally tolerable doses. No activity was exhibited against L1210 and P388 leukemias and Ridgway osteogenic sarcoma. Preclinical toxicologic evaluation in beagle dogs, rhesus monkeys, and BDF$_1$ mice revealed that the major toxicities are manifested mainly by reversible gastrointestinal and central nervous system signs and symptoms [PALA (NSC-224131) Clinical Brochure, 1977]. Effects on the hematopoietic system are marginal and not dose limiting.

Phase I studies are in progress in the United States.

VIII. MISCELLANEOUS

A. Bruceantin

Bruceantin, a new cytotoxic compound derived from the plant *Brucea antidysenterica* was selected for clinical trials because of its activity in P388 leukemia (Kupchan *et al.*, 1973). It has been reported that bruceantin showed significant activity against P388 over a 50- to 100-fold dose range at the μg/kg level (Kupchan *et al.*, 1973). Bruceantin interferes with some processes in the initiation step of protein synthesis (Liao *et al.*, 1976). The structural formula is shown in Fig. 6.

Dose-finding studies are being conducted at the Sidney Farber Cancer Institute

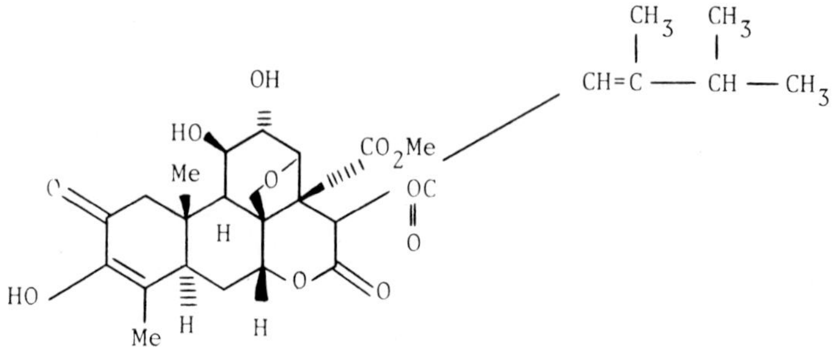

Fig. 6. Structure of bruceantin.

(SFCI) and M.D. Anderson Hospital (MDAH) [Bruceantin, Minutes of the Phase I Working Group Meeting, May 15, 1978]. In the SFCI study, a dose of 5 mg/m^2 administered once a week for 4 weeks has been reached with no significant toxicity observed. A daily dose schedule is being investigated at MDAH. Significant myelosuppression has been observed at 3 mg/kg daily × 5. In both studies no responses have been observed to date.

B. β-TGdR

β-TGdR, a nucleoside of thioguanine is an anomer of the parent compound deoxythioguanosine (TGdR) and was first synthesized by Iwamoto et al. (1963). Both the α and β anomers are produced in equal proportions but the β component was chosen for clinical investigation for the following reasons. First, it has been demonstrated that the α anomer was incorporated only at the terminal site of the DNA chain, whereas the β anomer was distributed evenly throughout (LePage and Junga, 1967; LePage, 1968). Second, the β anomer possesses more antitumor activity and less toxicity (LePage et al., 1964). The compound is active against L1210 leukemia and Walker 256 carcinosarcoma and appears to be active in animal tumors resistant to thioguanine (Rosenbaum and Carter, 1969).

A dose of 300 mg/m^2 per day × 5 given as a single agent has been recommended. When given in combination, it is suggested that the dose range should be between 60 mg/m^2 per day × 5 to 300 mg/m^2 per day × 5 [β-TGdR, Annual Report to the FDA, July 1977]. β-TGdRs primary effectiveness appears to be against acute leukemia and colorectal carcinoma but more studies are required to determine its true therapeutic value [β-TGdR, Annual Report to the FDA, July 1977].

C. Hexamethylmelamine

Hexamethylmelamine (HMM) is a cyanuric chloride derivative and is structurally related to triethylenemelamine (TEM) (Kaiser et al., 1951). The structural formulas of both compounds are shown in Fig. 7.

The exact mechanism of action of HMM is not known. Although very minor structural differences exist between the two compounds, studies have shown that each probably has a different mechanism of action. TEM has been demonstrated to be an alkylating agent, whereas HMM reacts negatively with the classical *in vitro* alkylating function test (Worzalla *et al.*, (1973). Further support to this is the cross-reactivity of HMM with other alkylating agents in clinical studies (Stolinsky and Bateman, 1973; Wampler *et al.*, 1972) [Hexamethylmelamine (NSC-13875) Clinical Brochure, 1974].

HMM has shown antitumor activity against mouse sarcoma 180, mouse adenocarcinoma 755, and Walker 256 rat carcinosarcoma [Hexamethylmelamine (NSC-13875) Clinical Brochure, 1974].

Clinical trials that consisted mostly of broad phase II studies have shown HMM to have antitumor activity against breast carcinoma, cervical cancer, ovarian cancer, malignant lymphomas, and lung cancer (Stolinsky and Bateman, 1973; Wampler *et al.*, 1972; Wilson and de la Garza, 1965; Wilson *et al.*, 1969, 1970; de la Garza *et al.*, 1968; Takita and Didolkar, 1974; Bergevin *et al.*, 1973; Blum *et al.*, 1973).

D. Gallium Nitrate

Gallium nitrate, a metal salt, has demonstrated preferential concentration in a number of human and animal tumors and has been used extensively as a diagnostic test in patients with neoplasms (Edwards and Hayes, 1969, 1970; Vaidya *et al.*, 1970). This had led to the expectation that it may also be useful therapeutically. Tumor uptake of radioactively labeled gallium nitrate has been reported in

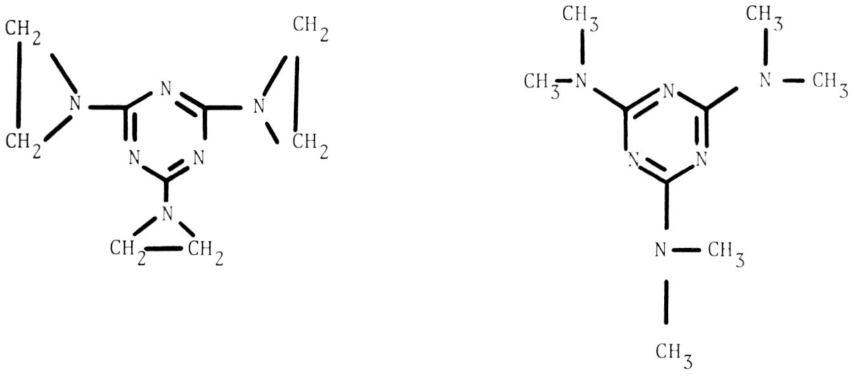

TRIETHYLENEMELAMINE   HEXAMETHYLMELAMINE

Fig. 7. Structure formula of triethylenemelamine and hexamethylmelamine.

malignant lymphomas, melanoma, and tissue myeloblastoma (Edwards and Hayes, 1969, 1970; Vaidya *et al.*, 1970; Arseneau *et al.*, 1972). The exact mechanism for this special affinity is not known.

Gallium nitrate appears most active against subcutaneously implanted Walker 256 carcinosarcoma in rats. It is also active in a number of solid tumors, including fibrosarcoma M-89, adenocarcinoma 755, reticulum cell sarcoma A-RCS, lymphosarcoma P1798, and osteosarcoma 124F (Adamson *et al.*, 1975; Hart *et al.*, 1971).

Twenty-one adults and 7 children were treated with gallium nitrate in a phase I study conducted at Memorial Sloan-Kettering Cancer Center (Brown *et al.*, 1978). Doses ranged from 400–600 mg/m^2 per week × 4 administered as a 90-min drug infusion. Dose-related (life threatening in one) nephrotoxicity was encountered. Minor tumor regression was observed in 2/6 Hodgkin's disease, 1/4 non-Hodgkin's lymphoma, and 1/3 ovarian cancer.

Valdivieso *et al.* (1978) also used gallium nitrate initially at a dose of 15 mg/m^2 per day × 3 every 2 weeks and then progressively increased to a maximum daily dose of 1350 mg/m^2. Dose-limiting and cumulative renal toxicity was likewise observed. Of the 43 evaluable patients treated, three responses were observed, one each with lymphoma, thyroid carcinoma, and melanoma.

E. *m*-AMSA

m-AMSA is one in a series of heteroaromatic compounds that have demonstrated high antitumor activity in the L1210 system (Cain *et al.*, 1969). The mechanism of action is described as inhibition of DNA synthesis by intercalation and external binding (Wilson, 1974). Studies on cycling and resting CHO Chinese hamster cells have revealed that cycling cells are more sensitive to *m*-AMSA than resting cells [*m*-AMSA (NSC-249992) Clinical Brochure, 1978]. The immunosuppressive activity of *m*-AMSA has likewise been studied. *m*-AMSA suppressed the direct plaque-forming cell response to sheep red blood cells in mice as well as in spleen cell culture systems (Baguley *et al.*, 1976).

In addition to the L1210 system, *m*-AMSA is highly active against B16 melanoma, p388 leukemia, and mouse colon tumor [*m*-AMSA (NSC-249992) Clinical Brochure, 1978]. Phase I studies of *m*-AMSA are in progress in the United States.

IX. SUMMARY

Available information on some of the anticancer drugs under clinical investigation both in the United States and abroad were reviewed. A summary of their administration schedules and clinical toxicities is shown in Table II. An intensive

TABLE II

New Anticancer Drugs: Dose, Administration, Potential Indications, Toxicity

Investigational Anticancer drugs	Chemical name	Dosage forms	Route of administration	Dosage regimens	Potentially responsive tumors	Clinical toxicity
Alkylating agents						
Isophosphamide (NSC-109724)	3-(2-Chloroethyl)-2-[(2-chloroethyl)-amino] tetrahydro-2H-1,3,2-oxazaphosphorine-2-oxide	3.0 g/vial.	Intravenous	4 g/m² I.V. q 3 weeks	Ovarian carcinoma Breast carcinoma Bronchogenic carcinoma	Nausea and vomiting Hemorrhagic cystitis Myelosuppression Alopecia
Dianhydrogalactitol (NSC-132313)	1,2,5,6-Dianhydro-galactitol	50 mg/vial	Intravenous	30–35 mg/m²/day × 5	Squamous cell carcinoma Oat cell carcinoma	Myelosuppression Transient liver function abnormalities Nausea and vomiting Skin eruptions
Prednimustine	11-Beta-17,21-trihydroxy-pregna-1,4-diene-3,20 dione, 21-(4-[N,N-bis (2-chloroethyl)-p-aminophenyl] butanoate)	20 mg/tablet 100 mg/tablet	Oral	20–30 mg/day 200 mg/day × 5 q 3 weeks	Chronic lymphocytic leukemia Non-Hodgkin's lymphoma Melanoma Breast cancer	Nausea and vomiting Myelosuppression Hyperglycemia Allergic reaction (rare)
Peptichemio	m-Dichlorodiethylamino-L-phenyl-alanine peptide complex	40 mg/vial	Intravenous	1–1.5 mg/kg/day × 5–6 q 1–2 weeks	Neuroblastoma Chronic myelogenous leukemia Lymphoma Cervical cancer	Nausea and vomiting Stomatitis Myelosuppression Phlebosclerosis
Tubulin binding agents						
Maytansine (NSC-153858)		0.25 mg/vial	Intravenous	0.6 mg/m² I.V. × 3 days q 2, 3, 4 weeks	Lung cancer Breast cancer	Nausea and vomiting Diarrhea Myelosuppression Neurotoxicity Phlebitis Alopecia Fever
VM-26 (teniposide) (NSC-122819)	Epipodophyllotoxin. 4'-demethyl-9-(4,6-0-2-thenylidene-β-D-glucopyranoside)	50 mg/ampule	Intravenous	100 mg/m² 2 × a week × 4 weeks 100–130 mg/m²/week	Neuroblastoma Acute lymphocytic leukemia Brain tumors	Nausea and vomiting Myelosuppression Diarrhea Stomatitis

(*continued*)

TABLE II (*Continued*)

Investigational Anticancer drugs	Chemical name	Dosage forms	Route of administration	Dosage regimens	Potentially responsive tumors	Clinical toxicity
				× 6–8 weeks	Bladder cancer	Alopecia Fever, phlebitis Anaphylaxis Hypotension
VP-16 (etoposide) (NSC-141540)	4′-Demethylepipodophyllo-toxin 9-(4,6-0-ethylidene-β-glucopyranoside)	100 mg/ampule	Intravenous, oral	100–125 mg/m² QOD q 4 weeks	Lung cancer Acute Nonlymphocytic leukemia Lymphomas	Nausea and vomiting Myelosuppression Diarrhea Stomatitis Allergic reaction
Vindesine	23-Amino-4-deacetoxy-23-demethoxy-4-hydroxy-vinca leuko blastine, sulfuric acid salt	10 mg/ampule	Intravenous	3 mg/m² once a week	Acute leukemia Lymphoma Melanoma Breast cancer	Nausea and vomiting Myelosuppression Neurotoxicity Phlebitis Alopecia
Anthracycline Analogues						
Rubidazone (NSC-164011)	Daunorubicin benzoyl-hydrazone hydrochloride	50 mg/vial	Intravenous	150–200 mg/m² q 3 weeks 4 mg/kg/day × 5	Acute myelogenous leukemia	Nausea and vomiting Mucositis Myelosuppression EKG changes
Carminomycin (NSC-180024)	5,12-Naphthacenedione, 8-acetyl-10 [(3-amino- 2,3,6-trideoxy-α-1-lyxo-hexo-pyranoxyl)oxy]-7,8,9,10-tetrahydro-1,6,8,11-tetrahydroxy	10 mg/vial	Intravenous, oral	7.5 mg/m² 2× a week × 3 weeks 5.5 mg/m² daily × 5 q 3 weeks	Soft tissue sarcoma Lymphoma Acute leukemia	Nausea and vomiting Myelosuppression Nonspecific EKG changes
Aclacinomycin	2-Ethyl-1,2,3,4,6,11-hexahydro-2,5,7-trihydroxy-	20 mg/vial	Intravenous	0.4 mg/kg I.V. daily	Lymphoma Breast cancer	Nausea and vomiting Myelosuppression

Antimetabolites

Drug (NSC)	Chemical name	Formulation	Route	Dose	Indications	Toxicity
	6.11-dioxo-4-[0-2,3,6-trideoxy-α-L-glycero-hexopyranos-4-ulosyl-(1,4)-0-2,6-dideoxy-α-L-lyxo-hexopyranosyl)-(1-4)-2,3,6-trideoxy-3-(dimethylamino)-α-L-lyxo-hexopyranosyl) oxy]-1-naphthacene-carboxylic acid methyl ester			0.4–1 mg/kg 2–3 ×/week	Lung carcinoma; Gastric cancer; Ovarian tumor	Liver toxicity
Florafur (NSC-148958)	5-Fluoro-1-(tetrahydro-2-furyl)-uracil	400 mg/ampule	Intravenous	2 g/m²/day × 5	GI malignancies; Breast cancer	Nausea and vomiting; Chills, fever; Ataxia, dizziness; Mucositis; Phlebitis; Myelosuppression
Baker's Antifol (NSC-139105)	Ethanesulfonic acid compounded with α-[2-chloro-4-(4,6,-diamino-32,2-dimethyl-s-triazin-1 (2H)-y 1) phenoxy]-N,N-dimethyl-m-toluamide (1:1)	100 mg/vial; 250 mg/vial	Intravenous	150–250 mg/m²/day × 3–5 q 2–3 weeks; 500 mg/m² single dose/week	Squamous cell carcinoma of the lung and tongue; Adenocarcinoma—lung; Renal cell carcinoma; Colorectal carcinoma	Nausea and vomiting; Myelosuppression; Mucositis, skin rash; CNS toxicity; Liver toxicity
Diglycoaldehyde (NSC-118994)	Diglycoaldehyde, α-(hydroxy-methyl)-α'-(6-hydroxy-9H-purine-9-yl)	500 mg/vial	Intravenous	2 g/m²/day × 3 q 4 weeks	Seminoma; Oat cell carcinoma	Nausea and vomiting; Myelosuppression; Renal toxicity; Coomb's (+) anemia; Phlebitis; Hypocalcemia
AAFC (NSC-166641)	2,2'-Anhydro-1-β-D-arabinofuranosyl-5-fluorocytosine		Intravenous	1200–1600 mg/m²/week; 15–20 mg/kg/day × 5 q 3 weeks	Nonlymphocitic leukemia; Gastric carcinoma	Nausea and vomiting; Myelosuppression; Conjunctivitis
5-Azacytidine (NSC-12816)	5-Triazine-2 (1H)-one, 4-amino-1-β-D-ribofuranosyl	100 mg/vial	Intravenous, subcutaneous	100–150 mg/m²/day × 5–10; 100 mg/m² q 12 h × 10	Acute myelogenous leukemia	Nausea and vomiting; Myelosuppression; Liver toxicity; Fever, diarrhea; Rash, hypotension

(continued)

TABLE II (*Continued*)

Investigational Anticancer drugs	Chemical name	Dosage forms	Route of administration	Dosage regimens	Potentially responsive tumors	Clinical toxicity
PALA (NSC-224131)	L-Aspartic acid, N-(phosphonoacetyl),-disodium salt	1 g/ampule	Intravenous	5–6 g/m²/day q 2 weeks		Neuromuscular side effects Mucositis Diarrhea Skin rash Mucositis Myelosuppression Nausea and vomiting
Nitrosoureas						
Streptozotocin (NSC-85998)	2-deoxy-2-(e-methyl-e-nitrosoureido)-D-glucopyranose	2 g/vial 100 mg/vial	Intravenous	1–2 g/m²/week ×4–5	Islet cell carcinoma of pancreas Malignant carcinoid Hodgkin's disease	Renal toxicity Liver toxicity Diabetogenic effect Nausea and vomiting Diarrhea Myelosuppression Insulin shock with hypoglycemia
Chlorozotocin (NSC-178248)	2-(((2-chloroethyl) nitrosoamino)carbonyl)-amino)-2-deoxy-D-Glucopyranose	50 mg/vial	Intravenous	120 mg/m² I.V. q 6 weeks 30–40 mg/m²/day × 5	Melanoma Lung adenocarcinoma Colorectal cancer	Nausea and vomiting Myelosuppression Liver toxicity
Antitumor antibiotics						
Neocarzinostatin (NSC-157365)		2000 units/ampule	Intravenous	3000–4500 U/m²/ week (pediatrics) 3000 U/m²/week	Acute leukemia Pancreatic cancer Gastric cancer	Nausea and vomiting Myelosuppression Skin rash Hypotension Chills and fever
Piperazinedione (NSC-135758)	2,5-Piperazinedione 3,6-bis-(5-chloro-2-piperidyl) dihydrochloride	5 mg/vial	Intravenous	12 mg/m² q 3–4 weeks I.V.	Lymphoma Cervical carcinoma Melanoma	Vomiting Myelosuppression Liver toxicity Coagulation abnormalities

Drug (NSC)	Chemical name	Supply	Route	Dose	Indications	Toxicity
Pepleomycin	3-[(S)-1'-phenylethyl amino]propylamino]bleomycin sulfate	10 mg/vial (freeze-dried powder)	Intravenous, intramuscular, intra-arterial local	10 mg 2-3 × a week (total dose-200 mg)	Lymphoma, Head and neck cancer, Squamous cell carcinoma—lung and skin	Fever, Stomatitis, Skin rash, Hyperkeratosis of the skin
Anguidine (NSC-141537)	Diacetoxyscirpenol	10 mg/vial	Intravenous	5-7.5 mg/m²/day × 5 q 3 weeks		Nausea and vomiting, Myelosuppression, Hypotension, Fever and chills, Somnolence
Miscellaneous						
m-AMSA (NSC-249992)	Methanesulfon-M-anisidide, 4'-(9-acridinylamino)	20 mg/ampule, 75 mg/ampule	Intravenous	120 mg/m² I.V. q 3 weeks	Acute leukemia, Ovarian cancer	Nausea and vomiting, Myelosuppression, Phlebitis, Elevation of alkaline phosphatase, Skin rash
β-TGdR (NSC-71261)	9H-Purine-6-thiol, 2-amino-9-(2-deoxy-β-D-erythro-pentafuranosyl) monohydrate	10 mg/vial, 50 mg/vial	Intravenous	300-500 mg/m²/day × 5	Acute leukemia, Colorectal cancer	Nausea and vomiting, Myelosuppression, Photosensitivity, Alopecia
Gallium nitrate (NSC-15200)	Gallium nitrate	100 mg/ampule	Intravenous	700 mg/m²/week	Cancer of the ovary and cervix, Melanoma, Lymphomas	Nausea and vomiting, Mucositis, Diarrhea, Nephrotoxicity, Metallic taste, Lethargy, Rash
Brucentin (NSC-165563)		3 mg/vial	Intravenous			Fever, Nausea and vomiting, Alopecia, Transient liver function abnormalities
Hexamethylmelamine (NSC-13875)	2,4,6-Tris (dimethylamine)-S-triazine	100 mg/capsule	Oral	12 mg/kg/day × 21 days q 4 weeks	Cancer of the ovary, lung, breast, and cervix, Lymphomas	Nausea and vomiting, Myelosuppression, Neurologic toxicity

search for more compounds with greater antitumor activity is being actively pursued. With further studies, a few of these compounds, used either singly or in combination with agents of known efficacy, may prove to be indispensable tools in certain types of human cancers. Moreover, for other tumor types, it is likely that one or more of these agents could be the "cure."

REFERENCES

Adamson, R. H., Canellos, G. P., and Sieber, S. M. (1975). *Cancer Chemother. Rep.* **59,** 599-610.

Arseneau, J., Adamson, R. H., Hart, M. M., Larson, S., Aamodt, R., Johnson, G., and Canellos, G. P. (1972). *Proc. Am. Assoc. Cancer Res.* **13,** 40.

Astaldi, G. (1975). *Wadley Med. Bull.* **5,** 303-326.

Astaldi, G., Meardi, G., Taverna, P. L., and Yallin, B. (1973). *In* "Leukamien und Maligne Lymphome. Pathophysiologic, Linik, Chemo-und Immunotherapie" (A. Stacher, ed.), pp. 379-383. Urban & Schwarzenberg, Munich.

Avery, T. L., Roberts, D., and Price, R. A. (1973). *Cancer Chemother. Rep.* **57,** 165-173.

Baguley, B. C., Falkenhaug, E. M., Rastrick, J. M., and Marbrook, J. (1976). *Eur. J. Cancer* **10,** 169-176.

Battelli, T., Bonsignori, M., and Manocchi, P. (1975). *Panminerva Med.* **17,** 262-264.

Beerman, T. A., and Goldberg, I. H. (1974). *Biochem. Biophys. Res. Commun.* **59,** 1254-1261.

Benjamin, R. S., Keating, M. J., McCredie, K. B., Luna, M. A., Loo, T. L., and Freireich, E. J. (1976). *Proc. Am. Assoc. Cancer Res.* **17,** 72.

Bergevin, P. R., Tormey, D. C., and Blum, J. (1973). *Cancer Res.* **57,** 51-58.

Bhuyan, B. K. (1970). *Cancer Res.* **30,** 2017-2023.

Bhuyan, B. K., and Fraser, T. J. (1974). *Cancer Chemother. Rep.* **58,** 149-155.

Bleyer, W. A., and Chard, R. (1978). *Proc. Am. Soc. Clin. Oncol.* **19,** 267.

Blokhina, N. G., Vozny, E. K., and Garin, A. M. (1972). *Cancer (Philadelphia)* **30,** 390-392.

Blum, R. H., and Kahlert, T. (1978). *Cancer Treat. Rep.* **62,** 435-438.

Blum, R. H., Livingston, R. B., and Carter, S. K. (1973). *Eur. J. Cancer* **9,** 977-979.

Bradner, W. T., and Hutchinson, D. J. (1966). *Cancer Chemother. Rep.* **50,** 79-84.

Bradner, W. T., and Rossomano, C. A. (1968). *Proc. Am. Assoc. Cancer Res.* **9,** 8.

Brian, P. W., Dawkins, A. W., and Grove, J. F. (1961). *J. Exp. Bot.* **12,** 1-12.

Brosky, G., and Logothetopoulos, J. (1969). *Diabetes* **18,** 606-611.

Brown, J., Santos, E., Rosen, G., Helson, L., Young, C., and Tan, C. (1978). *Proc. Am. Assoc. Cancer Res.* **19,** 198.

Bruckner, I., Gociu, M., and Berceanu, S. T. (1972). *Proc. Symp. Peptichemio, Milan.*

Buroker, T., Wojtaszak, B., Dindogru, A., DeMattia, M., Baker, L., Grother, C., and Vaitkevicius, V. K. (1978). *Cancer Treat. Rep.* **62,** 689-692.

Cabanillas, F., Rodriquez, V., Hall, S. W., Burgess, M. A., Bodey, G. P., and Freireich, E. J. (1978a). *Cancer Treat. Rep.* **62,** 425-428.

Cabanillas, F., Rodriquez, V., and Bodey, G. P. (1978b). *Proc. AACR/ASCO* **19,** 102.

Cain, B. F., Atwell, G. J., and Seelye, R. N. (1969). *J. Med. Chem.* **12,** 199.

Carella A. M., Giordano, D., and Santini, G. (1975). *Proc. Meet. Int. Soc. Haematol., 3rd, Eur. Afr. Div., London.*

Carter, S. K. (1978). *Cancer Chemother. Pharmacol.* **1,** 15-24.

Catane, R., Kaufman, J. H., Madajewicz, S., Mittelman, A., and Murphy, G. P. (1978). *Br. J. Urol.* **50,** 29-32.

Chabner, B. A., Levine, A. S., Johnson, B. L., and Young, R. C. (1978). *Cancer Treat. Rep.* **62**, 429-433.

Chakravorty, R., Serkar, S., Sen, S., and Mukeji, B. (1967). *Br. J. Cancer* **21**, 33-39.

Cihak, A., Tykva, R., and Sorm, F. (1966). *Collect. Czech. Chem. Commun.* **31**, 3015-3019.

Collins, K. D., and Stark, G. R. (1971). *J. Biol. Chem.* **246**, 6599-6605.

Cornman, I., and Cornman, M. E. (1951). *Ann. N.Y. Acad. Sci.* **51**, 1443-1487.

Costanzi, J. J., Gagliano, R., Loukas, D., Panettiere, F. J., and Hokanson, J. A. (1978). *Cancer (Philadelphia)* **41**, 1715-1719.

Crooke, S. T. (1977). *J. Med.* **8**, 295-316.

Daskal, Y., Merski, J., DuVernay, V., and Crooke, S. T. (1976). Unpublished observations.

Dawkins, A. W., Grove, J. F., and Tidd, B. K. (1965). *Chem. Commun.* **2**, 27.

DeBarbieri, A. (1968). *Acta Genet. Med. Gemellol.* **17**, 67-77.

DeBarbieri, A., DiVittorio, P., Maugeri, M., Mistretta, P., Perrone, F., Tassi, G. C., Temelcou, O., and Zapelli, P. (1970). *Proc. Int. Congr. Chemother., 6th,* **2**, *Tokyo* 146-152.

DeBernardi, B., Comelli, A., Cozzutto, C., Lamedica, G., Mori, P. G., and Massimo, L. (1978). *Cancer Treat. Rep.* **62**, 811-817.

de la Garza, J. G., Carr, D. T., and Bisel, H. F. (1968). *Cancer (Philadelphia)* **22**, 571-575.

Dombernowsky, P., and Nissen, N. I. (1973). *Arch. Pathol. Microbiol. Scand.* **81**, 715-724.

Dudnik, Y., Astorina, L. N., Kazmyan, L. J., and Gause, G. F. (1974). *Antibiotiki (Moscow)* **19**, 514-517.

Dyke, R. W. (1978). *Proc. Chemother. Found. Symp. III* p. 3.

Dyke, R. W., and Nelson, R. L. (1977). *Cancer Treat. Rev.* **4**, 135-142.

Eagan, R. T., Frytak, S., and Rubin, J. (1976). *Proc. Am. Assoc. Cancer Res.* **17**, 21.

Eagan, R. T., Ingle, J. N., Rubin, J., Frytak, S., and Moertel, C. G. (1978). *J. Natl. Cancer Inst.* **60**, 93-96.

Eckhardt, S. (1978). *Proc. Int. Cancer Congr., 10th, Washington, D.C.* **1**, 81-84.

Eckhardt, S., Selli, C., Horvath, I. P., and Institoris, L. (1963). *Cancer Chemother. Rep.* **33**, 57-61.

Eckhardt, S., Selli, C., Institoris, L., Fenyes, G., Karika, S., and Hartoi, F. (1964). *Congr. Hung. Ther. Invest. Pharmacol., Budapest* pp. 267-271.

Edwards, C. L., and Hayes, R. L. (1969). *J. Nucl. Med.* **10**, 103-105.

Edwards, C. L., and Hayes, R. L. (1970). *J. Am. Med. Assoc.* **212**, 1182-1190.

EORTC Clinical Screening Group (1975). *Sem. Hop.* **51**, 7-10.

EORTC Cooperative Group for Leukemias and Haematosarcomas (1972). *Br. Med. J.* **ii**, 744-748.

Falkson, G., VanDyk, J. J., VanEden, E. B., Van der Merwe, A. W., Van den Bergh, J. A., and Falkson, H. C. (1975). *Cancer (Philadelphia)* **35**, 1141-1144.

First All-Union Conference on the Chemotherapy of Malignant Tumors (1968). Riga pp. 624-625.

Flury, E., Mauli, R., and Sigg, H. P. (1965). *Chem. Commun.* **2**, 26.

Frei, E., III, Jaffe, N., Tattersall, M. H., Pitman, S., and Parker, L. (1975). *N. Engl. J. Med.* **292**, 846-851.

Furue, H., Komita, T., Nakao, I., Fururawa, I., Yakoyama, T., and Kanko, T. (1978). *Proc. Int. Cancer Congr., 12th, Buenos Aires* **2**, 9.

Gause, G. F., Brazhnikova, M. G., and Shorin, V. A. (1975). *Cancer Chemother. Rep.,* Part 2 **58**, 255-256.

Gingold, N., Pittermann, E., and Stacher, A. (1974). *Int. J. Clin. Pharmacol.* **10**, 190-202.

Goldin, A., and Johnson, R. K. (1975). *Proc. Int. Symp. Adriamycin, 2nd, Brussels* pp. 37-54.

Haas, C. D., Stephens, R. L., Hollister, M., and Hoogstraten, B. (1976). *Cancer Treat. Rep.* **60**, 611-614.

Hakansson, L., Konyves, I., Lindberg, L. G., and Moller, T. (1978). *Oncology* **35**, 103-106.

Handelsman, H., Broder, L., Slavik, M., and Carter, S. (1974). Streptozotocin (NSC-85998) Clinical Brochure. NCI Jan., 1974

Hanka, L. J., Evans, J. S., Mason, D. J., and Dietz, A. (1966). *Antimicrob. Agents Chemother.* (1961-70) pp. 619-624.

Harrap, K. R., Riches, P. G., Gilby, E. D., Sellwood, S. M., Wilkinson, R., and Konyves, I. (1977). *Eur. J. Cancer* **13**, 873-881.

Hart, M. M., Smith, C. F., Yanley, S. T., and Adamson, R. H. (1971). *J. Natl. Cancer Inst.* **47**, 1121-1127.

Hattori, T. (1973). *Jpn. J. Cancer Clin.* **19**, 50-53.

Helman, L., Henney, J., and Slavik, M. (1976). Anguidine (NSC-141537) Clinical Brochure.

Hoogstraten, B., O'Bryan, R., and Jones, S. (1978). *Cancer Treat. Rep.* **62**, 841-842.

Hoth, D., Schein, P., MacDonald, J., Buscaglia, D., and Haller, D. (1977). *Proc. Am. Soc. Clin. Oncol.* **18**, 309.

Hoth, D., Butler, T., Winokur, S., Kales, A., Woolley, P., and Schein, P. (1978). *Proc. Am. Soc. Clin. Oncol.* **19**, 381.

Ikeda, S., Nakayama, H., Miyasato, H., and Kobayashi, Y. (1978). *Proc. Int. Cancer Congr., 12th, Buenos Aires* **2**, 7-8.

Institoris, L., Horvath, I. P., and Csanyi, E. (1967a). *Arzneim.-Forsch.* **17**, 145-149.

Institoris, L., Horvath, I. P., Pethes, G., and Eckhardt, S. (1967b). *Cancer Chemother. Rep.* **51**, 261-270.

Inuyama, Y., Murakami, Y., and Asaoka, K. (1978). *Proc. Int. Cancer Congr., 12th, Buenos Aires* **2**, 192.

Ishibiki, K., Kumai, K., Kubota, T., Alkawa, N., and Abe, O. (1978). *Proc. Int. Cancer Congr., 12th, Buenos Aires* **2**, 249-250.

Ishida, N., Miyazaki, K., Kumagai, K., and Rikimaru, M. (1965). *J. Antibiot.* **18**, 68-76.

Issell, B. F., Prestayko, A. W., Comis, R. L., and Crooke, S. T. (1979). *Cancer Treat. Rev.* **6**, 239-249.

Iwamoto, R. H., Acton, E. M., and Goodman, L. (1963). *J. Med. Chem.* **6**, 684-688.

Jacquillat, C., Weil, M., Gemon, M. F., Izrael, V., Schaison, G., Boiron, M., and Bernard, J. (1972). *Br. Med. J.* **iv**, 468-469.

Jacquillat, C., Weil, M., Gemon-Auclerc, M. F., Izrael, V., Bussell, A., Boiron, M., and Bernard, J. (1976). *Cancer (Philadelphia)* **37**, 653-659.

Johnson, P., Randall, K., Inouye, T., Goldin, A., and Stark, G. (1976). *Cancer Res.* **36**, 2720-2725.

Jones, S. E., Tucker, W. G., Haut, A., Tranum, B. L., Vaughn, C., Chase, E. M., and Durie, B. G. M. (1977). *Cancer Treat. Rep.* **61**, 1617-1621.

Kaiser, D. W., Thurston, J. T., Dudley, J. R., Schaefer, F. C., Hechenbleikner, I., and Holm-Hansen, D. (1951). *J. Am. Chem. Soc.* **73**, 2984-2986.

Karev, N. I., Blokhina, N. G., Vozny, E. K., and Pershin, M. P. (1972). *Neoplasma* **19**, 347-350.

Karon, M., Sieger, L., Leimbrook, S., Finklestein, J. S., Nesbitt, M. E., and Swaney, J. J. (1973). *Blood* **42**, 359-365.

Kaufman, J. H., and Mittelman, A. (1975a). *Cancer Chemother. Rep.* **59**, 1007-1014.

Kaufman, J. H., and Mittelman, A. (1975b). *Proc. Am. Assoc. Cancer Res.* **16**, 51.

Kaufman, J. H., Hanjura, G. L., Mittelman, A., Aurgst, C. W., and Murphy, G. P. (1976). *Cancer Treat. Rep.* **60**, 277-279.

Kawai, Y., and Katoh, A. (1972). *J. Natl. Cancer Inst.* **48**, 1535-1538.

Keller, A. (1976). Dianhydrogalactitol (NSC-132313) Annual Report. To the Food and Drug Administration. NCI Report June 1, 1976.

Kelly, J., and Hartwell, J. (1954). *J. Natl. Cancer Inst.* **14**, 967-1010.

Konda, C., Kimura, K., Kumaoka, S., Niitani, H., Sakauchi, N., Suzuki, A., Sakai, Y., Sakano,

T., Shimoyama, M., and Kitachara, T. (1974). *Proc. Int. Congr. Chemother., 8th, Athens, 1973* **3**, 656–666.

Konno, K., Motomiya, M., Nakai, Y., and Koinumaru, S. (1978). *Cancer Chemother. Jpn.* **5**, 119–126.

Konyves, I., and Liljekvist, J. (1976). *Excerpta Med. Int. Congr. Ser.* No. 375, 98–105.

Konyves, I., Fex, H., and Hogberg, B. (1974). *Proc. Int. Congr. Chemother., 8th, Athens, 1973* **3**, 791–795.

Konyves, I., Nordenskjold, B., Forshell, G. P., DeSchryver, A., and Westerberg-Larsson, H. (1975). *Eur. J. Cancer* **11**, 841–844.

Koons, L. S., Bellet, R. E., and Mastrangelo, M. J. (1977). *Proc. Am. Soc. Clin. Oncol.* **18**, 299.

Kovach, J. S., Moertel, C. G., Schutt, A. J., and O'Connell, M. J. (1978). *Proc. Am. Assoc. Cancer Res.* **19**, 408.

Krishan, A., Paika, K., and Frei, E., III (1975). *J. Cell Biol.* **66**, 521–530.

Kubota, T., Shimosato, Y., Moon, Y. H., Matsumoto, S., Ishibiki, K., and Abe, O. (1978a). *Cancer Chemother. Jpn.* **5**, 55–63.

Kubota, T., Shimosato, Y., Moon, Y. H., Matsumoto, S., Miyahara, Y., Ishibiki, K., and Abe, O. (1978b). *Proc. Int. Cancer Congr., 12th, Buenos Aires* **1**, 281–282.

Kumagai, K., and Miyazaki, K. (1963). *J. Antibiot.* **16**, 55.

Kumagai, K., Koide, T., Kikuchi, M., and Ishida, N. (1970). *Int. Cancer Congr.* **10**, 401.

Kupchan, S. M. (1974). *Fed. Proc., Fed. Am. Soc. Exp. Biol.* **33**, 2288–2295.

Kupchan, S. M., Britton, R. W., Ziegler, M. F., and Sigel, C. W. (1973). *J. Org. Chem.* **38**, 178.

Kupchan, S. M., Komoda, Y., Branfman, A. R., Dailey, R. G., and Zimmerly, V. A. (1974). *J. Am. Chem. Soc.* **96**, 3706–3708.

Legha, S. S., Von Hoff, D. D., Slavik, M., and Muggia, F. M. (1976). *Oncology* **33**, 265–270.

LeLe, S. B., Piver, M. S., Barlow, J. J., and Murphy, G. P. (1978). *Oncology* **35**, 101–102

LePage, G. A. (1968). *Can. J. Biochem.* **46**, 655–661.

LePage, G. A., and Junga, I. G. (1967). *Mol. Pharmacol.* **3**, 37–43.

LePage, G. A., Junga, I. G., and Bowman, B. (1964). *Cancer Res.* **24**, 835–840.

Liao, L. L., Kupchan, S. M., and Horwitz, S. B. (1976). *Mol. Pharmacol.* **12**, 167.

Lichinitser, M. R., Assekritova, I. V., and Gorbunova, V. A. (1977). *Antibiotiki (Moscow)* **22**, 940–943.

Luporini, G. (1973). *In* "Leukamien und Maligne Lymphome. Pathophysiologie, Klinik, Chemo- und Immunotherapie"(A. Stacher, ed.), p. 384. Urban & Schwarzenberg, Munich.

McCredie, K. B., Bodey, G. P., Burgess, M. A., Gutterman, J. U., Rodriquez, V., Sullivan, M. P., and Freireich, E. J. (1973). *Cancer Chemother, Rep.* **57**, 319–323.

Maral, R., Ponsinet, G., and Jolles, G. (1972). *C. R. Acad. Sci., Ser. D* **275**, 301–304.

Marmont, A., Bordo, D., Damasio, E., Gori, G., and Rossi, F. (1973). *In* "Leukamien und Maligne Lymphome. Pathophysiologic, Klinik, Chemo-und Immunotherapie" (A. Stacher, ed.), pp. 371–378. Urban & Schwarzenberg, Munich.

Mathé, G., Misset, J. L., DeVassal, F., Gouveia, J., Hayat, M., Machover, D., Belpomme, D., Pico, J. L., Schwarzenberg, L., Ribaud, P., Musset, M., Jasmin, C., and DeLuca, L. (1978). *Cancer Treat. Rep.* **62**, 805–809.

Matsuda, A., Yoshioka, O., Takahashi, K., Yamashita, T., Ebihara, K., Ekimoto, H., Abe, F., Hashimoto, Y., and Umezawa, H. (1978). *Proc. Int. Cancer Congr., 12th, Buenos Aires* **2**, 7.

Meiren, D. V., and Belousova, A. K. (1972). *Vopr. Med. Khim.* **18**, 253–293.

Moller, T. R., Brand, T. L., Konyves, I., and Lindberg, L. G. (1978). *Acta Med. Scand.* 323–327.

Murphy, W. K., Burgess, M. A., Valdivieso, M., Livingston, R. B., Bodey, G. P., and Freireich, E. J. (1978). *Cancer Treat. Rep.* **62**, 1497–1502.

184   Manuel L. Gutierrez

Nemeth, L., Institoris, L., Somfai, S., Gal, F., Polyi, I., Sugar, J., Csuki, D., Szentirmey, Z., and
    Kellner, B. (1972). *Cancer Chemother. Rep., Part 1* **56**, 593-602.
Nishikawa, T., Kumagai, K., Kudo, A., and Ishida, N. (1965). *J. Antibiot., Ser. A* **18**, 223-227.
Nissen, N. I., Larsen, V., Pedersen, H., and Thomsen, K. (1972). *Cancer Chemother, Rep.* **56**,
    769-777.
Ohtsubo, K., Kaden, P., and Mittermayer, C. (1972). *Biochim. Biophys. Acta* **287**, 520-525.
Oki, T., Matsuzawa, Y., Yoshimoto, A., Numata, K., Kitamuara, I., Hori, S., and Takamatsu, A.
    (1975). *J. Antibiot.* **28**, 830-834.
Ono, Y., Ito, Y., Maeda, H., and Ishida, N. (1968). *Biochim. Biophys. Acta* **155**, 616-618.
Padilla, F., Correa, J., Buroker, T., and Vaitkevicius, V. K. (1978). *Cancer Treat. Rep.* **62**,
    553-554.
Palmer, R. L., Samal, B. A., Vaughn, C. B., and Tranum, B. L. (1977). *Cancer Treat. Rep.* **61**,
    1711-1712.
Pasmantier, M. W., Coleman, M., Kennedy, B. J., Eagan, R., Carolla, R., Weiss, R., Leone, L.,
    and Silver, R. T. (1977). *Cancer Treat. Rep.* **61**, 1731-1732.
Perevodchikova, N. I., Gorbunova, V. A., Lichinitser, M. R., Borisov, V. I., Alekseyev, N. A.,
    and Vygvskaya, Y. I. (1975). *Antibiotiki (Moscow)* **20**, 853-856.
Perevodchikova, N. I., Lichinitser, M. R., and Gorbunova, V. A. (1977). *Cancer Treat. Rep.* **61**,
    1705-1707.
Pittermann, E., Stacher, A., and Griendl, W. (1974). *Wien. Med. Wochenschr.* **124**, 216.
Posey, L. E., Morgan, L. R., Carter, R. D., Suterland, C., Krementz, E. T., and Bickers, J. (1978).
    Proc. Am. Assoc. Cancer Res. **19**, 388.
Pratt, C., Rivera, G., and Shanks, E. (1975). *Proc. Am. Assoc. Cancer Res.* **16**, 82.
Rakieten, N., Rakieten, M., and Nadkarni, M. (1963). *Cancer Chemother. Rep.* **29**, 91-98.
Raska, K., Jr., Jurovcik, M., Sormova, Z., and Sorm, F. (1965). *Collect. Czech. Chem. Commun.*
    30, 3001-3006.
Rauen, H. M., and Norpoth, K. (1966). *Arzneim.-Forsch.* **16**, 1001-1007.
Rivera, G., Avery, T., and Pratt, C. (1975). *Cancer Chemother. Rep.* **59**, 743-749.
Rodriquez, V., Gottlieb, J., Burgess, M. A., Livingston, R., Wheeler, W., Spitzer, G., Bodey, G.
    P., Blumenschein, G., and Freireich, E. J. (1976a). *Cancer (Philadelphia)* **38**, 690-694.
Rodriquez, Bodey, G. P., Freireich, E. J., McCredie, K. B., McKelvy, E. M., and Tashima, C. K.
    (1976b). *Cancer Res.* **36**, 2945-2948.
Rodriquez, V., Richman, S. P., Benjamin, R. S., Burgess, M. A., Murphy, W. K., Valdivieso, M.,
    Banner, R. L., Gutterman, J. U., Bodey, G. P., and Freireich, E. J. (1977). *Cancer Res.* **37**,
    980-983.
Rodriquez, V., McCredie, K. B., Keating, M. J., Valdivieso, M., Bodey, G. P., and Freireich, E. J.
    (1978). *Cancer Treat. Rep.* **62**, 493-497.
Rosenbaum, C., and Carter, S. K. (1969). *β-TGdR (NSC-71261) Clinical Brochure.*
Rosenkranz, H. S., and Carr, H. S. (1970). *Cancer Res.* **30**, 112-117.
Ruzicka, F., and Nowotny, H. (1973). *Int. J. Clin. Pharmacol.* **7**, 223-227.
Saito, T., and Yokoyama, M. (1974). *Proc. Int. Congr. Chemother., 8th, 1973, Athens* **3**, 631-636.
Sakano, T., Akawaki, N., Ise, T., Kitaoka, K., and Kimura, K. (1978). *Jpn. J. Clin. Oncol.* **8**,
    49-53.
Schein, P. S., Alberti, K. G. M., and Williams, D. (1971). *Endocrinology* **89**, 827-834.
Sklansky, B. D., Mann-Kaplan, R. S., Reynold, A. F., Jr., Rosenblum, M. L., and Walker, M. D.
    (1974). *Cancer (Philadelphia)* **33**, 460-467.
Skovsgaard, T. (1975). *Cancer Cheomther. Rep.* **59**, 301-308.
Skovsgaard, T., Hansen, H., Mouridsen, H., Nissen, N., and Pedersen-Bjergaard, J. (1978).
    Cancer Treat. Rep. **62**, 1053-1058.
Smart, C. R., Townsend, L. B., Rusho, W. J., Eyre, H. J., Quagliana, J. M., Wilson, M. L.,
    Edwards, C. B., and Mannings, S. J. (1975). *Cancer (Philadelphia)* **36**, 103-106.

Sonntag, R. W., Senn, H. J., Nagel, G., Giger, K., and Alberto, P. (1974). *Eur. J. Cancer* **10**, 93–98.

Sorm, F., and Vesely, J. (1964). *Neoplasma* **11**, 123–130.

Stahelin, H. (1970). *Eur. J. Cancer* **6**, 303–311.

Stahelin, H. (1973). *Eur. J. Cancer* **9**, 215–221.

Stolinsky, D. C., and Bateman, J. R. (1973). *Cancer Chemother. Rep.* **57**, 497–499.

Takita, H., and Didolkar, M. S. (1974). *Cancer Chemother. Rep.* **58**, 371–374.

Tan, C., Gralla, R., Steinherz, P., and Young, C. W. (1978). *Proc. Am. Assoc. Cancer Res.* **19**, 126.

Thigpen, J. T., O'Bryan, R. M., Benjamin, R. S., and Collman, C. A. (1977). *Cancer Treat. Rep.* **61**, 1485–1487.

Thigpen, J. T., Homesley, H., Prem, K., and Mladineo, J. (1978). *Proc. Am. Assoc. Cancer Res.* **19**, 162.

Tobey, R. A. (1972). *Cancer Res.* **32**, 309–316.

Tobey, R. A., Oka, M. S., and Crissman, H. A. (1975). *Eur. J. Cancer* **11**, 433–441.

Todd, G. C., Gibson, W. R., and Morton, D. M. (1976). *J. Toxicol. Environ. Health* **1**, 843–849.

Toguchi, T. (1972). *Jpn. J. Cancer Clin.* **18**, 550–553.

Tojo, S., Miura, T., Katayama, K., and Wada, T. (1978). *Proc. Int. Cancer Congr., 12th, Buenos Aires* **3**, 151.

Vadlamudi, S., Choudry, J. N., Waravdekar, V. S., Kline, I., and Goldin, A. (1970). *Cancer Res.* **30**, 362–369.

Vaidya, S. G., Chaudhri, M. A., Morrison, R., and Whait, D. (1970). *Lancet* **ii**, 911–914.

Vaitkevicius, V., and Reed, M. (1966). *Cancer Chemother. Rep.* **50**, 565–571.

Valdivieso, M., Bodey, G. P., Gottlieb, J. A., and Freireich, E. J. (1976). *Cancer Res.* **36**, 1821–1824.

Valdivieso, M., Bodey, G. P., and Freireich, E. J. (1978). *Proc. Am. Assoc. Cancer Res.* **19**, 215.

Vavra, J. J., DeBoer, C., Dietz, A., Hanka, J., and Sokolski, W. T. (1960). *Antibiot. Annu. 1959–1960* p. 230.

Venditti, J. M. (1971). *Cancer Chemother. Rep., Part 3* **2**, 35–59.

Vertogradova, T. P., Goldberg, L. Y., Filipposyants, S. T., Belova, I. P., Stepanova, E. G., and Shepelevtseva, N. G. (1974). *Antibiotiki (Moscow)* **19**, 50–57.

Vesely, J., Cihak, A., and Sorm, F. (1968). *Biochem. Pharmacol.* **17**, 519–524.

Vogler, W. R., Miller, D., and Keller, J. W. (1975). *Proc. Am. Assoc. Cancer Res.* **16**, 155.

Von Hoff, D., Handelsman, H., and Slavik, M. (1975). 5-Azacytidine Clinical Brochure. (NCI)

Wampler, G. L., Mellette, S. J., Kumperminc, M., and Regelson, W. (1972). *Cancer Chemother. Rep.* **56**, 505–514.

Wilson, W. L., and de la Garza, J. G. (1965). *Cancer Chemother. Rep.* **48**, 49–52.

Wilson, W. L., Schroeder, J. M., Bisel, H. F., Mrazek, R., and Hummel, R. P. (1969). *Cancer (Philadelphia)* **23**, 132–136.

Wilson, W. L., Bisel, H. F., Cole, D., Rochlin, D., Ramirez, G., and Madden, R. (1970). *Cancer (Philadelphia)* **25**, 568–570.

Wilson, W. R. (1974). *C.A.* **80**, 91332a.

Woolley, R., MacDonald, J., Rosenoff, S., Olmert, P., and Schein, P. (1977). *Proc. Am. Soc. Clin. Oncol.* **18**, 304.

Worzalla, J. F., Ramirez, G., and Bryan, G. T. (1973). *Cancer Res.* **33**, 2810–2815.

Zadrazil, S., Fucik, V., Bartl, P., Sormova, Z., and Sorm., F. (1965). *Biochim. Biophys. Acta* **108**, 701–703.

Zbinden, G., and Brandle, E. (1975). *Cancer Chemother. Rep., Part 1* **59**, 707–715.

11

HORMONE THERAPY
Elwood V. Jensen

I. BASIS OF ENDOCRINE THERAPY

The use of endocrine therapy in the treatment of human cancer is based on the fact that neoplasms derived from hormone-responsive tissues often retain the hormone sensitivity of their parent cells, even though the tumors may be growing widely dispersed throughout the body. The most common hormone-dependent cancers are those arising in tissues of the reproductive tract where growth and function require the continued presence of sex hormones, steroid substances produced predominantly, but not exclusively, by the ovary in the female and the testis in the male (Fig. 1). The ovary secretes two types of female sex hormones. Estrogens, represented by estradiol, are primarily responsible during puberty for the growth and development of the female reproductive organs (uterus, vagina, mammary glands) and for the subsequent maintenance of these tissues in their functional condition. Progestational hormones, represented by progesterone, induce further proliferation of the estrogen-stimulated uterine endometrium and mammary glands and play an important role during pregnancy in the nidation of the fertilized ovum and in preparing the breasts for milk secretion under the influence of prolactin, a protein hormone of pituitary origin. In postmenopausal

CANCER AND CHEMOTHERAPY, VOL. III
187

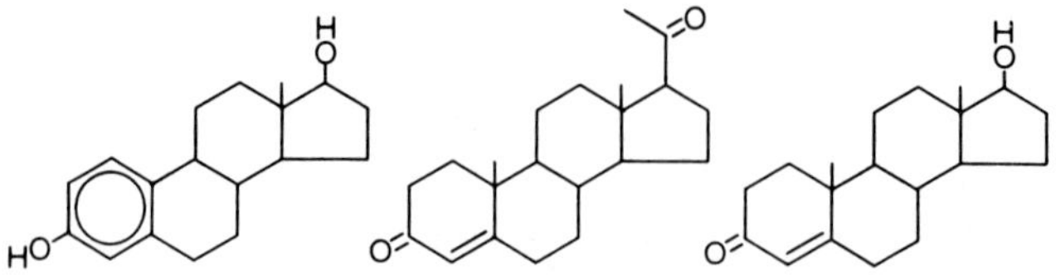

Fig. 1. The principal steroid sex hormones.

women, where ovarian production of sex hormones has declined to insignificant levels, the adrenal glands can serve as an indirect source of estrogenic hormones by their production of 4-androstene-3,17-dione, which is converted elsewhere in the body to the estrogenic substance estrone. The growth, development, and maintenance of the male accessory sex organs (prostate, seminal vesicles, penis) depend on androgenic hormones originating in the testis. The principal androgen secreted by the testis is testosterone, which in certain target tissues, such as the prostate, is converted to 5α-dihydrotestosterone before exerting its biological action.

The production of steroidal sex hormones by the gonads depends on their stimulation by protein hormones called gonadotrophins, which are secreted by the anterior lobe of the pituitary gland under regulation of peptides originating in the hypothalamus and known as gonadotrophin-releasing hormones. Synthesis of releasing factors by the hypothalamus and the ability of the pituitary to respond to them are inhibited by increased levels of the steroid sex hormones in the blood, so the gonadal hormones regulate their own levels by negative feedback control of the stimuli for their biosynthesis. In the case of the estrogen precursors produced by the adrenal glands, these, like the glucocorticoids themselves, depend on stimulation of the adrenal cortex by ACTH, another trophic protein hormone from the pituitary.

Cancers that depend on hormonal support for their continued proliferation may be deprived of this stimulation either by endocrine ablation or by additive hormone therapy. The first approach involves the surgical or radiological extirpation either of the hormone-secreting glands themselves or of the pituitary, which provides the trophic factors required for gonadal or adrenal hormone production. Alternatively, stimulation of the dependent cancer cells can be prevented by the administration of other steroid hormones, which inhibit the production and/or action of the supporting hormone, or of specific hormone antagonists that compete for the intracellular receptor proteins through which the biological actions of steroid hormones are mediated in target cells. Because of the side effects associated with prolonged administration of active hormonal agents and the more recent development of effective antiestrogens and antiandrogens with relatively minor side effects, additive antihormonal therapy is currently receiving increased application, especially in the use of tamoxifen as an estrogen antagonist in the treatment of advanced breast cancer.

In contrast to cancers of the reproductive organs, where endocrine therapy consists of deprivation or antagonism of a supporting hormone, the treatment of leukemias and other lymphomas with glucocorticoids is based on a primary action of these adrenal hormones to cause involution of lymphatic tissue. Some but not all malignancies of hematopoietic tissues retain this sensitivity to the lympholytic action of glucocorticoids.

II. PROSTATIC CANCER

Though the earliest example of response to endocrine ablation was observed with breast cancer (Beatson, 1896), the appreciation of endocrine manipulation for the treatment of malignant disease began with the classic studies of Huggins on carcinoma of the prostate (Huggins and Hodges, 1941; Huggins et al., 1941). Patients with widespread metastases were found to undergo striking remissions, either when deprived of androgenic hormones by orchiectomy (Fig. 2) or when large doses of estrogens (diethylstilbestrol) were given to counteract the action of endogenous androgens. These observations were widely confirmed (Nesbit and Baum, 1950; Burt, et al., 1957; Franks, 1958), and castration and/or estrogen therapy became the accepted treatment for inoperable prostatic carcinoma, with objective remissions observed in approximately 80% of the treated patients.

In many instances, an early indication of favorable response to endocrine treatment is provided by changes in the blood level of the enzyme acid phosphatase. The normal prostate gland produces substantial amounts of this enzyme, which are incorporated in the prostatic fluid. Most prostatic carcinomata continue to synthesize acid phosphatase; when the cancer has spread beyond the confines of the original gland, the enzyme is delivered to the blood resulting in an elevated level (Gutman and Gutman, 1938). Favorable response to endocrine therapy is usually reflected by a striking decrease in the serum level of acid phosphatase, detectable before actual regression of the tumor is evident (Huggins and Hodges, 1941; Johnson et al., 1976). Recent introduction of a sensitive radioimmunoassay procedure for measuring serum acid phosphatase offers promise for detecting prostatic cancer in early stages of its development (Foti et al., 1977).

In recent years, the use of endocrine therapy for prostatic cancer has undergone modification (Brendler, 1972; Catalona and Scott, 1978; Resnick and Grayhack, 1978; Flocks et al., 1978; Klein, 1979; Landau, 1979). With the advent of more precise techniques for determining various stages in the spread of the disease and the appreciation of deleterious side effects of large doses of estrogens on the cardiovascular system, which often negate any contribution of endocrine therapy to patient survival (Mellinger et al., 1967; Blackard, 1975),

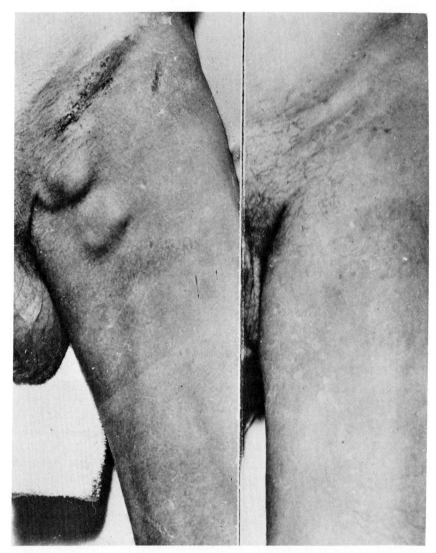

Fig. 2. Influence of orchiectomy on metastatic adenocarcinoma of the prostate in inguinal nodes. Left: preoperative. Right: same region 107 days after orchiectomy. (Reproduced from Huggins, 1942.)

there has been a trend toward reducing the amounts of estrogen administered and reserving endocrine therapy by itself for those cases in which the cancer is widely disseminated (stage D). For stage C cancers, which extend through the prostatic capsule but have not metastasized to distant sites, endocrine therapy may be employed in conjunction with radical prostatectomy (Scott and Boyd, 1969) or radiation therapy (Ray *et al.,* 1973; Hill *et al.,* 1974; Flocks *et al.,* 1978), and its use in stabe B carcinoma has been strongly criticized (Klein, 1979). With both stage C and D cancers, the former practice of administering diethylstilbestrol in oral doses of 5 mg or more per day has generally been replaced by the use of 1–2 mg per day (Resnick and Grayhack, 1978), an amount that does not completely suppress the testicular production of testosterone (Kent *et al.,* 1973) but that usually provides satisfactory control of the prostatic cancer without the vascular side effects associated with higher doses (Blackard, 1975).

Although the optimal therapeutic procedure may depend on the characteristics of the individual cancer, many authorities regard orchiectomy as the preferred initial treatment of stage D prostatic carcinoma, resorting to estrogen administration for those patients who either refuse this ablative procedure or do not respond well to it. As alternatives to diethylstilbestrol, other orally active estrogens, such as 17-ethinylestradiol and trianisylchlorethylene (Tace, chlorotrianisene), or long-acting injectables, such as polyestradiol phosphate (Estradurin), have been employed with essentially similar results. Androgen antagonists, such as flutamide and the progestational agents, cyproterone acetate, megestrol acetate (Megace), and medroxyprogesterone acetate (Provera), have been tried by a number of investigators, both as initial therapy and in patients who have become refractory to other treatment. Although these substances can cause remissions of prostatic cancer, no particular advantage over orchiectomy or diethylstilbestrol has been demonstrated (Catalona and Scott, 1978; Resnick and Grayhack, 1978).

Treatment of advanced prostatic carcinoma by either ablative or additive endocrine therapy effects objective remissions in 70–80% of the patients, usually persisting from 2 to 3 years, although remissions of 10 years or longer are not unknown. Survival in patients receiving large doses of estrogen is limited by treatment-induced pulmonary emboli and other cardiovascular problems (Mellinger *et al.,* 1967), but, properly applied, hormone manipulation has been found to improve the 5-year survival rate of stage D carcinoma from 6 to 40% (Blackard *et al.,* 1973).

In attempts to eliminate possible extratesticular sources of androgens, various investigators have examined the effect of adrenalectomy or hypophysectomy in patients who have relapsed or who failed originally to respond to orchiectomy. Although occasional beneficial effects have been noted (Scott and Schirmer, 1962; Brendler, 1973; Bhanalph *et al.,* 1974), the results in general have been disappointing, and these ablative procedures have found little place in the treatment of prostatic cancer. More promising and less traumatic has been "medical adrenalectomy," effected by the administration of large doses of dexamethasone or other glucocorticoids or by aminoglutethimide. Such treatment often is employed as a final attempt at endocrine therapy before resorting to the alternative of cytotoxic chemotherapy, which with most prostatic cancers is not highly effective.

Most patients with advanced prostatic cancer appear to have androgen-dependent tumors, but there is need for some means to identify the 20% who do not respond to endocrine therapy, as well as to determine whether patients who relapse after initial response still have hormone-dependent tumors that may be receiving supporting androgen from another source. A limited indication of responsiveness is provided by histological examination of the cancer tissue, well-differentiated cancers being more likely to be hormone sensitive than poorly differentiated ones. Following the success of estrogen receptor determinations in predicting hormone dependency of breast cancers (Section III, B), attempts have been made to use analogous assays of androgen receptors for prostatic cancers (Menon *et al.*, 1977). Because of technical difficulties in accurately measuring androgen receptors in prostatic cancer, correlations of receptor content with clinical response to endocrine therapy have not yet been established with certainty, although preliminary results suggest that receptor measurements may prove useful (Gustafsson *et al.*, 1978). Alternatively, the dihydrotestosterone content of prostatic cancer specimens, as determined by radioimmunoassay, appears to show a correlation with the response of the patient to endocrine therapy (Geller *et al.*, 1979).

III. BREAST CANCER

A. Endocrine Treatment of Advanced Breast Cancer

A relation between ovarian secretions and the growth of some human breast cancers was suggested as early as 1836 by observations of fluctuations in tumor growth rate during different phases of the menstrual cycle (Cooper, 1836). Direct evidence for supporting factors of ovarian origin was provided when Beatson (1896), with remarkable insight for the time, removed the ovaries from young women with advanced breast cancer and reported that some patients showed striking regression of their metastatic lesions. The introduction of orchiectomy for the treatment of prostatic cancer (Huggins and Hodges, 1941) reawakened interest in Beatson's observations, and ovarian ablation by oophorectomy or by radiation castration has become the generally accepted primary therapy for advanced breast cancer in premenopausal women.

The highest incidence of breast cancer is found in postmenopausal women, where the ovaries no longer produce significant amounts of steroid hormones. It was long suspected that, in the absence of ovarian function, the adrenal glands might serve as a source of estrogenic steroids. More recently it has been demonstrated that the adrenals do so indirectly by secreting androstenedione, which undergoes aromatization elsewhere in the body to produce estrone (Grodin *et al.*, 1973). After cortisol and other cortical hormones became available, so that adrenalectomized patients could be maintained by glucocorticoid replacement,

Huggins and Bergenstal (1951, 1952) removed the adrenals from post-menopausal women, as well as from men, with advanced breast cancer and found that some but not all experienced striking remission of their disease (Figs. 3 and 4). Shortly thereafter, it was shown by Luft, as well as by Pearson, that similar remissions can be achieved by surgical excision of the pituitary gland (Luft and Olivecrona, 1953; Luft et al., 1958; Pearson et al., 1956; Pearson and Ray, 1960). With the improved transsphenoidal surgical approach that provides essentially complete extirpation of the gland, some clinicians have come to regard hypophysectomy as the ablation of choice for postmenopausal breast cancer, since operative trauma is minimal, the patient is easily managed postoperatively,

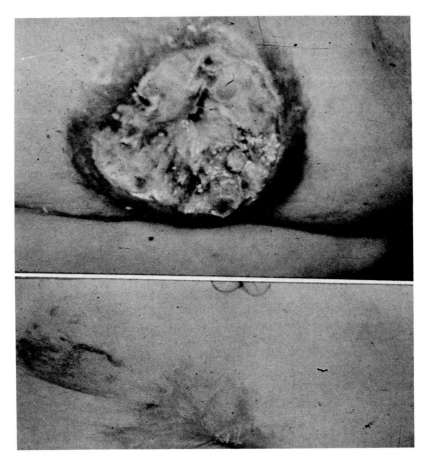

Fig. 3. Influence of bilateral adrenalectomy on mammary adenocarcinoma in a woman, age 62. Above: the primary tumor with extensive local spread. Below: same region 12 months after adrenalectomy. (Courtesy of Dr. C. Huggins.)

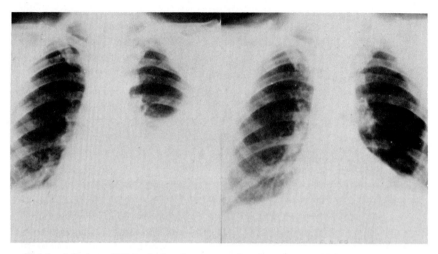

Fig. 4. Influence of bilateral adrenalectomy on pleural metastases with hydrothorax in a man, age 60, with cancer of the male breast. Left: preoperative. Right: 57 days after adrenalectomy. (Courtesy of Dr. C. Huggins.)

and instances have been reported in which hypophysectomy has led to remission in persons who have relapsed or failed to respond to adrenalectomy (Pearson and Ray, 1960).

The ability of ovariectomy, adrenalectomy, and hypophysectomy to effect striking remissions of some advanced breast cancers has been widely confirmed (Atkins *et al.*, 1957; Cade, 1962; Stoll, 1969; Landau, 1979). For those patients who respond, endocrine ablation represents the most effective therapy presently available in terms of both quality and duration of remissions, even though these usually do not exceed 2–3 years and sometimes are even less. But in contrast to cancer of the prostate, where the great majority of the patients are responsive to endocrine therapy, less than half the women with advanced breast cancer benefit from endocrine ablation, and the fraction of patients showing truly objective remissions for a period of 6 months or longer is closer to 25%.

Before means for predicting hormone dependency had been developed, there was reluctance on the part of many clinicians to subject patients to adrenalectomy or hypophysectomy when the probability of obtaining a remission was so low. As an alternative to these irreversible ablative procedures, additive hormone therapy has been used extensively (Nathanson, 1952; Stoll, 1969; Segaloff, 1975; Landau, 1979). The administration of androgens, either by injection (testosterone propionate) or by mouth (fluoxymestrone), to counteract or antagonize the action and/or production of estrogens has been widely employed (Goldenberg and Segaloff, 1973) and leads to remissions in 20–25% of the patients. However, the long-term use of these active male hormones is limited by their virilizing side effects. In an effort to find effective agents in which these side effects are minimized, many structural analogues of testosterone have been tested. 2α-Methyldihydrotestosterone propionate (Dromostanolone) elicits essentially the same pattern of tumor response as testosterone propionate but is significantly less virilizing (Blackburn and Childs, 1959), whereas 1-dehydrotestololactone (Δ^1-testololactone, Teslac), though showing a somewhat lower response rate, is essentially devoid of androgenic activity and is well tolerated on continued therapy (Volk *et al.*, 1974). Although the extremely high response rates originally reported (Gordan *et al.*, 1970) have not been confirmed by others (Goldenberg *et al.*, 1973), $7\beta,17\alpha$-dimethyltestosterone (calusterone) appears to be an especially favorable androgen analogue for the treatment of breast cancer, with only moderate androgenicity and hepatotoxicity.

Although the growth of hormone-dependent breast cancers is stimulated by physiological amounts of estrogenic substances, it was first shown by Haddow and associates (1944) that massive doses of estrogens can cause regression of some breast cancers. Till now, high-dose estrogen therapy has been the most widely used medical treatment for advanced breast cancer in postmenopausal women. It is commonly held that estrogens are less effective than androgens in treating the younger patient, although remissions in premenopausal women have been described (Kennedy, 1962). Estrogens appear to be especially effective against soft tissue metastases, whereas androgen therapy may be superior for bone metastases. Estimates of remission rates (38%) run somewhat higher than with other types of additive hormone therapy (Landau, 1979), but whether this means that there are patients who respond only to estrogen therapy remains to be established with certainty. Prolonged estrogen administration is associated with side effects, in particular the cardiovascular problems mentioned under prostatic cancer, as well as nausea, vomiting, breast soreness, uterine bleeding, and stress incontinence. In general these effects can be fairly well controlled, and with most patients estrogens are tolerated better than androgens.

The estrogen used most commonly for breast cancer therapy, at least in the United States, is diethylstilbestrol, usually given orally as three 5-mg doses per day. Comparable doses of orally active steroidal estrogens, such as 17-ethinylestradiol or its 3-methyl ether (mestranol), are also used with generally similar results. Such amounts of hormone are from 50 to 100 times those usually administered as replacement therapy. Whether these massive doses of estrogen cause tumor regression by a direct action on the cancer cell or by some indirect mechanism, possible involving the pituitary gland or the immune system, has not been established.

In general, progestational hormones have not enjoyed wide success in the treatment of breast cancer, but there are reports that highly potent, orally active progestins, such as medroxyprogesterone acetate (Provera) and megestrol acetate (Megace), produce remissions in approximately 25% of the patients, with a remarkable absence of side effects (Stoll, 1969; Ansfield *et al.*, 1974). There are also studies indicating that treatment with a combination of estrogen and progestin may cause remissions in patients who have proved refractory to estrogen alone (Landau *et al.*, 1962; Crowley and McDonald, 1965). Attempts to effect "medical adrenalectomy" with large doses of glucocorticoids have caused regressions of breast cancer (Nissen-Meyer and Vogt, 1959), but these remissions are not as satisfactory or extensive as those produced by adrenalectomy itself (Dao *et al.*, 1961).

At the present time the most promising approach for the medical treatment of hormone-dependent breast cancers appears to be the use of estrogen antagonists. A number of such substances, with similar basic chemical structures (Fig. 5), have been known for some time. Compounds of this type are themselves weak estrogens, but when present in excess they compete with the natural estrogens for the receptor proteins in target cells (Section III,B). Although the antiestrogens also effect translocation of the receptor to the nucleus, the interaction there is somehow different from that of the true estrogens, for it appears to block the replenishment of the depleted extranuclear receptor necessary for the sustained hormonal support of growth (Clark *et al.*, 1974).

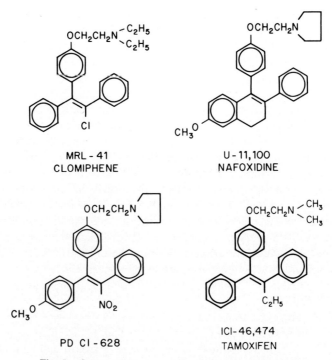

Fig. 5. Structures of some common estrogen antagonists.

Initial attempts to use nafoxidine for the treatment of breast cancer were limited by the dermatologic side effects (photosensitivity, icthyosis) produced on prolonged administration. More recently tamoxifen (Nolvadex), which shows similar antagonism of estrogenic action in rats (Harper and Walpole, 1966), was found to cause remissions of human breast cancers without inducing undesirable side effects (Cole *et al.*, 1971; Ward, 1973). These observations have been widely confirmed (Henningsen, *et al.*, 1980). Because of its low toxicity, tamoxifen is rapidly becoming the agent of choice for the medical treatment of hormone-dependent breast cancers in postmenopausal women, and it provides an attractive alternative to the more aggressive ablative techniques of adrenalectomy and hypophysectomy.

Breast cancer in the male, which occurs with about 1% the frequency seen in the female, appears to be hormone dependent in the majority of cases. Approximately two-thirds of the men with metastatic breast cancer are reported to show regression after orchiectomy (Farrow and Adair, 1942), and similar remissions are observed with adrenalectomy (Fig. 4), hypophysectomy, or the administration of estrogens, progestins, or estrogen–progestin combinations (Stoll, 1969). It is not certain whether the primary effect of castration is to deprive the tumor of androgen or of estrogen derived from it. Observations that administration of androgens to patients after castration-induced remission exacerbates the disease have been taken to suggest that cancer of the male breast may be androgen dependent (Landau, 1979).

B. Prediction of Hormone Dependency

Because most patients with advanced mammary carcinoma do not respond favorably to endocrine manipulation, clinicians have sought ways to distinguish between responding and nonresponding cancers, so that endocrine therapy, especially adrenalectomy and hypophysectomy, could be reserved for those patients who have a reasonable chance of benefit. On the basis of clinical experience, a number of guidelines were developed. Patients who enjoyed a long disease-free interval between mastectomy and the appearance of distant metastases were more likely to respond to endocrine therapy than those in whom recurrence was rapid. Skin and lymph node metastases were more likely to regress than bone metastases, whereas prognosis was especially unfavorable with lesions in the brain or viscera. Response was more probable if the patient had responded earlier to another type of endocrine therapy. Cancer in very young women usually progressed extremely rapidly and rarely responded to hormonal treatment.

In an attempt to predict hormone dependency with greater accuracy, Bulbrook and his associates have carried out extensive and elegant studies of the pattern of steroid hormone metabolites excreted in the urine of breast cancer patients, in particular the relation between metabolites of adrenal and gonadal origin (Atkins *et al.*, 1968). Although some relation with clinical response was suggested, the degree of correlation was not sufficient to exert a major influence on therapy decisions.

A more satisfactory means for predicting hormone dependency of mammary cancer is provided by determination of the estrogen receptor content of an excised specimen of the tumor. It was observed that administration of radioactive hexestrol (Glascock and Hoekstra, 1959) or estradiol (Jensen and Jacobson, 1960) to experimental animals led to a striking concentration of radioactive hormone in the uterus and other reproductive tissues and that, on similar administration of labeled hexestrol to breast cancer patients about to undergo adrenalectomy, more radioactivity was taken up by the tumors in those women who responded favorably than in those who did not (Folca *et al.*, 1961). After techniques were devised for the study of estradiol binding *in vitro* (Jensen *et al.*, 1967), and the accumulation of hormone in the nucleus was shown (Gorski *et al.*, 1968; Jensen *et al.*, 1968) to depend on its initial reaction with an extranuclear receptor protein (Fig. 6), the uptake of estradiol by tumor slices, and later the presence of receptor in the cytosol fraction of a tumor homogenate, was correlated with the response of the patient to endocrine therapy. It was found that

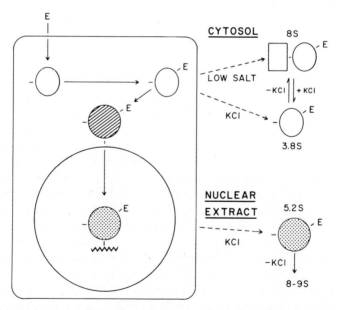

Fig. 6. Schematic representation of interaction pathway of estrogen in target cell. Diagram at left indicates estrogen (E) combining with native receptor protein to induce its conversion to active form and translocation of the activated complex to bind to chromatin in the nucleus. Diagram at right indicates sedimentation properties of complexes extracted from cell after homogenization.

patients whose tumors contained little or no estrogen receptor rarely responded to any type of endocrine treatment, whereas most but not all patients with receptor-containing cancers showed objective remission to such therapy (Jensen *et al.*, 1971). These observations were soon confirmed (Maass *et al.*, 1972; Engelsman *et al.*, 1973), and analysis of human breast cancers for their content of estrogen receptor (estrophilin) was widely investigated (Wittliff, 1974; McGuire *et al.*, 1975; Jensen *et al.*, 1976; McGuire, 1978). As methods for detecting and measuring estrophilin became more sensitive, it became evident that many tumors have a low content of receptor but that such cancers resemble those with no detectable receptor in their lack of response to endocrine treatment. Many investigators now use the terms ''receptor-rich'' and ''receptor-poor'' instead of positive and negative, using a dividing line determined empirically on the basis of clinical experience (Jensen *et al.*, 1976).

Table I shows the correlation of receptor analysis with clinical response for women treated by endocrine ablation at the University of Chicago. It is evident that approximately two-thirds of the patients with receptor-rich tumors will respond to one or another type of endocrine therapy, whereas those with receptor-poor cancers have little chance of benefit from endocrine manipulation and are better treated directly with cytotoxic chemotherapy. The results with additive hormone therapy are essentially similar, except that, in our experience, the response rate seen with the receptor-rich patients is about 60%. Of the more than 1300 primary and metastatic breast cancers we have analyzed, most contain some detectable estrophilin, but 60–70% can be classified as receptor-poor, as defined empirically on the basis of the experience with treated patients. Because the estrogen receptor assay predicts clinical response correctly in approximately two-thirds of the patients with receptor-rich tumors and in essentially all those of the receptor-poor group, its overall accuracy is approximately 85%.

The failure of one-third of the patients with receptor-rich cancers to respond to endocrine treatment is probably due in some cases to tumor heterogeneity and in

TABLE I

Objective Remissions to Endocrine Ablation

Treatment	ER-Rich	ER-Poor
Adrenalectomy	4/6	0/20
Adrenalectomy and oophorectomy	14/19	1/17
Hypophysectomy	2/4	0/9
Castration	9/12	1/30
Total: 117 cases	29/41	2/76
	71%	3%

others to the fact that receptor may be present but nonfunctional. Some human breast cancers and their metastases appear to be multiclonal; if a receptor-rich specimen is taken for assay but the patient also contains appreciable amounts of receptor-poor metastases, she will fail to show objective remission, although subjective remissions, in which some metastases regress, are often observed. In an effort to identify breast cancers with nonfunctioning estrogen receptor, Horwitz et al. (1975) have suggested determining the tumor content of progesterone receptor, which in normal reproductive tissues is known to depend on estrogen stimulation and thus on functioning estrogen receptor. Subsequent experience has established that breast cancers that contain significant amounts of both estrogen receptor and progesterone receptor show a significantly higher response rate than those containing only estrogen receptor, so that measuring both receptors can increase the accuracy of the predictive assay (McGuire, 1978). However, some cancers with high levels of both receptors still do not respond to hormonal therapy, and many containing only estrogen receptor do respond. At the present state of knowledge, progesterone receptor assay can complement but not substitute for estrogen receptor determination.

In many patients with metastatic breast cancer, assay of hormone receptors is precluded by the lack of a readily accessible tumor specimen. Thus it has been of considerable interest to know whether estrogen receptor determination on the primary tumor at the time of mastectomy will predict response to endocrine therapy if metastatic disease appears at a later time. Preliminary findings suggest that the primary tumor can be used for this purpose (Jensen et al., 1976; Block et al., 1978). In our most recent experience we have found that of 20 patients with receptor-rich primary cancers, 15 responded favorably to endocrine therapy, in contrast to only one response among 25 patients with receptor-poor primary tumors, when metastases appeared from 1 month to 67 months after mastectomy.

It was further observed that receptor analysis of the primary tumor provides valuable prognostic information concerning the probability of recurrence of metastatic disease. For patients with comparable lymph node involvement, those with receptor-rich primary tumors showed a lower recurrence rate and a significantly longer disease-free interval after mastectomy than patients with receptor-poor cancers (Knight et al., 1977). These observations have been widely confirmed; at present there is general agreement that estrogen receptor determinations should be carried out on all primary breast cancers to provide information relevant both to the prognosis for cancer recurrence and to the selection of optimal therapy when metastases appear.

IV. CANCER OF THE UTERINE ENDOMETRIUM

Though the uterus has long been recognized to depend on steroid sex hormones for its growth and function, surprisingly little work has been reported concerning the effect of endocrine ablation on metastatic cancer of the uterine endometrium. The pioneer work in the hormonal therapy of endometrial cancer is that of Kelley and Baker (1961, 1965), who showed that the administration of progestional hormones effects striking regressions in about 30% of the patients with advanced disease. These observations have been widely confirmed (Reifenstein, 1974), and progestational therapy has become the method of choice for the treatment of advanced endometrial carcinoma. In general, the remissions last from 1 to 3 years, but some patients show essential "cure" for periods exceeding 13 years (Reifenstein, 1974).

The earliest studies were carried out with daily intramuscular injections of 50–200 mg of progesterone in oil, but most later therapy has used the long-acting substance, 17α-hydroxyprogesterone caproate (Delalutin), given intramuscularly in amounts of 500 mg twice a week or 1 g once a week. More recently, orally active progestins, such as medroxyprogesterone acetate (Provera) and megestrol acetate (Megace), have also been found to be effective. These amounts of progestational agents cause essentially no adverse side effects.

A number of studies are currently under way to correlate the clinical response of endometrial cancers with their content of either estrogen or progesterone receptors in an effort to identify which patients will or will not benefit from progestin therapy. It is still too early to draw definite conclusions concerning the prediction of hormone dependency in endometrial cancer.

V. LYMPHOMAS

Although detailed discussion of the clinical management of leukemias and other lymphomas is beyond the scope of this survey, it should be mentioned that these malignancies represent another example of the use of steroid hormones in the therapy of human cancer. The use of glucocorticoids for treating lymphomas is based on their long-recognized ability to cause involution of the thymus gland and other lymphoid tissues (Selye, 1937; Ingle, 1938). Because lymphoid cancers in general are highly sensitive to the action of cytotoxic chemotherapeutic agents, corticosteroids (usually prednisone) are rarely given alone but are used in conjunction with a cytotoxic drug or with a combination of such agents (Goldin et al., 1971).

The most extensive use of glucocorticoid therapy is in chronic lymphocytic leukemia (CLL), where the effectiveness of corticosteroids is clearly established and prednisone is routinely included in the treatment regimen. In addition to its direct lympholytic action, prednisone can exert a secondary beneficial effect in those cases of CLL that involve severe anemia or thrombocytopenia. Glucocorticoids are of probable benefit in the treatment of multiple myeloma and in some cases of acute lymphoblastic leukemia, although their use in the latter condition has decreased somewhat as other therapies have become available. Corticoids appear to contribute little to the treatment of acute myeloblastic or chronic myelocytic leukemias. For Hodgkin's disease and other lymphomas, prednisone is included in most but not all the currently employed treatment regimens, but sound experimental evidence to justify its use is lacking.

Because of its administration in combination with other agents, it is difficult to know what contribution the corticosteroid makes to clinical responses seen in the patients. Thus, there is uncertainty as to what proportion of lymphoid cancers are sensitive to hormone, but it is generally considered that various lymphomas may include both glucocorticoid-sensitive and glucocorticoid-resistant types (Claman, 1972). Because of their inhibitory effect on the immune system, increasing the susceptibility to infections, it would be preferable not to administer prednisone or other glucocorticoids unless there was evidence that the patient had a corticoid-sensitive cancer. Attempts have been made to use the glucocorticoid-binding properties of lymphoma cells as an indication of their hormone sensitivity, but at present there is no general agreement on the ability of glucocorticoid receptor measurements to predict clinical response (Thompson, 1979). Although there are reports of correlations between receptor content and steroid responsiveness in acute lymphoblastic leukemias (Lippman *et al.*, 1973, 1978), acute myelogenous leukemias (Lippman *et al.*, 1975), and non-Hodgkin's lymphomas (Bloomfield *et al.*, 1980), corticoid-resistant cell lines of human and mouse leukemias have been found to contain high levels of receptor (Gailani *et al.*, 1973; Lippman *et al.*, 1974) and several investigators could find little correlation between glucocorticoid receptors and clinical or biochemical responses of various types of human lymphomas (Bird *et al.*, 1976; Duval and Homo, 1978; Crabtree *et al.*, 1978). Some of the disagreement appears to result from technical difficulties in studying the rather unstable glucocorticoid receptor protein in broken cell systems. Evaluation of the utility of receptor assays in predicting hormone sensitivity in human leukemias and lymphomas must await the results of experimentation that is now in progress in many laboratories.

VI. SUMMARY

Endocrine therapy finds its principal application with cancers of the prostate, breast, uterine endometrium, and lymphoid tissues, although there have also been attempts to use hormones or their antagonists in the treatment of malignancies of the ovary, kidney, and larynx. Endocrine manipulation may consist either of removing or destroying the hormone-producing glands or the stimuli that control them, or of administering hormonal or antihormonal agents that inhibit the cancer cell directly or interfere with the action of the supporting hormone. Though most prostatic cancers appear to be hormone dependent, most mammary and endometrial cancers do not respond to endocrine therapy, and the relative proportion of hormone-sensitive and hormone-resistant lymphomas and leukemias is difficult to ascertain. Determination of the estrogen and progesterone receptor contents of breast cancers has proved useful in predicting which patients will or will not respond to endocrine therapy. It is hoped that analogous studies on hormone receptors in prostatic and endometrial carcinomas and in leukemias and lymphomas will also prove helpful in selecting the proper type of therapy for the individual patients.

REFERENCES

Ansfield, F. J., Davis, H. L., Jr., Ellerby, R. A., and Ramirez, G. (1974). *Cancer (Philadelphia)* **33,** 907–910.

Atkins, H. J. B., Falconer, M. A., Hayward, J. L., and MacLean, K. S. (1957). *Lancet* **i,** 489–496.

Atkins, H., Bulbrook, R. D., Falconer, M. A., Hayward, J. L., MacLean, K. S., and Schurr, P. H. (1968). *Lancet* **ii,** 1255–1260, 1261–1263.

Beatson, G. T. (1896). *Lancet* **ii,** 104–107, 162–165.

Bhanalph, T., Varkarakis, M. J., and Murphy, G. P. (1974). *Ann. Surg.* **179,** 17–23.

Bird, C. C., Waddel, A. W., Robertson, A. M. G., Currie, A. R., Steel, C. M., and Evans, J. (1976). *Br. J. Cancer* **33,** 700–707.

Blackard, C. E. (1975). *Cancer Chemother. Rep.* **59,** 225–227.

Blackard, C. E., Byar, D. P., and Jordan, W. P., Jr. (1973). *Urology* **1,** 553–560.

Blackburn, C. M., and Childs, D. S., Jr. (1959). *Mayo Clin. Proc.* **34,** 113–126.

Block, G. E., Ellis, R. S., DeSombre, E., and Jensen, E. (1978). *Ann. Surg.* **188,** 372–376.

Bloomfield, C. D., Peterson, B. A., Zaleskas, J. A., Frizzera, G., Smith, K. A., Hildebrandt, L., Gajl-Peczalska, K. J., and Munck, A. (1980). *Lancet* **i,** 952–956.

Brendler, H. (1972). *In* "Current Controversies in Urologic Management" (R. Scott, Jr., ed.), pp. 99–102. Saunders, Philadelphia, Pennsylvania.

Brendler, H. (1973). *Urology* **2,** 99–102.

Burt, F. B., Finney, R. P., and Scott, W. W. (1957). *J. Urol.* **77,** 485–491.

Cade, S. (1962). *In* "On Cancer and Hormones" pp. 121–134. Univ. of Chicago Press, Chicago, Illinois.

Catalona, W. J., and Scott, W. W. (1978). *J. Urol.* **119,** 1–8.

Claman, H. N. (1972). *N. Eng. J. Med.* **287,** 388–397.

Clark, J. H., Peck, E. J., Jr., and Anderson, J. N. (1974). *Nature (London)* **251,** 446–448.

Cole, M. P., Jones, C. T. A., and Todd, I. D. H. (1971). *Br. J. Cancer* **25,** 270–275.

Cooper, A. P. (1836). "The Principles and Practice of Surgery," Vol. I, pp. 333–335. Cox, London.

Crabtree, G. R., Smith, K. A., and Munck, A. (1978). *Cancer Res.* **38,** 4268–4272.

Crowley, L. G., and McDonald, I. (1965). *Cancer (Philadelphia)* **18,** 436–446.

Dao, T. L., Tan, E., and Brooks, V. (1961). *Cancer (Philadelphia)* **14,** 1259–1265.

Duval, D., and Homo, F. (1978). *Cancer Res.* **38,** 4263–4267.

Engelsman, E., Persijn, J. P., Korsten, C. B., and Cleton, F. J. (1973). *Br. Med. J.* **ii,** 750–752.

Farrow, J. H., and Adair, F. E. (1942). *Science* **95,** 654.

Flocks, R. H., O'Donoghue, E. P. N., Milleman, L. A., and Culp, D. A. (1978). *Urol. Clin. North Am.* **2,** 163–179.

Folca, P. J., Glascock, R. F., and Irvine, W. T. (1961). *Lancet* **ii,** 796–798.

Foti, A. C., Cooper, J. F., Herschman, H., and Malvaez, R. R. (1977). *N. Engl. J. Med.* **297,** 1357–1361.

Franks, L. M. (1958). *Br. J. Urol.* **30,** 383–388.

Gailani, S., Minowada, J., Silvernail, P., Nussbaum, A., Kaiser, N., Rosen, F., and Shimaoka, K. (1973). *Cancer Res.* **33,** 2653–2657.

Geller, J., Albert, J., and Loza, D. (1979). *J. Steroid Biochem.* **11,** 631–636.

Glascock, R. F., and Hoekstra, W. G. (1959). *Biochem. J.* **72,** 673–682.

Goldenberg, I. S., and Segaloff, A. (1973). *In* "Cancer Medicine" (J. F. Holland and E. Frei, III, eds.), pp. 929–933. Lea & Febiger, Philadelphia, Pennsylvania.

Goldenberg, I. S., Waters, M. N., Ravdin, R. S., Ansfield, F. J., and Segaloff, A. (1973). *J. Am. Med. Assoc.* **223,** 1267–1268.

Goldin, A., Sandberg, J. S., Henderson, E. S., Newman, J. W., Frei, E., III, and Holland, J. F. (1971). *Cancer Chemother. Rep.* **55,** 309–507.

Gordan, G. S., Halden, A., and Walter, R. M. (1970). *Calif. Med.* **113,** 1–10.

Gorski, J., Toft, D., Shyamala, G., Smith, D., and Notides, A. (1968). *Recent Prog. Hormone Res.* **24,** 45–80.

Grodin, J. M., Siiteri, P. K., and MacDonald, P. C. (1973). *J. Clin. Endocrinol. Metab.* **36,** 207–214.

Gustafsson, J. Å., Ekman, P., Snochowski, M., Zetterberg, A., Pousette, Å., and Högberg, B. (1978). *Cancer Res.* **38,** 4345–4348.

Gutman, A. B., and Gutman, E. B. (1938). *J. Clin. Invest.* **17,** 473–478.

Haddow, A., Watkinson, J. M., and Patterson, E. (1944). *Br. Med. J.* **ii,** 393–398.

Harper, M. J. K., and Walpole, A. L. (1966). *Nature (London)* **212,** 87.

Henningsen, B., Linder, F., and Steichele, C., eds. (1980). *Recent Results Cancer Res.* **71.**

Hill, D. R., Crews, Q. E., Jr., and Walsh, P. C. (1974). *Cancer (Philadelphia)* **34,** 156–160.

Horwitz, K. B., McGuire, W. L., Pearson, O. H., and Segaloff, A. (1975). *Science* **189,** 726–727.

Huggins, C. (1942). *Ann. Surg.* **115,** 1192–1200.

Huggins, C., and Bergenstal, D. M. (1951). *J. Am. Med. Assoc.* **147,** 101–106.

Huggins, C., and Bergenstal, D. M. (1952). *Cancer Res.* **12,** 134–141.

Huggins, C., and Hodges, C. V. (1941). *Cancer Res.* **1,** 293–297.

Huggins, C., Stevens, R. E., Jr., and Hodges, C. V. (1941). *Arch. Surg.* **43,** 209–223.

Ingle, D. J. (1938). *Proc. Soc. Exp. Biol. Med.* **38,** 443–444.

Jensen, E. V., and Jacobson, H. I. (1960). *In* "Biological Activities of Steroids in Relation to Cancer" (G. Pincus and E. P. Vollmer, eds.), pp. 161–178. Academic Press, New York.

Jensen, E. V., DeSombre, E. R., and Jungblut, P. W. (1967). *In* "Endogenous Factors Influencing Host Tumor Balance" (R. W. Wissler, T. L. Dao, and S. Wood, Jr., eds.), pp. 15–30. Univ. of Chicago Press, Chicago, Illinois.

Jensen, E. V., Suzuki, T., Kawashima, T., Stumpf, W. E., Jungblut, P. W., and DeSombre, E. R. (1968). *Proc. Natl. Acad. Sci. U.S.A.* **59,** 632–638.

Jensen, E. V., Block, G. E., Smith, S., Kyser, K., and DeSombre, E. R. (1971). *Natl. Cancer Inst., Monogr.* **34,** 55–70.

Jensen, E. V., Smith, S., and DeSombre, E. R. (1976). *J. Steroid Biochem.* **7,** 911–917.

Johnson, D. E., Scott, W. W., Gibbons, R. P., Prout, G. R., Schmidt, J. D., and Murphy, G. P. (1976). *Urology* **8,** 123–126.

Kelley, R. M., and Baker, W. H. (1961). *N. Engl. J. Med.* **264,** 216–222.

Kelley, R. M., and Baker, W. H. (1965). *Cancer Res.* **25,** 1190–1192.

Kennedy, B. J. (1962). *Cancer (Philadelphia)* **15,** 641–648.

Kent, J. R., Bischoff, A. J., Arduino, L. J., Mellinger, G. T., Byar, D. P., Hill, M., and Kozbur, X. (1973). *J. Urol.* **109,** 858–860.

Klein, L. A. (1979). *N. Engl. J. Med.* **300,** 824–833.

Knight, W. A., III, Livingston, R. B., Gregory, E. J., and McGuire, W. L. (1977). *Cancer Res.* **37,** 4669–4671.

Landau, R. L. (1979). *In* "Endocrinology" (L. J. DeGroot, ed.), Vol. 3, pp. 2111–2124. Grune & Stratton, New York.

Landau, R. L., Erlich, E. N., and Huggins, C. B. (1962). *J. Am. Med. Assoc.* **182,** 632–636.

Lippman, M. E., Halterman, R. H., Leventhal, B. G., Perry, S., and Thompson, E. B. (1973). *J. Clin. Invest.* **52,** 1715–1725.

Lippman, M. E., Perry, S., and Thompson, E. B. (1974). *Cancer Res.* **34,** 1572–1576.

Lippman, M. E., Perry, S., and Thompson, E. B. (1975). *Am. J. Med.* **59,** 224–227.

Lippman, M. E., Yarbro, G. K., and Leventhal, B. G. (1978). *Cancer Res.* **38,** 4251–4256.

Luft, R., and Olivecrona, H. (1953). *J. Neurosurg.* **10,** 301–316.

Luft, R., Olivecrona, H., Ikkos, D., Nilsson, L. B., and Mossberg, H. (1958). *In* "Endocrine Aspects of Breast Cancer" (A. R. Currie, ed.), pp. 27–35. Livingstone, Edinburgh.

Maass, H., Engel, B., Hohmeister, H., Lehmann, F., and Trams, G. (1972). *Am. J. Obstet. Gynecol.* **113,** 377–382.

McGuire, W. L. (1978). *Semin. Oncol.* **9,** 428–433.

McGuire, W. L., Carbone, P. P., and Vollmer, E. P., eds. (1975). "Estrogen Receptors in Human Breast Cancer." Raven, New York.

Mellinger, G. T., Bailar, J. D., III, and Arduino, L. J. (1967). *Surg., Gynecol. Obstet.* **124,** 1011–1017.

Menon, M., Tananis, C. E., McLaughlin, M. G., and Walsh, P. C. (1977). *Cancer Treat. Rep.* **61,** 265–271.

Nathanson, I. T. (1952). *Cancer (Philadelphia)* **5,** 754–762.

Nesbit, R. M., and Baum, W. C. (1950). *J. Am. Med. Assoc.* **143,** 1317–1320.

Nissen-Meyer, R., and Vogt, J. H. (1959). *Acta Unio Int. Contra Cancrum* **15,** 1140–1143.

Pearson, O. H., and Ray, B. S. (1960). *Am. J. Surg.* **99,** 544–552.

Pearson, O. H., Ray, B. S., Harrold, C. C., West, C. D., Li, M. C., Maclean, J. P., and Lipsett, M. B. (1956). *J. Am. Med. Assoc.* **161,** 17–21.

Ray, G. R., Cassady, J. R., and Bagshaw, M. A. (1973). *Radiology* **106,** 407–418.

Reifenstein, E. C., Jr. (1974). *Gynecol. Oncol.* **2,** 377–414.

Resnick, M. I., and Grayhack, J. T. (1978). *Urol. Clin. North Am.* **2,** 141–161.

Scott, W. W., and Boyd, H. L. (1969). *J. Urol.* **101,** 86–92.

Scott, W. W., and Schirmer, H. K. A. (1962). *In* "On Cancer and Hormones," pp. 175–204. Univ. of Chicago Press, Chicago, Illinois.

Segaloff, A. (1975). *Cancer Treat Rev.* **2,** 129–135.

Selye, H. (1937). *Endocrinology* **21,** 169–188.

Stoll, B. A. (1969). "Hormonal Management in Breast Cancer." Lippincott, Philadelphia, Pennsylvania.

Thompson, E. B. (1979). *Cancer Treat. Rep.* **63,** 189–195.

Volk, H., Deupree, R. H., Goldenberg, I. S., Wilde, R. C., Carabasi, R. A., and Escher, G. C. (1974). *Cancer (Philadelphia)* **33,** 9–13.

Ward, H. W. C. (1973). *Br. Med. J.* **i,** 13–14.

Wittliff, J. L. (1974). *Semin. Oncol.* **1,** 109–118.

12

A HUMAN TUMOR STEM CELL SYSTEM: CONCEPTS, METHODOLOGY, AND APPLICATION
Daniel D. Von Hoff

I. INTRODUCTION

A. The Stem Cell Concept

Work on the cell kinetics of normal tissues has led to the concept that for every renewal tissue in an adult there is a subpopulation of stem cells. These stem cells are defined as cells that can reproduce themselves (capacity of self-renewal) and also give rise to a differentiating line of mature and functional cells (Steel, 1975). In many tissues the identity and properties of stem cells have not been elucidated but for the bone marrow and intestinal epithelium there has been intense investigation (Steel, 1975; Pike and Robinson, 1970: Metcalf, 1977). It has been shown that the marrow stem cells make up a very small percentage (1%) of the marrow population (Pike and Robinson, 1970). Under normal circumstances they prolif-

CANCER AND CHEMOTHERAPY, VOL. III

erate rather slowly. In intestinal epithelium, most of the cells in the crypts of Lieberkuhn proliferate and rapidly migrate as a sheet onto the intestinal villi. Under normal circumstances only cells near the base of the crypts are the "effective" stem cells because all the progeny cells that are higher up on the villi are eventually lost by exfoliation (Steel, 1975). It is not known what proportion of the crypt cells is made up of stem cells.

Bearing in mind that many tumors retain some of the structural and morphological characteristics of the tissue of origin, it is possible to conceptualize that tumors may also have stem cell populations. A *tumor stem cell* is defined as a cell that gives rise to large numbers of tumor specific progeny cells and still has the ability to renew itself (make other stem cells). These tumor stem cells may be only a small proportion of the total number of tumor cells and they may be kinetically different from the majority of tumor cells (Steel, 1975).

It should be pointed out that at present the view that only a small proportion of of cells in primary tumors are potential stem cells is only a hypothesis. However, it is an attractive hypothesis which is gaining some scientific basis (Wilcox *et al.*, 1965; Bruce and Lin, 1969; Hill and Bush, 1969; Hewitt and Wilson, 1959; Brown and Carbone, 1971; Bruce *et al.*, 1966; Park *et al.*, 1971; Ogawa *et al.*, 1973; Roper and Drewinko, 1976; Preisler and Shoham, 1978; Hamburger *et al.*, 1979). If the tumor stem cell population is *the* important population that is responsible for tumor growth and if it is only a small percentage of the total number of tumor cells, it may explain a variety of phenomena:

1. The transplantation of experimental tumors into syngeneic recipients commonly requires much in excess of 10 cells for 50% takes (the TD_{50} inoculum). Tumors that have been frequently passaged in syngeneic recipients sometimes achieve TD_{50} values with as low as 1–2 cells but this could be due to the progressive selection of clonogenic cells. In contrast, primary tumors invariably have high TD_{50} values often *in excess of 10 cells* needed to start a tumor in another animal. This information (Steel, 1975) implies that only a small percentage of cells (possibly tumor stem cells) from a primary tumor have the ability to grow in another animal.

2. There is a very poor correlation between the labeling index of experimental tumors and the actual lethality of anticancer drugs for cells *in vitro* (Steel, 1975; Roper and Drewinko, 1976). It may be that labeling index data are dominated by cells that are incapable of contributing to regrowth and that the cells with the regrowth potential (i.e., the tumor stem cells) may form a kinetically atypical minority (Steel, 1975).

3. When the thymidine suicide index for human leukemic cells that produce clones *in vitro* was compared to the tritiated thymidine labeling index of the leukemic cells, the suicide index was five times greater than the thymidine labeling index. This important piece of work by Preisler and Shoham (1978) has

demonstrated that there is indeed a highly proliferative subpopulation of leukemic cells (*in vitro* colony-forming units) among the relatively slowly proliferating leukemic cells. This leads to speculation that there may be a similar subpopulation of cells in human solid tumors.

4. The *in vitro* colony-forming technique which purportedly grows the stem cells of a tumor was shown by Roper and Drewinko (1976) to be the most reliable dose-dependent index of cell lethality. Dye excretion, ^{51}Cr release, labeling index, and rate of [^{3}H]thymidine uptake (scintillation index), all tests that measure metabolic death, ''grossly overestimate or underestimate'' killing activity induced by anticancer drugs. They therefore found those techniques unreliable and not useful to predict loss of proliferative capacity. However, the *in vitro* colony-forming assay technique was a reliable index of cell lethality.

Since anticancer drugs that are useful in man have to cause sufficient injury to tumor cells that they lose their ability to regenerate, the human tumor stem cell assay, which is capable of measuring viable clones, should be a better way to assay for cells having regenerative capacity (i.e., those that survive chemotherapy).

In summary, there is increasing evidence that tumors do indeed have stem cell populations. A better understanding of the biology of these stem cells for solid tumors could have widespread therapeutic implications.

B. Specific Stem Cell Assay Systems

Clonogenic or stem cells may be detected in animal tumors by a variety of transplantation techniques, including the end-point dilution method (Hewitt and Wilson, 1959), the spleen colony or lung colony methods (Hill and Bush, 1969; Bruce *et al.*, 1966), regrowth assays (Wilcox *et al.*, 1965), and *in vitro* cloning (Brown and Carbone, 1971; Hermans and Barendsen, 1969). It is uncertain whether these various techniques measure the same population of cells (Steel, 1975). Because of recent developments outlined below, methods are now available to grow human tumor stem cells directly from biopsies in a clonogenic assay in semisolid media.

About 13 years ago Bruce and colleagues at the Ontario Cancer Institute demonstrated the potential for studying tumor stem cells from transplantable murine neoplasms by using a spleen colony assay (Bruce *et al.*, 1966). Subsequently, investigators from the same institute developed and tested an *in vitro* agar colony assay for transplantable BALB/c mouse myeloma which used irradiated tumor-inoculated spleen cells as a feeder layer (Park *et al.*, 1971). They further showed that the results obtained for drug assays against the tumor *in vitro* were predictive for *in vivo* results (Ogawa *et al.*, 1973). Unfortunately, primary explanation of human tumors for colony formation has met with little success; the major problems being the creation of an environment that gives tumor cells a selective advantage over normal cells (Hamburger and Salmon, 1977b). Two groups of investigators did have some success in obtaining colony growth in a soft agar system with pediatric solid tumors (rhabdomyosarcomas and hepatoblastomas) (McAllister and Reed, 1968; Altman *et al.*, 1975).

The major breakthrough in culturing progenitor cells of human tumors came with the work of Hamburger and Salmon (1977a,b; Hamburger *et al.*, 1978, 1979; Jones *et al.*, 1979; Salmon *et al.*, 1978). They devised a system using soft agar (with a bottom layer containing conditioned media from spleens of BALB/c mice primed with mineral oil) for assay of human myeloma stem cells (Hamburger and Salmon, 1977a,b; Hamburger *et al.*, 1979). Using this method they have been able to grow colonies from 75% of 70 patients with multiple myeloma or related monoclonal disorders (Hamburger and Salmon, 1977a,b). The number of colonies that grew was proportional to the number of cells plated (making a quantitative test of drug sensitivity a possibility). Morphological, histochemical, and functional criteria (including the presence of intracytoplasmic immunoglobulin) showed the colonies growing in the agar were myeloma cells. Clearly the methodology had now become available to grow human tumor stem cells in a soft agar system.

II. METHODOLOGY

The methodology for performing the human tumor stem cell assay system has been described by Hamburger and Salmon (1977a,b). Briefly (see Fig. 1), after appropriate informed consent is obtained according to institutional and federal guidelines malignant pleural fluid, malignant ascites, bone marrow containing tumor, or solid tumor specimens are collected in bottles or syringes containing preservative-free heparin (100 units/ml). Single-cell suspensions are made from

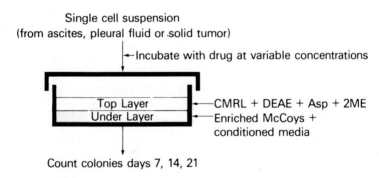

Fig. 1. Technique for human tumor stem cell assay (see text for complete description).

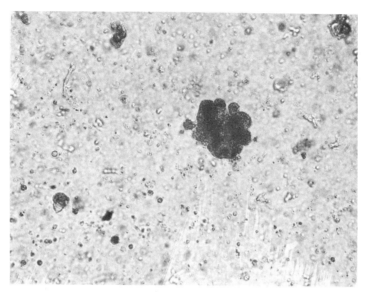

Fig. 2. Human squamous cell lung cancer colony growing in soft agar (inverted) miscroscope, 60× magnification.

the solid tumors by mincing them with a scalpel, teasing apart with needles, and passing through 20, 22, and 25 gauge needles. The cells are washed twice in Hank's balanced salt solution (Grand Island Biological Co., Grand Island, N.Y.) with 10% heat-inactivated fetal calf serum (Grand Island Biological Co., Grand Island, N.Y.). The viability of bone marrow, ascites, and solid tumor specimens is determined in a hemocytometer with trypan blue.

Cells to be tested are suspended in 0.3% agar in enriched CMRL 1066 medium (Grand Island Biological Co.) supplemented with 15% horse serum, penicillin (100 units/ml), streptomycin (2 mg/ml), glutamine (2 mM), CaCl$_2$ (4 mM), and insulin (3 units/ml). Just prior to plating, asparagine (0.6 mg/ml) DEAE-dextran (0.5 mg/ml) (Pharmacia Fine Chemical, Div. of Pharmacia, Inc., Piscutaway, N.J.), and freshly prepared 2-mercaptoethanol (final concentration 50 uM) are added to the cells. One milliliter of the resultant mixture is pipetted onto 1-ml feeder layers in 35-mm plastic petri dishes. The final concentration of cells in each culture is 5 × 10^3 cells in 1 ml of agar–medium mixture. The feeder layer consists of McCoy's 5A medium plus 15% heat-inactivated fetal calf serum and variety of nutrients as described by Pike and Robinson (1970). Immediately before use, 10 ml of 3% tryptic soy broth (Grand Island Biological Co.), 0.6 ml of asparagine, and 0.3 ml of DEAE-dextran are added to 4.0 ml of the enriched medium. Agar (0.5% final concentration) is added to the enriched medium and underlayers are poured in 35-mm petri dishes.

The feeder layer used by Hamburger and Salmon (1977a,b) consists of 1 ml of the enriched McCoy's 5A medium as described above along with 0.5% agar and with varying concentrations of millipore-filtered medium conditioned by the adherent spleen cells of mineral-oil-primed BALB/c mice.

After preparation of both bottom and top layers, cultures are incubated at 37° in a 7.5% CO_2 humidified atmosphere.

Cultures are examined with an inverted-phase microscope at ×20, ×100, and ×200. Colony counts are made 5, 10, 15, and 20 days after plating. Aggregates of 50 or more cells are considered colonies (see Fig. 2) (Salmon and Buick, 1979).

For drug studies, single-cell suspensions of tumor cells are incubated with clinically achievable concentrations of an anticancer drug for 1 hr at 37°C. A control tube without drug is also incubated. After incubation, the cells are washed twice to remove the drug and the cells are plated in a top layer of agar over a bottom layer of media-containing agar. All plating is done in triplicate. The plates are incubated at 37°, 7% CO_2, and 100% humidity. Plates are examined at 7 and 14 days. On day 14 the number of colonies on drug-treated plates

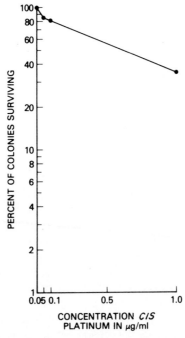

Fig. 3. Drug sensitivity (survival) curve. This curve represents *in vitro* survival of ovarian carcinoma stem cell colonies after incubation with *cis*-platinum. Only a 61% kill of colonies was noted. The patient did not respond clinically to the drug.

will be determined and compared to the number of colonies on control plates. Results are plotted as percent colonies surviving versus concentration of drug (see Fig. 3).

III. APPLICATIONS

A. Type of Tumors That Can Be Grown

Using the system described earlier (along with the use of conditioned media in the bottom layer of agar) Hamburger and Salmon attempted to grow a variety of metastatic cancers with some success, including oat cell carcinoma of the lung, non-Hodgkin's lymphoma, adenocarcinoma of the ovary, melanoma, and neuroblastoma (Hamburger and Salmon, 1977b). They have recently extended their observations in ovarian carcinoma with 85% of 31 ovarian cancer biopsy and effusion specimens forming tumor colonies *in vitro* (Hamburger *et al.*, 1978). Morphological and histochemical criteria confirmed that the colonies consisted of cells with the same characteristics as the original tumor. Results of cytogenetic studies were also consistent with a malignant origin for the tumor colonies.

A number of additional studies have been done to document that the colonies growing in the agar are the same as the tumor in the patient. Studies in our laboratories have confirmed that histologies of the tumor colonies *in vitro* are similar to the tumor in man for colon and breast carcinoma, melanoma, ovarian carcinoma, and neuroblastoma. In addition, we have found that the tumor colonies secrete a number of tumor markers such as melanogens, catecholamines, somatostatin, and acid phosphatase (Von Hoff and Johnson, 1979).

From the preliminary studies there is good evidence that the tumor cells grown in culture are producing the same tumor markers that they are producing in the patient. This information provides additional evidence that the human tumor stem cell culture system reflects the *in vivo* situation.

The human tumor stem cell system has also been more extensively studied in non-Hodgkin's lymphoma. Lymphoid colony growth was obtained in 11 (61%) of 18 bone marrows microscopically involved by tumor and in 3 (50%) of 6 lymph nodes histologically involved by lymphocytic lymphoma. Conversely, colony growth was observed in only a single instance from 49 bone marrows without overt lymphoma and was not observed in cultures of 4 normal lymph nodes, 2 normal spleens, 10 normal bone marrows, and 6 peripheral blood specimens (Jones *et al.*, 1979).

Our laboratory has also developed extensive experience with the human tumor stem cell assay system (Von Hoff and Johnson, 1979). As noted in Table I, we have been able to grow a wide variety of malignancies, including some of the most common tumor types (lung cancer, colon cancer, breast cancer, etc.).

TABLE I

Growth of Tumor Stem Cell Colonies from Various Human Neoplasms

Type of tumor (source of sample)[a]	Number of patients with + culture/total tested
Ovarian (A,T,P)	27/35
Neuroblastoma (M)	21/26
Melanoma (P,N,T)	10/16
Colorectal (A)	7/10
Breast (A,T,P)	8/12
Lung cancer (T,M,P)	
Oat cell	11/14
Squamous cell	12/13
Adenocarcinoma	6/7
Head and neck	7/16
Testicular (T)	2/4
Multiple myeloma	3/5
Osteogenic sarcoma (T)	3/5
Rhabdomyosarcoma (M,T)	3/6
Islet cell carcinoma (T)	3/3
Endometrial	3/3
Pancreatic carcinoma	4/4
Cervix	3/3
Ewing's sarcoma (M)	2/2
Renal	2/3
Thyroid (T)	1/2
Hepatoma	2/2
Prostate	3/5
Wilms	1/2
T cell lymphoma (P)	1/1
Parathyroid	1/1
Burkitt's lymphoma (T)	0/1
Hodgkin's disease (T)	0/1
CML	0/1
Glioma (T)	0/1
Thymoma	0/1
Undifferentiated sarcoma (P)	0/1
CLL	0/2
Malignant fibrous histio. (T)	0/1
Hairy cell leukemia	0/1
Normal marrow (M)	0/6

[a] A—ascites, P—pleural fluid, T—solid tumor, M—marrow, N—lymph node. Overall, 146 of the 209 tumors attempted have grown (70%).

Both adult and pediatric malignancies have been grown. Clearly, a large spectrum of tumor types can be grown from a variety of sources using the human tumor stem cell assay system described by Hamburger and Salmon (1977b).

B. Determining Chemosensitivity of an Individual Patient's Tumor

The most important clinical development with the *in vitro* stem cell assay came from Salmon and colleagues with their report of using the system to quantitate the differential sensitivity of human tumors to various anticancer agents (Salmon *et al.*, 1978). Using the *in vitro* stem cell assay they performed 32 retrospective or prospective clinical studies in nine patients with myeloma and nine with ovarian cancer. These patients were treated with standard anticancer drugs which were also tested *in vitro*. Each tumor was cultured using the stem cell assay technique after incubation of the single-cell suspension with various drug concentrations for 1 hr. The number of colonies that eventually grew out on drug-treated specimens was compared to the number of colonies on control plates. The data were expressed as colonies surviving versus drug concentration. In eight cases of myeloma and in three cases of ovarian carcinoma *in vitro* sensitivity* corresponded with *in vivo* sensitivity whereas in one case of myeloma it did not. *In vitro* resistance correlated with clinical resistance in all 5 comparisons in myeloma and all 15 in ovarian cancer. They concluded that the assay warranted larger-scale testing to determine its efficacy for selection of new agents and for individualization of cancer chemotherapy regimens.

Their experience was recently updated (Salmon *et al.*, 1979). There have been 92 *in vitro–in vivo* correlations available for 20 patients with ovarian cancer and 16 patients with multiple myeloma. Sixteen correlations demonstrated sensitivity *in vitro* and *in vivo,* eight showed sensitivity *in vitro* and resistance *in vivo* (false positive test), one was resistant *in vitro* and sensitive *in vivo* (false negative test), and 67 showed both *in vivo* and *in vitro* resistance. Overall, then, in myeloma and ovarian cancer the false positive rate for the system is 8/92 (9%) and the "false negative" rate is 1/92 (1%). These early correlations are impressive and certainly warrant rapid, well-designed follow-up studies.

C. Screening for New Antineoplastics

The human tumor stem cell assay system provides a unique method to screen for new antineoplastic agents. Recently our laboratory has been screeening a number of "high-priority" agents that have been found active in conventional

---

*As defined by area under the drug sensitivity curve.

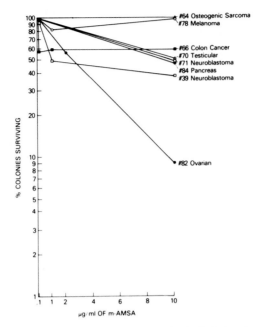

Fig. 4. Effect of *m*-AMSA on a variety of tumors growing in the human tumor stem cell assay system.

animal tumor screens. Currently some of these compounds include ICRF-187, methly GAG, *m*-AMSA, and PALA. Figure 4 shows the results from a number of tumors that *m*-AMSA has been tested against *in vitro*. One patient's tumor (ovarian cancer) (number 82) showed a significant response to *m*-AMSA *in vitro*. She received the drug and attained a partial response. The other tumors tested were refractory *in vitro*.

It is possible that in the near future the human tumor stem cell assay systems will be used to choose new antineoplastics for clinical development as well as to screen for new analogues of compounds with clinically established antitumor activity (Von Hoff and Bradley, 1979).

IV. CONCLUSIONS

From the preceding discussion it is clear that there is mounting evidence that tumors have self-renewing populations of cells that have the capacity both to make other self-renewing cells or to give rise to large numbers of tumor-specific progeny cells. These tumor stem cells may be the important cells against which cytotoxic chemotherapy should be directed. Recent developments have made it possible to culture human tumor progenitor or stem cells.

As noted in the earlier discussion, it is clear that a large spectrum of tumor types can be grown from a variety of sources using the human tumor stem cell assay system designed by Hamburger and Salmon (1977a, 1977b). Not all tumors of a given type of tumor will grow, and additional work to improve success rates is needed.

From the preliminary studies presented earlier there is good evidence that the tumor cells growing in culture are producing the same markers that they are producing in the patient. This information provides additional evidence that the human tumor stem cell assay system closely reflects the *in vivo* situation.

The questions of specificity for tumor growth, low plating efficiency, time and resource consumption, and other difficulties for clinical application remain problems. At this point none of these problems seem insurmountable given additional targeted research in those areas.

Finally, two examples of possible clinical applications of the human tumor stem cell assay system are detailed. These examples showed the potential utility of the system for predicting the response or lack of response of an individual patient's tumor to a particular drug. They also showed that the system can be used to screen new compounds for antineoplastic activity.

The initial experience with the human tumor stem cell assay suggests that the clinical and basic science applications of the system are of potential significance.

REFERENCES

Altman, A. J., Crussi, F. G., Rierden, W. J., and Baehner, R. L. (1975). *Cancer Res.* **35,** 1809–1811.

Brown, C. H., and Carbone, P. P. (1971). *J. Natl. Cancer Inst.* **46,** 989–996.

Bruce, W. R., and Lin, H. (1969), *Cancer Res.* **29,** 2308–2310.

Bruce, W. R., Meeker, B. E., and Valeriote, F. A. (1966). *J. Natl. Cancer Inst.* **37,** 233–243.

Hamburger, A. W., and Salmon, S. E. (1977a). *J. Clin. Invest.* **60,** 846–854.

Hamburger, A. W., and Salmon, S. E. (1977b). *Science* **197,** 461–463.

Hamburger, A. W., Salmon, S. E., Kim, M. B., Trent, J. M., Soehnlen, B. J., Alberts, D. S., and Schmidt, H. J. (1978). *Cancer Res.* **38,** 3438–3444.

Hamburger, A. W., Kim, M. B., and Salmon, S. W. (1979). *J. Cell. Physiol,* **98,** 371–376.

Hermans, A.F., and Barendsen, G. W. (1969). *Eur. J. Cancer* **5,** 173–176.

Hewitt, H. B., and Wilson, C. W. (1959). *Br. J. Cancer* **13,** 69–75.

Hill, R. P., and Bush, R. S. (1969). *Int. J. Radiat. Biol.* **15,** 435–437.

Jones, S. E., Hamburger, A. W., Kim, M. B., and Salmon, S. E. (1979). *Blood,* **53,** 294–303.

McAllister, R. M., and Reed, G. (1968). *Pediat. Res.* **2,** 356–360.

Metcalf, D. (1977). *Ann. Intern. Med* **87,** 483–488.

Ogawa, M., Bergsagel, D. E., and McCulloch, E. A. (1973). *Blood* **41,** 7–15.

Park, C. H., Bergsagel, D. E., and McCulloch, E. A. (1971). *J. Natl. Cancer Inst.* **46,** 411–420.

Pike, B. L., and Robinson, W. A. (1970). *J. Cell. Physiol.* **76**, 77–81.

Preisler, H., and Shoham, D. (1978). *Cancer Res.* **38**, 3681–3684.

Roper, P. R., and Drewinko, B. (1976). *Cancer Res.* **36**, 2182–2188.

Salmon, S. E., and Buick, R. M. (1979). *Cancer Res.* **39**, 1133–1136.

Salmon, S. E., Hamburger, A. W., Soehnlen, B., Durie, B. G., Alberts, D. S., and Moon, T. E. (1978). *N. Eng. J. Med.* **298**, 1321–1327.

Salmon, S. W., Soehnlen, B.J., Durie, B. G. M., Alberts, D. S., Meyskens, F. L., Chen, H. S. G., and Moon, T. E. (1979). *Proc. AACR/ASCO* **20**, 340.

Steel, G. G. (1975). *In* "Medical Oncology—Medical Aspects of Malignant Disease" (K. D. Bagshawe, ed.) p. 49. Blackwell, Oxford.

Von Hoff, D. D., and Bradley, E. C. (1979). *Proc. Int. Cong. Antimicrobials and Chemoth., IX.* Abstract #920.

Von Hoff, D. D., and Johnson, G. E. (1979). *Proc. AACR/ASCO* **20**, 51.

Wilcox, W. S., Griswald, D. P., Laster, W. R., Schabel, F. M., and Skipper, H. F. (1965). *Cancer Chemother. Rep.* **47**, 27–39.

Part II
Molecular
Pharmacology of
Selected Antineoplastic
Agents

13

THE MOLECULAR PHARMACOLOGY
OF BLEOMYCIN
Stanley T. Crooke

I. INTRODUCTION

Since its discovery by Umezawa and colleagues in 1966 (Umezawa *et al.*, 1966), bleomycin has proven of value in the treatment of several human malignancies; however, at least as interesting as its clinical activities has been the molecular pharmacology of bleomycin. Its unique structure and unusual effects on DNA and the cell not only have proven of interest relative to bleomycin but have introduced a variety of questions concerning the mechanism of several other antineoplastic agents.

CANCER AND CHEMOTHERAPY, VOL. III

II. CHEMISTRY

The structures of bleomycin and several analogues of interest are shown in Fig. 1. Bleomycin analogues may be divided into two groups of molecular pharmacological interest. The first group, and by far the largest, is the group in which the belomycinic acid portion of the molecule is constant, and the terminal amine varies. The second group is composed of compounds that vary in the bleomycinic acid portion of the molecule. Compounds that have minor modifications include phleomycin, isobleomycin A_2, desamidobleomycin, and zorbamycin and zorbonamycin (Crooke and Bradner, 1977). Compounds in which the bleomycinic acid portion is modified significantly include tallysomycin and the various degradative products of tallysomycin and bleomycin such as W_a and W_b peptides. These analogues have been employed extensively in the evolution of the understanding of the molecular pharmacology of bleomycin.

III. THE INTERACTIONS OF METALS WITH BLEOMYCIN AND ANALOGUES

It is now clearly established that bleomycin can chelate a variety of divalent cations and that metal chelation has pronounced effects on the conformation and activities of bleomycin. Thus a discussion of bleomycin molecular pharmacology must include a discussion of the effects of metals on bleomycin.

Bleomycin and analogues bind avidly to Co(II), Cu(II), Zn(II), Fe(II), and Fe(III). They do not bind to Mg(II) or Mn(II) (Dabrowiak *et al.*, 1978a,b).

The site at which Fe(II), Cu(II), and Zn(II) bind has been defined by several types of experiments. The site proposed by Dabrowiak and colleagues for bleomycin A_2 and tallysomycin (Dabrowiak *et al.*, 1978a,b) is a four-coordination site that is comprised of the primary amine of the β-aminoalanine, the N_1 of the pyrimidine, N_1 of the imidazole, and the amino group of the carbamoyl group and is shown in Fig. 2. A slightly different complex structure (square pyramidal geometry) has recently been proposed (Takita *et al.*, 1978). In this complex structure the N^π and the deprotonated amide nitrogens of histidine, the N(1) of the pyrimidine and the secondary amine serve as the square coordination sites. The α-NH_2 of the β-aminoalanine serves as the apical site, and the sixth site may be ligated with the carbamoyl group in the Cu(II) complex or molecular oxygen in the Fe(II) complex.

Although Fe(II) binds to approximately the same site as Cu(II), Zn(II), and Fe (III), the effects are distinctly different. When Fe(II) is added to bleomycin A_2 in the presence of oxygen, it is very rapidly oxidized to Fe(III), which evidently remains bound to bleomycin A_2 (Sausville *et al.*, 1976). In the absence of DNA the oxidation of Fe(II) bound to bleomycin has been reported to fragment some of

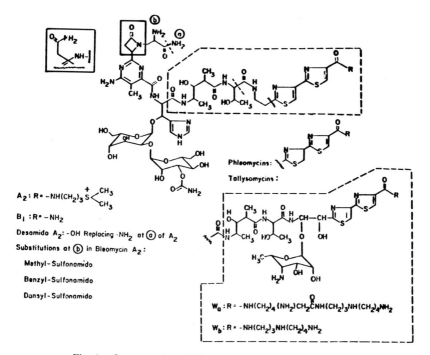

A₂ : R = $-NH(CH_2)_3\overset{+}{S}\underset{CH_3}{\overset{CH_3}{\diagdown}}$

B₁ : R = $-NH_2$

Desamido A₂ : $-OH$ Replacing $-NH_2$ at (a) of A₂

Substitutions at (b) in Bleomycin A₂ :

  Methyl-Sulfonamido

  Benzyl-Sulfonamido

  Dansyl-Sulfonamido

Phleomycins :

Tallysomycins :

Wₐ : R = $-NH(CH_2)_4(NH_2)CH_2\overset{O}{\overset{\|}{C}}NH(CH_2)_3NH(CH_2)_4NH_2$

W_b : R = $-NH(CH_2)_3NH(CH_2)_4NH_2$

Fig. 1.   Structure of tested bleomycin-related drug compounds.

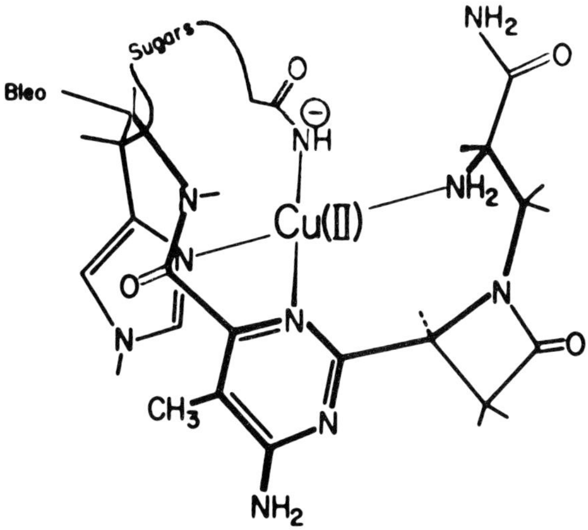

Fig. 2.   Metal-binding site of bleomycin.

the bleomycin molecules (Umezawa, 1979). Furthermore, the oxidation of Fe(II) attached to bleomycin has been shown to generate free radicals (Sausville *et al.*, 1978; Lown and Sim, 1977).

The bleomycins are fluorescent, and the predominant source of fluorescence is the bithiazole (Chien *et al.*, 1977; Strong and Crooke, 1978). The addition of various cations to bleomycin analogues results in quenching of fluorescence. However, the fluorescence quenching induced by Fe(II) is much greater than that of other ions for active bleomycin analogues. Moreover, the quenching induced by Fe(II) is significantly greater in active analogues than in inactive analogues, and no other ion tested behaves similarly. Table I presents a summary of these results (Huang *et al.*, 1979). The fact that metal binding at a site distant from the bithiazole fluor induces quenching of the fluorescence spectrum suggests that significant conformational changes result in the bleomycin molecule on binding a cation (Huang *et al.*, 1979).

The effects of various metals on the DNA degradative activity of bleomycin analogues have been studied and suggest that metals play a key role in the mechanism of action of bleomycin. Copper (II) and Zn(II) have been reported to inhibit degradation of DNA by bleomycin and analogues (Suzuki *et al.*, 1968;

TABLE I

A Comparison of the DNA Breakage Activity with the Maximal Fluorescence Quenching by Fe(II) of Various Bleomycin-Related Compounds. The Reaction Conditions for the Fluorescence Quenching and the DNA Breakage Were as Described in the Section on Materials and Methods

	EC_{50} for DNA breakage[a] (ng/ml)	Residual fluorescence after quenching[b] (%)
Bleomycin A_2	78	20
Phleomycin D_1	80	37
Tallysomycin A	80	49
Bleomycin $B_1{}'$	135	25
Desamido-bleomycin A_2	220	20
Methylsulfonamido-bleomycin A_2	3900	80
Benzylsulfonamido bleomycin A_2	2500	70
Dansylsulfonamido-bleomycin A_2	2500	77
W_a	inactive	82
W_b	inactive	82

[a] Concentration for drugs to cause breaks of 50% DNA molecules.
[b] The residual fluorescence level after maximal quenching by Fe(II).

Nagai *et al.*, 1969; Ishida and Takahashi, 1975; Lown and Sim, 1977; Dabrowiak *et al.*, 1978a,b; Takita *et al.*, 1978; Sausville *et al.*, 1976; Sleight, 1976). The addition of Fe(II) salts to bleomycin has been reported to stimulate markedly the DNA degradative activity of bleomycin (Lown and Sim, 1977; Sausville *et al.*, 1976, 1978). Indeed, it has been proposed (as will be discussed) that bleomycin degrades DNA via an Fe(II) oxidation-dependent reaction (Lown and Sim, 1977; Sausville *et al.*, 1978). Other metals have also been reported to have no effect or to stimulate or inhibit degradation indirectly by affecting the conformation of the DNA (Takashita *et al.*, 1976).

IV. EFFECTS OF BLEOMYCIN ON ISOLATED DNA

A. Binding

That bleomycin and analogues bind to DNA has been demonstrated by several techniques, including experiments employing radioactively labeled bleomycin (Suzuki *et al.*, 1969), ultraviolet and circular dichroic spectroscopy (Krueger *et al.*, 1973), equilibrium dialysis (Chien *et al.*, 1977), perturbed gamma-ray angular correlations (Sastry *et al.*, 1978), fluorescence quenching (Chien *et al.*, 1977; Strong and Crooke, 1978; Povirk *et al.*, 1977). Although the bithiazole portion of the molecule appears to be most intimately involved in DNA binding, the precise nature of this interaction is poorly understood. Currently, the consensus is that the bithiazole portion of the molecule binds to DNA via an intercalative interaction (Mvrakami *et al.*, 1976, Taira, 1976; Povirk *et al.*, 1977; Müller and Zahn, 1977; Chien *et al.*, 1977). The terminal amine structure appears to enhance binding via ionic interactions with the negatively charged phosphate groups in the DNA.

B. Excision of Bases

During the reaction of bleomycin with DNA *in vitro*, free bases are released. At lower concentrations, thymine is released selectively; at high concentrations, all four bases are released (Haidle *et al.*, 1972; Haidle, 1971; Ishida and Takahashi, 1975; Takashita *et al.*, 1976; Müller and Zahn, 1976; Müller *et al.*, 1972). A variety of experiments have suggested that the release of free bases is due to the hydrolysis of *N*-glycosidic bonds in DNA (Müller *et al.*, 1972; Haidle *et al.*, 1972; Müller and Zahn, 1977). The amount of release of free bases is directly proportional to the adenosine and thymidine content of the DNA, and also appears to be affected by molecular topology of the DNA (Müller and Zahn, 1977). Other factors that affect the extent and specificity of the reaction include bleomycin concentration and the presence of reducing agents.

Removal of bases results in alkali lability, that is, the induction of sites in DNA that on treatment with alkali become sites of strand scission (Ross and Moses, 1978; Strong and Crooke, 1978). It has been suggested that the alkali lability induced is due to intercalation of bleomycin rather than alkylation (Ross and Moses, 1978).

C. Strand Scission

In addition to excission of bases and induction of alkali labile sites, bleomycin induces single- and double-strand breaks in DNA. The reaction is highly substrate specific. Although it binds to RNA, bleomycin does not degrade RNA (Umezawa, 1976; Müller *et al.*, 1972; Haidle *et al.*, 1972). Moreover, bleomycin has been shown to be capable of selectively degrading the DNA strand in a DNA–RNA copolymer (Haidle and Bearden, 1975). It has been suggested that this specificity results from the presence of deoxyribose moieties in DNA (Haidle and Bearden, 1975) and is not due to the presence of uracil or the less secondary structure in RNA relative to DNA.

Single-strand DNA has been shown to be approximately as sensitive as double-strand DNA (Kuo *et al.*, 1973; Umezawa, 1973). Incubation of DNA with relatively high concentrations of bleomycin has been reported to result in limit degradation products with a molecular weight of approximately 4000 daltons that are resistant to degradation by bleomycin (Kuo *et al.*, 1973; Crooke *et al.*, 1975). The bleomycin-resistant DNA has been reported to have a base composition approximately equivalent to that of bleomycin-sensitive DNA, and the number of nucleotides (12–13) is larger than the number of nucleotides per bleomycin binding sites (3–4) (Strong and Crooke, 1978; Sastry *et al.*, 1978). Thus there is no apparent explanation for the resistance of these fragments to degradation by bleomycin.

Bleomycin has been demonstrated to induce degradation selectively at certain sites within DNA determined by the nucleotide sequence. The nucleotide sequence specificity was first suggested by studies comparing the sensitivity of nucleolar and extranucleolar DNA to degradation by bleomycin (Crooke *et al.*, 1975). More recently, a total of 11 discrete sites in the PM-2 DNA genome have been shown to be susceptible to cleavage by bleomycin (Fig. 3) (Lloyd *et al.*, 1978a,b). It has also been shown to cleave DNA preferentially at G-C and G-T sites (and to a much less degree, TA)(D'Andrea and Haseltine, 1978).

Various factors alter the rate and extent of DNA degradation in addition to the effects of variations in the substrate previously discussed. Divalent cations affect the reaction. Fe(II) has been shown to stimulate the reaction markedly. Cu(II) and Zn(II) have been shown to inhibit DNA degradation. Fe(III) and Mg(II) have been shown to have little effect on the reaction. EDTA inhibits degradation

(Muller and Zahn, 1978, for review). The pH and temperature of incubation affect degradation with the optimal pH being approximately 9 and the optimum temperature being 37° (Strong and Crooke, 1978). The presence of reducing or oxidizing agents stimulates the reaction.

D. Proposed DNA Degradative Reaction Mechanism

As a result of studies demonstrating the effects of Fe(II) and reducing agents on degradation of DNA by bleomycin, two groups have proposed that bleomycin degrades DNA via oxidation of Fe(II) to Fe(III) and generation of free radicals. Thus bleomycin has two functions: (1) to bind to DNA and (2) to bind to Fe(II) and facilitate its oxidation in the presence of DNA. A mechanism has been proposed for DNA degradation by Lown and Sim. (Lown and Sim, 1977; Sausville *et al.*, 1976). It is unclear whether the excision of bases and DNA degradation are independent processes or are linked.

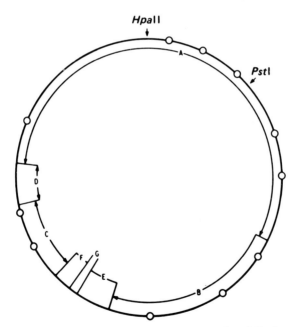

Fig. 3.   Map of regions on the PM-2 DNA genome that are preferentially cleaved by bleomycin (open circles). A–G indicate the fragments formed by *Hind* III action on PM-2 DNA. *HPA* II and *Pst*I sites are indicated by arrows. (Adapted from Haidle *et al.*, 1979.)

V. CELLULAR EFFECTS

A. Degradation of Intracellular DNA

Bleomycin has been shown to bind to the DNA of hepatoma cells in tissue culture. Approximately 30–50% of the radioactive bleomycin that was taken up by sensitive cells was found in nuclei, and approximately 0.7% was found in DNA. Sensitive cells were reported to bind 8.7 times as much bleomycin to DNA and to experience 8 times as many breaks in DNA as resistant cells (Miyaki *et al.*, 1975).

Bleomycin treatment of a variety of cells has been shown to result in DNA degradation. Treatment of hepatoma cells, L cells, and fibroblasts has been reported to induce breakage demonstrable by alkaline sucrose density centrifugation, and double-strand breaks have also been demonstrated (Cox *et al.*, 1975; Miyaki *et al.*, 1973, 1975; Saito and Andoh, 1973). Repair of DNA has been shown to be stimulated by bleomycin in a number of cell lines (Sartiano *et al.*, 1973, 1975; Saito and Andoh, 1973). Alkaline elution has also been employed to show that bleomycin degrades intracellular DNA and that both DNA degradation and cytotoxicity are enhanced when the pH of the tissue culture medium is increased above pH 7.3 (Iqbal *et al.*, 1976; Kohn and Wig, 1976). The treatment of isolated nuclei from Chinese hamster cells was reported to release nucleosomes by selectively degrading linker DNA at or near nucleosomes (Kuo and Hsu, 1978). Furthermore, bleomycin treatment of tumor cells has been shown to result in chromosomal damage (Hittleman and Rao, 1974; Paika and Krishan, 1973).

B. Effects on Macromolecular Syntheses

DNA synthesis has been shown to be inhibited in all cells sensitive to bleomycin and is the most sensitive of the macromolecular syntheses to the effects of bleomycin (Crooke and Bradner, 1977). Bleomycin also inhibits the synthesis of RNA, but only at much higher concentrations than those required to inhibit DNA synthesis (Crooke and Bradner, 1977; Suzuki *et al.*, 1968). The inhibition of RNA synthesis is apparently nonspecific and no effects on the functionality of messenger RNA were detected (Kuo *et al.*, 1973), although atypically small fragments of nucleolar RNA were reported, probably because of abortive synthesis from nicked template (Crooke *et al.*, 1975). Protein synthesis is also inhibited but little information is available about the specificities of the inhibitory effects of bleomycin.

C. Other Effects

Bleomycin has been shown to inhibit DNA-dependent DNA polymerase activity. The inhibition is preceded by a brief phase of stimulation. The stimulation is probably due to induction of nicks allowing more initiation sites for DNA polymerase, and inhibition is probably due to more extensive DNA degradation (Müller and Zahn, 1977). DNA-dependent RNA polymerase is also inhibited again probably by degradation of the DNA template. Deoxyribonucleases have been reported to be inhibited by effects of bleomycin on DNA (Müller et al., 1973). Ribonucleases and phosphodiesterases were unaffected.

VI. EFFECTS ON THE CELL CYCLE

Bleomycin is cytotoxic to dividing and nondividing cells in vitro. It is also cytotoxic during all phases of the cell cycle. However, nondividing or plateau phase cells of several lines have been shown to be most sensitive to bleomycin (Barranco, 1978). Moreover, dividing cells are most sensitive during early G_2 and M phases of the cell cycle (Terasima and Umezawa, 1970; Barranco and Humphrey, 1971).

Bleomycin also blocks cell cycle progression, and progression delay is specific for cells in the G_2 phase of the cell cycle (Kunimoto et al., 1967; Baranco and Humphrey, 1971; Tobey and Crissmen, 1972). Cells treated in mitosis, G_1, or S have been shown to experience no delay in cell cycle traverse. The effects of bleomycin on cell cycle traverse have not been correlated with inhibition of macromolecular syntheses however (Tobey and Crissman, 1972).

Bleomycin has also been reported to induce potentially lethal damage (PLD). It has been reported that when cells were treated with bleomycin, then held for 2–6 hr prior to plating, survival was greater than for cells that were plated immediately (Barranco et al., 1975). Furthermore, cells in mitosis did not demonstrate this phenomenon (Barranco and Bolton, 1977). These studies suggest that cells treated with bleomycin can recover, perhaps by repair DNA synthesis, and that cells in mitosis may be more sensitive to bleomycin because they cannot recover from potentially lethal damage (Barranco, 1978; Terasima et al., 1976).

VII. MORPHOLOGICAL EFFECTS

Bleomycin-treated cells have been shown to be larger than untreated cells and to have multiple nuclei that were often bizzare and enlarged (Krishan, 1973; Daskal et al., 1975). The predominant morphological lesion however, has been observed to be alterations in nucleolar morphology, including segregation, extrusion of fibrillar components, and induction of microspherules (Daskal et al., 1975; Madreiter et al., 1976). These effects have also been observed in human beings treated with bleomycin (Yasuzumi et al., 1976; Daskal and Gyorkey,

1978). Other effects include chromosomal aberrations (Paika and Krischan, 1973; Hittleman and Rao, 1974; Daskal and Gyorkey, 1978).

VIII. INTRACELLULAR FATE AND METABOLISM

Relatively little is understood about the intracellular fate and metabolism of bleomycin. Although bleomycin sensitive cells have been reported to incorporate greater amounts of bleomycin into cells, and DNA, and to experience more DNA breakage than a resistant cell line (Miyaki *et al.*, 1975), these studies have not been reproduced, and in other cell lines, much lower uptake of bleomycin has been observed. Once taken up by cells, bleomycin has been reported to localize to the nucleus and/or nuclear membrane.

Bleomycin hydrolase, an enzyme that metabolizes bleomycin, has been reported. It is an aminopeptidase that cleaves the amide group of the β-amino alanine moiety (Umezawa *et al.*, 1974). The product of that reaction, desamidobleomycin, has been reported to be one-twentieth as active as its parent compound in DNA breakage antibacterial activities (Umezawa, 1976). However, in other systems desamidobleomycin A_2 has been found to be more active than previously reported.

Bleomycin hydrolase is localized to the 105,000 g supernatant, and the content of the enzyme varies, depending on the cell type and tissue studied (Yoshioka *et al.*, 1978). It has been suggested that the sensitivity to the toxicities and antitumor activities of bleomycin is inversely proportional to the level of this enzyme (Yoshioka *et al.*, 1978).

Bleomycin has also been reported to be degraded by a low-molecular-weight fraction obtained from the 105,000 g supernatant of tumor cells, and this inactivation was directly proportional to the ascorbic acid concentration (Onishi *et al.*, 1975; Yoshioka *et al.*, 1978). The low-molecular-weight fraction-induced degradation apparently is independent of bleomycin hydrolase and varies, depending on the tissue studied. Thus both mechanisms may be important in the intracellular degradation of bleomycin.

It has also been proposed that there is an intracellular system that removes copper from bleomycin and thus activates it to induce DNA degradation and presumably induce cytotoxicity (Umezawa, 1976). Essentially nothing is known about further metabolic interactions or potential receptors other than DNA.

IX. CONCLUSIONS

The bleomycins are a group of glycopeptides that chelate metal ions and interact with DNA. They also facilitate the oxidation of Fe(II). It is thought that these two capacities allow the bleomycins to degrade isolated DNA and intracellular DNA resulting in inhibition of replication. Bleomycin is most effective in M and G_2 phases of the cell cycle and against nondividing cells. Intracellular metabolism and distribution are complex and only poorly understood.

REFERENCES

Barranco, S. C. (1978). *In* "Bleomycin—Current Status and New Developments" (S. K. Carter, S. T. Cooke, and H. Umezawa, eds.), pp. 81–90. Academic Press, New York.

Barranco, S. C., and Bolton, W. E. (1977). *Cancer Res.* **32**, 2726–2732.

Barranco, S. C., and Humphrey, R. M. (1971). *Cancer Res.* **31**, 1218–1223.

Barranco, S. C., Novack, J. K., and Humphrey, R. M. (1975). *Cancer Res.* **35**, 1194–1204.

Chien, M., Grollman, A. P., and Horwitz, S. B. (1977). *Biochemistry* **16**, 3641–3646.

Cox, R., Daoud, A. H., and Irving, C. C. (1974). *Biochem. Pharmacol.* **23**, 3147–3151.

Crooke, S. T., and Bradner, W. T. (1977). *J. Med. (Basel)* **7**, 333–428.

Crooke, S. T., Sitz, T. O., Bannon, M., and Busch, H. (1975). *Physiol. Chem. Phys.* **7**, 177–190.

Dabrowiak, J. C., Greenaway, F. T., Longo, W. E., VanHusen, M., and Crooke, S. T. (1978a). *Biochim. Biophys. Acta* **517**, 517–526.

Dabrowiak, J. C., Greenaway, F. T., and Grulich, R. (1978b). *Biochemistry* **17**, 4090–4094.

D'Andrea, F. O., and Haseltine, W. A. (1978). *Proc. Natl. Acad. Sci. U.S.A.* **75**, 3608–3612.

Daskal, Y., and Gyorkey, F. (1978). *In* "Bleomycin—Current Status and New Developments" (S. K. Carter, S. T. Crooke, and H. Umezawa, eds.), pp. 57–71. Academic Press, New York.

Daskal, Y., Crooke, S. T., Smetana, K., and Busch, H. (1975). *Cancer Res.* **35**, 374–381.

Haidle, C. W. (1977). *Mol. Pharmacol.* **7**, 645–652.

Haidle, C. W., and Bearden, J. (1975). *Biochem. Biophys. Res. Commun.* **65**, 815–821.

Haidle, C. W., Weiss, K. K., and Kuo, M. T. (1972). *Mol. Pharmacol.* **8**, 531–537.

Haidle, C. W., Lloyd, R. S., and Robberson, D. L. (1979). *In* "Bleomycin, Chemical, Biochemical, and Biological Aspects" (S. M. Hecht, ed.), pp. 222–243. Springer-Verlay, Berlin and New York.

Hittleman, W. N., and Rao, P. N. (1974). *Cancer Res.* **34**, 3422–3439.

Huang, C. H., Galvan, L., and Crooke, S. T. (1979). *Biochemistry* **18**, 2880–2887.

Iqbal, Z. M., Kohn, K. W., Ewig, R. A. G., and Fornace, A. J. (1976). *Cancer Res.* **36**, 3834–3838.

Ishida, R., and Takahashi, T. (1975). *Biochem. Biophys. Res. Commun.* **66**, 1432–1435.

Kohn, K. W., and Ewig, R. A. G. (1976). *Cancer Res.* **36**, 3839–3841.

Krishan, A. (1973). *Cancer Res.* **33**, 777–785.

Krueger, W. C., Pschigoda, L. M., and Reusser, F. (1973). *J. Antibiot.* **26** 424–428.

Kunimoto, T., Hori, M., and Umezawa, H. (1967). *J. Antibiot., Ser. A* **20**, 277–281.

Kuo, M. T., and Hsu, T. L. (1978). *Nature (London)* **271**, 83–84.

Kuo, M. T., Haidle, C. W., and Inners, L. D. (1973). *Biophys. J.* **13**, 1296–1305.

Lloyd, R. S., Haidle, C. W., and Robberson, D. L. (1978a). *Biochemistry* **17**, 1890–1896.

Lloyd, R. S., Haidle, C. W., Robberson, D. L., and Dobson, M. L. (1978b). *Curr. Microbiol.* **1**, 45–50.

Lown, J. W., and Sim, S. K. (1977). *Biochem. Biophys. Res. Commun.* **77**, 1150–1157.

Madreiter, H., Oseika, R., Kaden, P., Rombach, A., and Mittermyer, C. (1976). *Z. Zellforsch. Mikrosk. Anat.* **85**, 63–80.

Miyaki, M., Morohashi, S., and Ono, T. (1973). *J. Antibiot.* **26**, 369–373.

Miyaki, M., Ono, T., Hori, S., and Umezawa, H. (1975). *Cancer Res.* **35**, 2015–2019.

Müller, W. E. G., and Zahn, R. K. (1976). *In* "Fundamental and Clinical Studies of Bleomycin" (S. K. Carter, T. Ichikawa, G. Mathe, and H. Umezawa, eds.), Gann Monograph, No. 19, pp. 51–62. Univ. of Tokyo Press, Tokyo.

Müller, W. E. G., and Zahn, R. K. (1977). *Prog. Nucleic Acid Res. Mol. Biol.* **20**, 21–32.

Müller, W. E. G., Rohde, H. J., and Zahn, R. K. (1972). *Eur. J. Biochem.* **31**, 518–524.

Müller, W. E. G., Yamazaki, Z., Zollner, J., and Zahn, R. K. (1973). *FEBS Lett.* **31**, 217–223.

Murakami, H., Mori, H., and Taira, S. (1976). *J. Theor. Biol.* **59**, 1–23.

Nagai, K., Yamaki, H., Suzuki, H., Tanaka, N., and Umezawa, H. (1969). *Biochim. Biophys. Acta* **179**, 165–171.

Onishi, T., Iwata, H., and Takagi, Y. (1975). *Biochim. Biophys. Acta* **378**, 438–449.

Paika, K. D., and Krishan, A. (1973). *Cancer Res.* **33**, 961–965.

Povirk, L. F., Wubker, W., Kohnlein, W., and Hutchinson, F. (1977). *Nucleic Acids Res.* **4**, 3578–3580.

Ross, S. L., and Moses, R. E. (1978). *Biochemistry* **17**, 581–586.

Saito, M., and Andoh, T. (1973). *Cancer Res.* **33**, 1696–1700.

Sartiano, G. P., Winkelstein, A., Lynch, W., and Boggs, S. S. (1973). *J. Antibiot.* **26**, 437–443.

Sartiano, G. P., Lynch, W., and Boggs, S. S. (1975). *Proc. Soc. Exp. Biol. Med.* **150**, 718–727.

Sastry, K. S. R., Haller, G. J., Ottlinger, M. E., and Westhead, E. W. (1978). *Hyperfine Interact.* **4**, 891–905.

Sausville, E. A., Peisach, J., and Horwitz, S. B. (1976). *Biochem. Biophys. Res. Commun.* **73**, 806–814.

Sausville, E. A., Peisach, J., and Horwitz, S. B. (1978). *Biochemistry* **17**, 2740–2745.

Sleight, M. J. (1976). *Nucleic Acids Res.* **3**, 891–896.

Strong, J. E., and Crooke, S. T. (1978). *Cancer Res.* **38**, 3322–3326.

Suzuki, H., Nagai, K., Yamaki, H., Tanaka, N., and Umezawa, H. (1968). *J. Antibiot.* **21**, 379–386.

Suzuki, H., Nagai, K., Yamaki, H., Tanaka, N., and Umezawa, H. (1969). *J. Antibiot.* **22**, 446–449.

Taira, S. (1976). *J. Theor. Biol.* **59**, 1–23.

Takashita, M., Grollman, A. P., and Horwitz, S. B. (1976). *Virology* **69**, 453–463.

Takita, T., Muraoka, Y., Nakatani, T., Fujii, A., Iitaka, Y., and Umezawa, H. (1978). *J. Antibiot.* **31**, 1070–1073.

Terasima, T., and Umezawa, H. (1970). *J. Antibiot.* **23**, 300–304.

Terasima, T., Watanabe, M., Takabe, Y., and Miyamoto, T. (1976). *In* "Fundamental and Clinical Studies of Bleomycin" (S. K. Carter, T. Ichikawa, G. Mathe, and H. Umezawa, eds.), Gann Monograph, No. 19, pp. 63–81. Univ. of Tokyo Press, Tokyo.

Tobey, R. A., and Crissmen, H. A. (1972). *Cancer Res.* **32**, 2726–2732.

Umezawa, H. (1973). *Biomedicine* **18**, 459–475.

Umezawa, H. (1976). *In* "Fundamental and Clinical Studies of Bleomycin" (S. K. Carter, T. Ichikawa, G. Mathe, and H. Umezawa, eds.), Gann Monograph, No. 19, pp. 3–37. Univ. of Tokyo Press, Tokyo.

Umezawa, H. (1979). Unpublished observations.

Umezawa, H., Maeda, K., Takeuchi, T., and Akami, Y. (1966). *J. Antibiot., Ser. A.* **19**, 200–209.

Umezawa, H. (1974). *Fed. Prod. Fed. Am. Soc. Exp. Biol.* **33**, 2296–2301.

Yasuzumi, G., Hyo, Y., Hoshiya, T., and Yasuzumi, F. (1976). *Cancer Res.* **36**, 3574–3583.

Yoshioka, O., Amano, N., Takahashi, K., Matsuda, A., and Umezawa, H. (1978). *In* "Bleomycin—Current Status and New Developments" (S. K. Carter, S. T. Crooke, and H. Umezawa, eds.), pp. 35–56. Academic Press, New York.

14

MOLECULAR PHARMACOLOGY OF ANTHRACYCLINE ANTITUMOR ANTIBIOTICS

Virgil H. DuVernay

CANCER AND CHEMOTHERAPY, VOL. III

233

I. INTRODUCTION

Anthracyclines represent a major class of antitumor antibiotics. Their importance in modern cancer chemotherapy has grown significantly since the discovery of daunomycin (DNM) (DiMarco *et al.*, 1964) and adriamycin (ADM) (Arcamone *et al.*, 1969), the two prototype anthracyclines. Recent advances in the use of combination chemotherapy have resulted in significant improvements in long-term survival rates of several types of cancer. The clinical introduction of the anthracycline antitumor antibiotic ADM has contributed significantly to these advances. The spectrum of activity of DNM is limited to acute leukemias and lymphomas. Both compounds are natural products of the soil fungus Streptomycetes (See Fig. 1, Crooke, Chapter 8).

ADM was first isolated from fermentation cultures of the soil fungus *Streptomyces peucetius* var. *caecius* by DiMarco and co-workers (1969) and was found to have a broader spectrum of antitumor activity than the closely related analogue DNM. ADM differs only slightly from DNM by the presence of a hydroxyl group at the C-14 position. This minor structural alteration appears to confer a broader spectrum of activity and a longer biological half-life. Consequently, ADM has proved to be effective in the treatment of osteogenic sarcoma, Hodgkin's disease, non-Hodgkin's lymphoma, adenocarcinoma of the breast, leukemias, and adenocarcinomas of other sites (Blum and Carter, 1974; Gottlieb and Hill, 1974; Carter, 1975). Because of the fact that ADM is active against a wide range of solid tumors, many of which are poorly responsive or nonresponsive to other drugs, it is probably the single most important antitumor agent on the market today (Henry, 1975).

Of major concern in the use of ADM is the potentially fatal, dose-limiting toxicities associated with its therapy (Isetta *et al.*, 1971; Massimo *et al.*, 1971; Lefrak *et al.*, 1973; Buyniski, and Hirth, 1980; Schurig *et al.*, 1980). The acute dose-limiting toxicity of ADM is myelosuppression (Isetta *et al.*, 1971; Massimo *et al.*, 1971). The chronic dose-limiting toxicity is cumulative, irreversible cardiomyopathy, which occurs with relatively high frequency in patients exposed to greater than 450 mg/m^2 total dose of ADM (Lefrak *et al.*, 1973). The cardiomyopathy is exacerbated by radiotherapy to the mediastinum and perhaps by other cytotoxic agents (e.g., cyclophosphamide).

As a result of the significant activity and spectrum of ADM, an analogue development effort is directed toward the acquisition of new anthracyclines possessing less cardiotoxicity and myelosuppression at effective doses while achieving greater potency and broader spectrum of activity. Notable results of several laboratories working in this area include the compound *N*-trifluoroacetyladriamycin-14-valerate (AD-32) (Israel *et al.*, 1975), *N*-trifluoroacetyladriamycin (AD-41) (Israel *et al.*, 1975), rubidazone (Moral *et al.*, 1972), and carminomycin

(CMM) (Brazhnikova *et al.,* 1974; Gause *et al.,* 1974), the structures of which are shown in Fig. 1 (see Crooke, Chapter 8).

Some recent data have been acquired on a series of new anthracycline glycosides, the majority of which are derivatives of the aglycone pyrromycinone (see Fig. 2, Crooke, Chapter 8). These pyrromycinone-based anthracyclines differ structurally from the DNM–ADM group in a number of ways, including the lack of a carbonyl group at position C-13, the presence of a carbomethoxy-($COOCH_3$) group at position C-10, and the presence of a glycosidic side chain containing up to three sugar residues. Additional structural differences at positions C-1, C-4, C-11, C-3' amino group, and C-4' exist; however, these differences are relatively minor as can be seen by comparing the compounds in Fig. 1 (ADM and DNM) with those in Fig. 2 in Chapter 8.

II. CHEMISTRY

Anthracycline antibiotics are structurally characterized by the presence of a substituted tetrahydronaphthacene quinone (aglycone) moiety conjugated via glycosidic linkages to a side chain containing one or more sugar groups. Most clinically important anthracyclines contain an aminosugar attached to the aglycone portion of the molecule as indicated for ADM is Fig. 1, Chapter 8. Anthracycline glycosides are relatively stable crystalline compounds, usually orange-red, soluble in water, methanol, and aqueous alcohols but insoluble in most organic solvents. Solutions of anthracyclines absorb strongly in the ultraviolet as well as the visible regions of the spectrum (DiMarco, 1975a&b; DuVernay *et al.,* 1979b). Anthracyclines are fluorescent compounds, possessing fluorescence maxima at wavelengths greater than 500 nm. This property of anthracyclines can be effectively exploited for a variety of studies, including pharmacokinetic studies (Wilkinson *et al.,* 1979) and biochemical analyses (DiMarco *et al.,* 1977; DuVernay *et al.,* 1979b,c). The lability of the glycosidic linkages is indicated by the fact that mild acid hydrolysis will cleave the anthracycline molecule into an aqueous insoluble aglycone portion and an aqueous soluble sugar portion. It has been demonstrated that anthracycline antitumor activity is adversely affected by the removal of the sugar group and that this activity cannot be reconstituted by a mixture of the free aglycone and free sugar residue (DiMarco, 1975a; Henry, 1975).

Anthracycline compounds can be classified according to the structures of their aglycones, as previously described by Oki (1977). Accordingly, several groups of anthracyclines were described, four of which are shown in Fig. 1. These include the daunomycinone, the adriamycinone, the carminomycinone, the pyrromycinone, and the aklavinone groups of anthracyclines. The first three groups

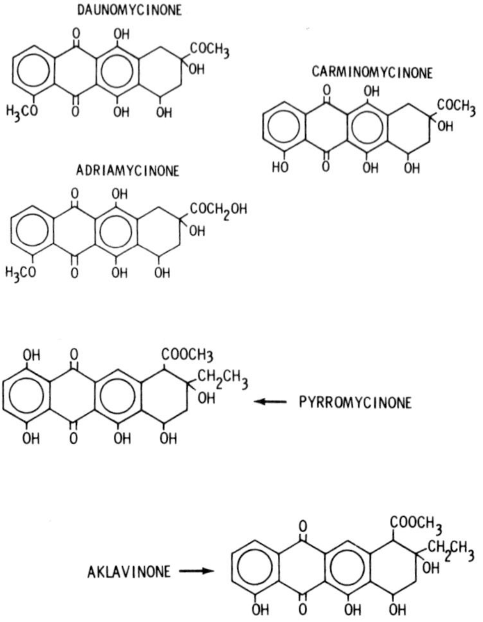

Fig. 1. Structures of the aglycones of several groups of anthracyclines, including adriamycinone, daunomycinone, carminomycinone, ε-pyrromycinone, and aklavinone.

are closely related structurally, differing only at positions 4 and 14 of the aglycone. These three groups fall under the general heading of the ADM–DNM family of anthracyclines. Included in this group is the agent CMM a new anthracycline that has been recently isolated and characterized (Brazhnikova *et al.*, 1974; Gause *et al.*, 1974). Also included in this group are the two clinically important semisynthetic analogues rubidazone and AD-32. Rubidazone is the benzoylhydrazone of DNM, modified at position 13 of the aglycone (Moral *et al.*, 1972), and AD-32 is an ADM analogue modified at position 14 of the aglycone and the C3′ amino group of the daunosamine sugar (Israel *et al.*, 1975). These analogues will be discussed in detail.

Oki and co-workers (1975) reported on the isolation of aclacinomycin A (ACM) from the soil fungus *Streptomyces galilaeus*. Structural characterization revealed ACM to be a trisaccharide derivative of the aglycone aklavinone. The aklavinone aglycone differs from that of ε-pyrromycinone by the absence of a hydroxyl group at position 1. Also shown in Fig. 2, Chapter 8, is the structure of cinerubin A, the ε-pyrromycinone analogue of ACM.

Several new anthracycline glycoside derivatives of the ε-pyrromycinone family have been recently isolated and structurally characterized (Nettleton *et al.*, 1977; Doyle *et al.*, 1978, 1979). These include marcellomycin (MCM), muset-

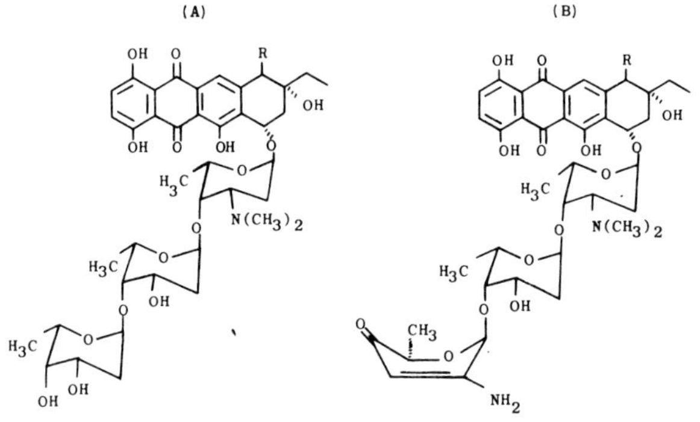

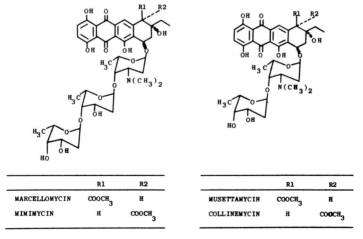

(A) (B)

Marcellomycin,   R = COOCH$_3$

10-Descarbomethoxy-
    marcellomycin,   R = H

Rudolfomycin,   R = COOCH$_3$

10-Descarbomethoxy-
    rudolfomycin   R = H

Fig. 2. Structures of marcellomycin, 10-descarbomethoxymarcellomycin, rudolfomycin, and 10-descarbomethoxyrudolfomycin.

tamycin (MSM), and rudolfomycin (RDM). Pyrromycin (PYM), an agent that had been previously studied (Brockmann *et al.*, 1957; Brockmann and Lenk, 1959; Brockmann and Brochmann, 1960), was also present. Subsequently, analogues of several of these anthracyclines modified at position 10 of the aglycone were obtained. These include the 10-descarbomethoxy analogues of MCM and RDM (DuVernay *et al.*, 1979a) shown in Fig. 2, which lack the ester

	R1	R2			R1	R2
MARCELLOMYCIN	COOCH$_3$	H		MUSETTAMYCIN	COOCH$_3$	H
MIMIMYCIN	H	COOCH$_3$		COLLINEMYCIN	H	COOCH$_3$

Fig. 3. Structures of marcellomycin, mimimycin, musettamycin, and collinemycin.

function, and the C-10 epimers of MSM and MCM (Doyle *et al.*, 1979) shown in Fig. 3. The C-10 epimers of MSM and MCM are collinemycin (CLM) and mimimycin (MIMI), respectively. It should become obvious that a parallel plot to the operetta *La Bohème* is slowly unfolding in this chapter.

III. STUDIES ON THE MECHANISM OF ACTION OF ANTHRACYCLINES

A. Nucleic Acid Synthesis Inhibitory Effects

ADM has been reported to exert a variety of effects on cells and cellular metabolism. These actions include cell surface effects (Murphree *et al.*, 1976), antimitotic effects (Silvestrini *et al.*, 1970), effects on mitochondrial function (Thayer, 1977), and DNA strand breakage effects (Schwartz, 1975). However, it is generally accepted that anthracyclines exert their antitumor effect by inhibiting normal nucleic acid synthesis and metabolism as a result of the drug's interaction with cellular DNA (DiMarco *et al.*, 1965a, 1975; Silvestrini *et al.*, 1970; Danø *et al.*, 1972; Meriwether and Bachur, 1972; Tatsumi *et al.*, 1974; Crooke *et al.*, 1978; DuVernay *et al.*, 1979a).

Ever since the isolation and identification in the mid-1960s of the two prototype compounds ADM and DNM, anthracyclines were all thought to fall into one large homogeneous class of agents. This view persisted until new information began to emerge in the early to mid-1970s, on anthracycline glycosides that were distant relatives of ADM and DNM. Both ADM and DNM inhibited whole cellular DNA and RNA synthesis at approximately equivalent concentrations (e.g., when comparing 50% inhibitory concentrations–IC_{50} values). These results suggested a lack of specificity of the nucleic acid synthesis inhibitory pattern for these agents. However, in 1975 Oki and co-workers reported an intriguing finding for a new anthracycline glycoside, aclacinomycin A (ACM). The structures of ACM and ADM differ at a number of sites, including the presence of a longer sugar side chain on ACM. Oki and colleagues (1975) demonstrated the selective inhibition of whole cellular RNA synthesis, at a 10-fold lower concentration than that needed for DNA synthesis inhibition. Similar findings were obtained for the anthracyclines cinerubins A and B (close structural analogues of ACM), nogalamycin, and rhodomycin B (Henry, 1975). A comparison of the structures of these latter agents with that of ADM suggests structural features that may be important in determining the RNA specificity of nucleic acid synthesis inhibition. However, no clear structure activity relationships were developed regarding RNA selectivity until the definitive study carried out by Crooke and co-workers (1978). In this study the whole cellular nucleic acid synthesis effects of ADM and CMM were compared with those of PYM,

MSM, RDM, ACM, and MCM. The results obtained are summarized in Table I. As indicated, Crooke and colleagues (1978) repeated the earlier findings of Oki and co-workers (1975). Furthermore, the anthracyclines studied were divided into two groups based on the selectivity for the inhibition of whole cellular RNA synthesis. ADM and two newer anthracyclines, PYM and CMM, showed no preference for the inhibition of RNA synthesis. To contrast, ACM, MSM, MCM, and RDM selectively inhibited whole cellular RNA synthesis at concentrations six to eight times lower than those required to inhibit DNA synthesis (Crooke et al., 1978; DuVernay et al., 1979a).

Finally, as indicated in Table I, protein synthesis is much less sensitive to the inhibitory effects of anthracyclines (Crooke et al., 1978). This is an agreement with the earlier studies of Kitaura and co-workers (1972) and others (Wang et al., 1972).

B. Nucleolar RNA Synthesis Inhibitory Effects

Several early studies were carried out (DiMarco et al., 1965a,b; Rusconi and Calendi, 1966) to examine the effects of DNM on nucleolar RNA synthesis. DiMarco and co-workers (1965a,b), employing autoradiographic studies with in vitro cultures of HeLa cells, demonstrated a higher susceptibility to DNM of [^{3}H]uridine incorporation into nucleolar RNA than into extra-nucleolar RNA. Rusconi and Calendi (1966) reported a high degree of inhibition of the synthesis of ribosomal RNA by DNM, whereas a "messenger RNA" fraction appeared to be less sensitive. Similar results were obtained by Perry (1963) with the nucleolar

TABLE I

IC$_{50}$ Values of Anthracyclines for DNA, RNA, and Protein Synthesis in Cultured Novikoff Hepatoma Ascites Cells[a]

	IC$_{50}$ Values (μM)			Ratios	
Anthracycline	DNA synthesis	RNA synthesis	Protein synthesis	$\dfrac{IC_{50} \text{ DNA}}{IC_{50} \text{ RNA}}$	$\dfrac{IC_{50} \text{ DNA}}{IC_{50} \text{ protein}}$
Adriamycin	6.1	3.2	18.0	1.91	0.34
Carminomycin	14.7	8.9	10.0	1.65	1.47
Pyrromycin	5.7	4.5	22.0	1.27	0.26
Musettamycin	10.0	1.5	10.0	6.67	1.00
Aclacinomycin	6.3	0.83	12.0	7.59	0.52
Marcellomycin	11.3	1.70	10.0	6.65	1.13
Rudolfomycin	69.7	3.65	–	19.10	1.13

[a] IC$_{50}$ values (50% inhibitory concentrations) were determined using probit analyses as reported previously (Crooke et al., 1978; DuVernay et al., 1979a).

specific antibiotic actinomycin D. The findings of Rusconi and Calendi (1966) were subsequently confirmed by Crooke and co-workers (1972) and others (Kann and Kohn, 1972; Danø et al., 1972), working with DNM, and by Ellen and Rhode (1970), studying nogalamycin. At concentrations of drug that did not completely suppress RNA synthesis, DNM inhibited ribosomal RNA synthesis but only partially inhibited the synthesis of "heterogeneous RNA" (DiMarco et al., 1975). No detectable inhibition of the processing of 45S preribosomal RNA was detected with DNM (Snyder et al., 1971).

The first systematic investigation of the inhibitory effects of anthracyclines on nucleolar RNA synthesis in cultured mammalian tumor cells was reported by Crooke and colleagues (1978). Nucleolar RNA synthesis was assayed by purifying nucleolar RNA from control and drug-treated cells and analyzing the extracted RNA by linear sucrose density gradient centrifugation. A typical sucrose density gradient profile of nucleolar RNA extracted from control and drug-treated cells is shown in Fig. 4. The newly synthesized 45S nucleolar preribosomal RNA (pre-rRNA) appears near the bottom of the gradient. This species is rapidly processed to lower-molecular-weight species with the end products being the mature 18 S and 28 S rRNA molecules. The anthracycline-

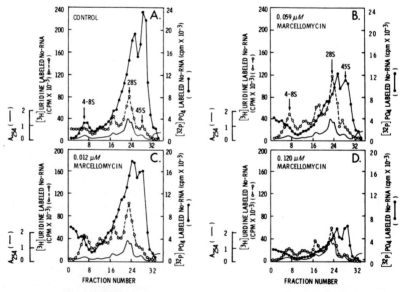

Fig. 4. Sedimentation profiles of nucleolar RNA extracted from control and marcellomycin-treated cells. Procedures are as described previously (Crooke et al., 1978). Gradients were fractionated into 1.0-ml fractions while monitoring A_{254}, ^{3}H-radioactivity (uniformly labeled nucleolar RNAs), and ^{32}P-radioactivity (de novo synthesized RNA-labeled postdrug treatment). The four patterns represent the results of a single experiment with the bottoms of the gradients to the right of each pattern.

induced inhibitory effects on nucleolar RNA synthesis were quantitated by measuring the changes in specific activity of the newly synthesized 45S nucleolar RNA at each drug concentration and comparing these values with those of the control (Crooke *et al.*, 1978). Probit analysis (Litchfield and Wilcoxon, 1949; DuVernay *et al.*, 1979a) was applied to the data and the IC_{50} values determined (Crooke *et al.*, 1978; DuVernay *et al.*, 1979a).

Table II summarizes the nucleolar RNA synthesis inhibitory potencies obtained for the several anthracyclines studied. The whole cellular RNA selective anthracyclines ACM, MSM, RDM, and MCM were shown to selectively inhibit nucleolar RNA synthesis at concentrations from 200 to 1300 times lower than those required to inhibit DNA synthesis. In contrast, ADM, CMM, and PYM inhibited DNA, RNA, and nucleolar RNA syntheses at approximately equivalent concentrations (Crooke *et al.*, 1978). Based on these results, the anthracyclines were divided into two classes. Class II or nucleolar selective anthracyclines include ACM, MSM, RDM, and MCM. Class I or nucleolar nonselective anthracyclines include ADM, CMM, and PYM. This study suggested that at least one structure activity relationship regarding nucleolar selectivity is localized in the glycosidic sidechain (Crooke *et al.*, 1978; DuVernay *et al.*, 1979a).

As previously reported by Snyder and co-workers (1971) for DNM, the processing of 45 S preribosomal RNA to the mature lower-molecular-weight species was not inhibited by the anthracyclines studied (Crooke *et al.*, 1978; DuVernay *et al.*, 1979a).

TABLE II

Inhibition of Nucleolar RNA Synthesis Relative to Whole Cellular DNA Synthesis

Anthracycline	IC_{50} No-RNA[a] synthesis (μM)	Ratio: IC_{50} DNA synthesis / IC_{50} No-RNA synthesis
Adriamycin	6.00	1.02
Carminomycin	13.06	1.12
Pyrromycin	6.15	0.93
Musettamycin	0.014	714
Rudolfomycin	0.290	240
Aclacinomycin	0.037	170
Marcellomycin	0.009	1256

[a] The IC_{50} values for nucleolar RNA synthesis were estimated by determining the ratio of $[^{32}P]PO_4$ cpm in the 45 S peak (see Fig. 4) to the $[^3H]$uridine cpm in the 28 S peak at each drug concentration, comparing with that of the control, and plotting versus drug concentration for probit analysis as previously described (DuVernay *et al.*, 1979a).

C. Electron Microscopic Observations of the Ultrastructural and Morphological Effects of Anthracyclines on the Nucleolus

Morphological effects of anthracyclines have been reported by Daskal and co-workers (1978). Their comparative study of the three anthracyclines ADM, CMM, and MCM revelaed that one distinctive ultrastructural change caused by these agents was the production of nucleolar lesions. A series of nucleolar structural changes that increased to complete segregation of granular and fibrillar components was observed to occur at higher doses and longer treatment times. Although the end results were the same, when comparing MCM with ADM and CMM, the mechanism(s) involved in the segregation phenomenon was somewhat different and thought to be related to the structural characteristics of the anthracyclines (Daskal et al., 1978).

ADM and CMM induced nucleolar segregation at equivalent concentrations by initially forming conspicuous fibrillar centers. This is followed by the collapse and fusion of the fibrillar centers. The doses required for MCM-induced segregation were significantly lower than those of ADM and CMM, and nucleolar fragmentation into micronucleoli was observed (Daskal et al., 1978). The considerably lower doses at which complete nucleolar segregation was observed and the formation of microspherules (Unuma and Busch, 1967), also produced on treatment with actinomycin D, may indicate a different mode of action and/or specificity of this analogue (Daskal et al., 1978). The difference in pathways leading to nucleolar segregation for MCM versus ADM and CMM may reflect the morphological component of the nucleolar specific actions of MCM and the class II anthracyclines.

D. DNA Binding Characteristics of Anthracyclines

Early studies on the prototype anthracyclines DNM and ADM demonstrated the importance of DNA binding in the mechanism of action of these agents (Calendi et al., 1965). Subsequent studies from a number of laboratories (Gabbay et al., 1976; Waring, 1970; Zunino et al., 1972, 1977; DiMarco et al., 1977) have added substantially to our understanding of characteristics of the anthracycline–DNA interaction. As a result, it is generally accepted that a major portion of the anthracycline–DNA interaction involves the insertions of the anthracycline aglycone between adjacent nucleotide bases of the DNA-duplex by an intercalation mechanism (Lerman, 1961). This argument was further substantiated by the findings of Pigram and co-workers (1972). The interaction of DNM with DNA involves a strong intercalative binding process, occurring at low DNA-to-drug ratios, and a weaker binding process, occurring at high DNA-to-drug ratios involving electrostatic interactions between the phosphate group of

DNA and the ammonium group of the amino-sugar of DNM (Pigram *et al.*, 1972). Studies demonstrating the intercalative binding interaction between anthracyclines and native DNA have been reported by several groups (Waring, 1970; DiMarco *et al.*, 1975; Gabbay *et al.*, 1976; Böhner and Hagen, 1977; Zunino *et al.*, 1977). The result of this interaction is an alteration in the secondary structure of the DNA molecule resulting in a decreased template activity and an altered sensitivity to nucleases. Moreover, a reduction in the whole cellular nucleic acid synthesis inhibitory activity of ADM obtained as a result of the addition of exogenous DNA to an *in vitro* assay system suggests that DNA binding is important in the mechanism of action of anthracyclines (Goodman *et al.*, 1974; Momparler *et al.*, 1976). Gabbay and co-workers (1976) demonstrated that the biological activity of DNM, ADM, and a series of analogues was directly related to the degree of intercalative binding with DNA.

The *in vitro* anthracycline–DNA interaction has been studied by a variety of techniques, including equilibrium dialysis (Zunino *et al.*, 1972; Arlandini *et al.*, 1977), spectrophotometric methods (Calendi *et al.*, 1965; Gabbay *et al.*, 1976), and viscometric methods (Arlandini *et al.*, 1977; Zunino *et al.*, 1977). However, the generally preferred method of analysis currently is the fluorescence titration method (Tsou and Yip, 1976; Zunino *et al.*, 1976, 1977; DiMarco *et al.*, 1977; DuVernay *et al.*, 1979b,c). This method takes advantage of the

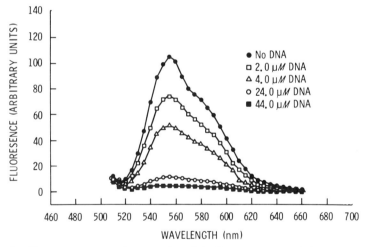

Fig. 5. Fluorescence spectra of pyrromycin and the fluorescence spectral changes that occur on interaction with salmon sperm DNA. Spectra were taken on 5 μM anthracycline solutions in 0.05 M sodium phosphate buffer, pH 6.2, 0.05 M NaCl, 0.001 M EDTA. Spectra were obtained, as previously reported (DuVernay *et al.*, 1979b), by using the excitation wavelength of 490 nm and recording drug fluorescence at wavelengths in the low-energy region of the spectrum (longer wavelengths). Increasing concentrations of DNA were obtained by addition of microliter volumes of a concentrated solution of salmon sperm DNA in the preceding buffer.

fluorescence properties of the anthracyclines and the fact that fluorescence spectral changes occur on the interaction of these compounds with DNA. An example of these changes is shown in Fig. 5 for PYM (DuVernay et al., 1979b). Here the fluorescence spectrum of PYM is progressively quenched by addition of increasing concentrations of DNA. These results are typical of the anthracyclines.

By titrating a fixed concentration of anthracycline with increasing concentrations of DNA, while monitoring the emissions changes that occur at the peak of fluorescence, the fluorescence quench curves shown in Fig. 6 are obtained. The levels of bound and free anthracycline are then calculated and the Scatchard analysis of the anthracycline–DNA interaction obtained, two typical curves of which are shown in Fig. 7. From these curves the apparent association constant (Kapp) and the apparent binding site (napp) parameters were determined (DuVernay et al., 1979b,c).

The anthracyclines shown in Table II were divided into two groups based on the selectivity for the inhibition of nucleolar RNA synthesis. One possible explanation of the nucleolar selectivity of class II anthracyclines is the preferential

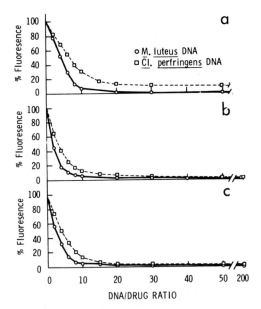

Fig. 6. Fluorescence quenching of anthracyclines in the presence of increasing concentrations of *M. luteus* DNA and *Cl. perfringens* DNA. To a series of glass tubes containing increasing concentrations of nucleic acid in DNA binding buffer, 0.05 M sodium phosphate buffer, pH 6.2, 0.05 M NaCl, 0.001 M EDTA, a fixed concentration of each anthracycline was added. The tubes were incubated at 25°C for 1 hr, and fluorescence measurements were taken using the fluorescence parameters as previously determined (DuVernay, 1979). The results of duplicate experiments, each of which contained duplicate or triplicate values at each DNA concentration, are shown: (a) adriamycin; (b) pyrromycin; (c) musettamycin.

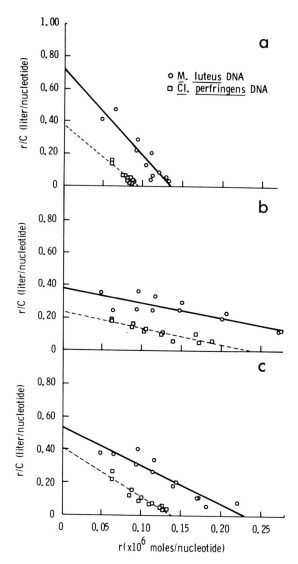

Fig. 7.   Scatchard plots of the binding data for the interaction of anthracyclines with *M. luteus* DNA and *Cl. perfringens* DNA. The Scatchard parameters *r* (moles ligand bound per nucleotide), *C* (moles per liter of free ligand), and *r/C* were calculated from the data presented in Fig. 6 as previously reported (DuVernay, 1979; DuVernay *et al.*, 1979b). (a)Adriamycin; (b) pyrromycin; (c) musettamycin.

binding of these agents to GC-rich regions of DNA as for actinomycin D (Gellert
et al., 1965; Hyman and Davidson, 1971). Therefore DuVernay and co-workers
(1979b) used DNAs of varying GC content in order to study the sequence
specificities of DNA binding by these anthracyclines. The synthetic copolymers
poly (dAdT)–poly (dAdT) and poly(dGdC)–poly(dGdC) were taken as limits of
either extreme of GC content. In addition, three naturally occurring DNA's with
varying base compositions were employed. These included calf thymus DNA
(43% GC), *Micrococcus luteus* DNA (72% GC), and *Clostridum perfringens*
DNA (28% GC) (DuVernay *et al.*, 1979b). Figure 8 summarizes the results
obtained with regard to the sequence specificity of DNA binding of these agents.
This figure compares the effects of changes in the base composition of DNA on
the association constants of these anthracyclines. As indicated, the sequence
specificities of ADM differ from those of MCM and its analogues. ADM demonstrated a definite GC requirement for binding to DNA, whereas the
pyrromycinone-based anthracyclines showed no base specificity for binding to
DNA (DuVernay, 1979; DuVernay *et al.*, 1979b). In fact, an increase in avidity
for binding to poly(dAdT)–poly(dAdT) was observed. These findings support
similar findings for nogalamycin, steffimycin B (two closely related anthracyclines) (Bhuyan and Smith, 1965, 1975; Ward *et al.*, 1965; Reusser, 1975), and
DNM (Ward *et al.*, 1965; DiMarco, 1975a).

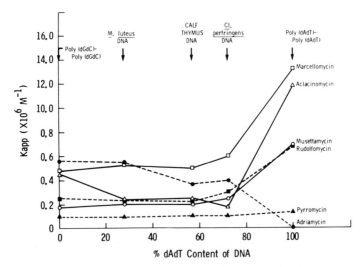

Fig. 8.   The effect of varying DNA base compositions on the apparent association constants of
anthracyclines. Results obtained from previous reports (DuVernay, 1979; DuVernay *et al.*, 1979b).
The % dAdT sequences varied, depending on the DNAs studied: poly (dGdC)–poly (dGdC) (0%); *M.
luteus* DNA (28%); calf thymus DNA (57%); *Cl. perfringens* DNA (72%); and poly (dAdT)–poly
(dAdT) (100%).

The demonstration of selective nucleolar RNA synthesis inhibition is difficult to explain in light of the finding of AT specificity of MCM and its analogues. The electron micrographic demonstration of regional disruption of the nucleolar transcriptional apparatus by RDM (Daskal, 1979) suggests that spacer or promoter regions, known to have high AT content, may be targets of anthracycline binding.

E. DNA Strand Breakage Effects of Anthracyclines

In order to examine the direct DNA strand breakage effects of anthracyclines, workers in several laboratories have studied the effects of these compounds on isolated DNA as well as on intact cellular chromosomal DNA (Hittleman and Rao, 1975; Schwartz, 1975; DuVernay, 1979). Studies demonstrating extensive chromosomal damage in cells treated with ADM have been reported by Schwartz (1975) and DuVernay (1979), using alkaline sucrose gradient techniques, and Hittleman and Rao (1975), using premature chromosome condensation methods. The latter method suggests direct DNA strand breakage, without the generation of alkaline-labile sties (Hittleman and Rao, 1975). These results include a broad banding of whole cellular DNA, indicative of heterogeneous size classes of DNA and probably resulting from random DNA degradation. Similar results were obtained with actinomycin D (Pater and Mak, 1974). The degradation patterns produced by neocarzinostatin (Beerman and Goldberg, 1977) and bleomycin A_2 (Strong and Crooke, 1978), known DNA breakage agents, do not resemble those of the anthracyclines. Thus, for the anthracyclines, these findings are in agreement with studies suggesting an induction of nucleases or a stimulation of nuclease activity *in vivo* (Hittleman and Rao, 1975; Schwartz, 1975; DuVernay, 1979).

The level of contribution of DNA breakage to the mechanism of action of ADM and other anthracyclines is not known, and the nature of the DNA distortion that may lead to DNA degradation is not understood, Lown and co-workers (1977) have reported that one result of the ADM–DNA interaction *in vitro* is DNA strand breakage. However, this effect could only be accomplished under harsh conditions (96°C, in the presence of sodium borohydride) and at extremely high concentrations of ADM (0.2 mM). Furthermore, as reported by Mong and co-workers (1980), this effect required the presence of reducing agents, e.g., 2-mercaptoethanol and sodium borohydride. By employing milder conditions and lower drug concentrations, which are more likely to be obtained *in vivo*, Lee and Byfield (1976), using isolated mouse L1210 DNA, and Mong and co-workers (1980), employing superhelical PM-2 DNA, could not demonstrate DNA breakage by ADM *in vitro*. In fact, the major effect of the binding of anthracyclines on PM-2 DNA is the induction of significant conformational changes readily demonstrable in several systems (Mong *et al.*, 1980). Furthermore, treatment of this anthracycline–PM-2 DNA complex with the DNA breakage agent bleomycin A_2 generated the typical bleomycin A_2 DNA breakage patterns previously demonstrated (Strong and Crooke, 1978; Mong et al., 1980). The results suggest that the anthracycline-induced diffuse staining regions were not due to random breakage, since posttreatment with bleomycin A_2 would not be expected to produce this banding pattern of relaxed circular (form II) DNA, and linear duplex (form III) DNA (Strong and Crooke, 1978; Mong et al., 1980). In addition, no DNA breakage action could be demonstrated for ADM (up to 50 μM) by employing PM-2 DNA and analyzing on alkaline-sucrose density gradients (Mong et al., 1980). Hence the evidence to date shows no direct DNA strand breakage effect of the anthracyclines.

F. Anthracyclines Whose Mechanism of Action Does Not Appear to Depend on Interaction with DNA

Although most anthracyclines studied thus far possess significant avidity for binding to DNA and thus depend on the interaction with DNA as a part of their mechanism of action, several analogues have been recently studied that do not require DNA interactions to exert their effects. These analogues include the natural product CMM and the semisynthetically modified agents carminomycin-11-methylether (CMM-OMe) (Fig. 9) and AD-32. The synthesis of AD-32 (Israel et al., 1975) and of CMM-OMe (Essery and Doyle, 1979) has been recently described.

Despite the reported aqueous solubility problems of AD-32, and the attendant

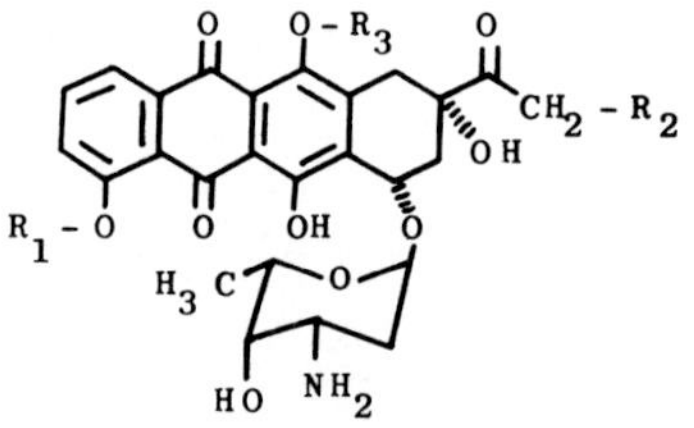

	R_1	R_2	R_3
Adriamycin	CH_3	OH	H
Carminomycin	H	H	H
Carminomycin-11-methyl ether	H	H	CH_3

Fig. 9.   Structures of adriamycin, carminomycin, and carminomycin-11-methyl ether.

difficulties encountered in administration, AD-32 represents the first anthracycline analogue that appears to act differently from ADM and that possesses significant clinical potential. AD-32 exhibited markedly higher antitumor efficacies against P388 and L1210 leukemias at significantly reduced antitumor potencies (Table III) (Israel *et al.*, 1975). Similar results have been reported by a number of groups employing a variety of tumors (Parker *et al.*, 1978; Vecchi *et al.*, 1978; Pratesi *et al.*, 1978). The lack of appreciable DNA binding ability (Sengupta *et al.*, 1976; Facchinetti *et al.*, 1978) and the absence of subcellular nuclear localization of AD-32 (Krishan *et al.*, 1976, 1978) suggest that the DNA template may not be the subcellular target of AD-32. Thus this indicates a differing mechanism of action from ADM.

Other anthracyclines that fall into this group of non-DNA binding agents include CMM and CMM-OMe. The close structural similarity of these agents with ADM is shown in Fig. 9. Previous studies employing a variety of systems have suggested a similarity of action for ADM and CMM (Crooke, 1977; Crooke *et al.*, 1978; Daskal *et al.*, 1978; Merski *et al.*, 1979). The *in vivo* antitumor activities of ADM, CMM, and CMM-OMe against mouse L1210 leukemia are summarized in Table IV. Although ADM exhibited a higher efficacy than CMM or CMM-OMe in this system, when given in single doses (cf. maximum %T/C values from Table IV), CMM was significantly more potent than ADM when comparing maximum effective doses (DuVernay *et al.*, 1980). Thus CMM was approximately 20 times more potent than ADM, the latter agent being roughly equipotent with CMM-OMe. Similar results were obtained *in vitro* against cultured Novikoff ascites cells when comparing IC_{50} values for cell viability inhibition (see Table IV).

Previous studies have shown that ADM and CMM inhibit DNA, whole cellular RNA, and No-RNA syntheses at approximately equal concentrations (Crooke *et al.*, 1978). CMM-OMe was markedly less potent against whole cellular nuc-

TABLE III

In Vivo **Antitumor Activity of Ad-32 and Adriamycin**[a]

Anthracycline	Tumor	Optimal[b] dose (mg/kg)	Increase in survival time (%)	60-day survivors
Adriamycin	P388	4.0	132	0/6
AD-32	P388	40	429	3/5
Adriamycin	L1210	4.0	42	0/7
AD-32	L1210	50	400	5/7

[a] Data obtained from Israel *et al.* (1975).

[b] Schedule: qd 1–4, i.p.

TABLE IV

In Vivo and in Vitro Activities of Carminomycin and Carminomycin-11-Methylether as Compared to Adriamycin

Anthracycline	IC$_{50}$ Values (μM)[a]		Antitumor activity		In vitro IC$_{50}$ value (μM)	Ratio[d] $\dfrac{\text{IC}_{50}\ \text{DNA}}{\text{IC}_{50}\ \text{cell viability}}$	K_{app} ($\times\ 10^6\ M^{-1}$)[e]	
	DNA synthesis	RNA synthesis	In vivo[b] dose (mg/kg)	% T/C[c]			Salmon sperm DNA	Calf thymus DNA
Adriamycin	8.52	2.91	15	207	0.39	21	11.68	3.67
			12	164				
			9	171				
			6	193				
			4	157				
			2	157				
			1	143				
			0.5	129				
			0.25	114				
Carminomycin	10.14	4.87	1.6	143	0.09	112	0.15	0.26
			0.8	157				
			0.4	150				
			0.2	114				
			0.1	100				
			0.05	107				
Carminomycin-11-methylether	>80	>25	32	114	0.52	>160	–	–
			16	136				
			8	129				
			4	114				
			2	100				
			1	100				
			0.5	114				

[a] Values obtained by probit analysis of results obtained in vitro, employing Novikoff hepatoma ascites cells, as previously reported (DuVernay et al., 1980). [b] In vivo antitumor activity against mouse L1210 leukemia. Drug was administered i.p. once on day 1 as previously reported (DuVernay et al., 1980). [c] % T/C = (MST treated/MST control) × 100. % T/C > 125 is considered significant antitumor activity. [d] This ratio reflects the relative cytotoxic potencies of these compounds. [e] K_{app} (apparent association constants) were obtained by Scatchard analyses of fluorescence titration results as previously described (DuVernay et al., 1980).

leic acid syntheses (DuVernay *et al.*, 1980). The ratios of the IC_{50} values for DNA synthesis to that for cell viability inhibition for ADM (21) differ significantly from those of CMM (112) and CMM-OMe (> 160). Thus the antitumor activity of CMM and CMM-OMe is difficult to explain on the basis of nucleic acid synthesis inhibition.

Further evidence that CMM and CMM-OMe differ mechanistically from ADM derives from studies examining the DNA binding affinities of these compounds for three natural DNAs, including superhelical covalently closed circular (ccc-) PM-2 DNA. As illustrated in Fig. 10, titration of superhelical ccc-DNA with intercalating agents results in an initial relaxation or uncoiling of the negatively supercoiled DNA followed by a reversal of the supercoiling, producing a positively supercoiled DNA molecule at saturating concentrations of intercalator (Waring, 1970; Revet *et al.*, 1971; Mong *et al.*, 1980). If these molecules are subjected to electrophoresis, the order of anodal migration is the superhelical form DNA (molecules A and E) migrating fastest, followed by the partially relaxed form DNA (molecules B and D), with the fully relaxed form DNA (molecule C) migrating the slowest.

Figure 11 shows the results obtained by titrating fixed concentrations of PM-2 DNA with increasing concentrations of ADM, CMM, and CMM-OMe. That this binding probably involves an intercalative mechanism is suggested by the genera-

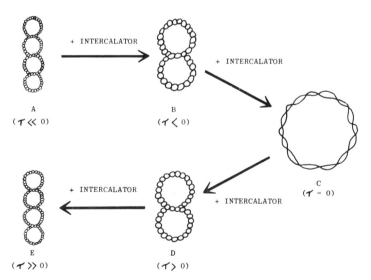

Fig. 10. Diagrammatic representation of the effects of intercalating agents on superhelical covalently closed circular DNA. A, naturally isolated supercoiled ccc-DNA (negative supercoiled); B, partially relaxed ccc-DNA; C, completely relaxed ccc-DNA; D, partially reverse coiled ccc-DNA; E, completely reverse-coiled ccc-DNA (positively supercoiled). τ represents the superhelix density of a given species of ccc-DNA, which is a measure of the extent of supercoiling of the DNA duplex.

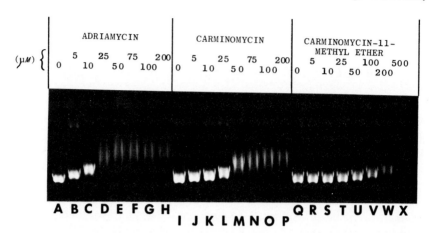

Fig. 11. Agarose gel electrophoretic separations of anthracycline–PM-2 DNA reaction products. Reactions were performed and agarose gel electrophoresis conducted as previously reported (DuVernay *et al.*, 1980). Direction of electrophoresis is from top to bottom, with the fastest-migrating band being the superhelical ccc–PM-2 DNA and the slowest-migrating band (faintly visible) being the relaxed form DNA. Lanes A through H correspond to increasing concentrations of adriamycin of 0, 5, 10, 25, 50, 75, 100, and 200 μM, respectively. Lanes I through P correspond to identical concentrations of carminomycin. Lanes Q through X correspond to increasing concentrations of carminomycin-11-methyl ether of 0, 5, 10, 25, 50, 100, 200, and 500 μM, respectively. Electrophoresis was at 5 V/cm for 10 hr at room temperature. Gels were stained with 0.5 μg/ml of ethidium bromide.

tion of "smear patterns" of diffuse staining regions (lanes D–H, M–P, W, and X) representing gradations of relaxed ccc–PM-2 DNA (DuVernay, 1979; DuVernay *et al.*, 1980). The order of the potencies for the binding and generation of conformational changes in the superhelical PM-2 DNA was ADM > CMM >> CMM-OMe.

Scatchard analyses of the interactions of these agents with calf thymus DNA and salmon sperm DNA revealed a similar ordering of the DNA binding abilities (see Table IV). Therefore a correlation exists between the DNA binding abilities and the nucleic acid synthesis inhibitory activities of these anthracyclines. Thus CMM and CMM-OMe are much more potent antitumor agents than can be accounted for on the basis of their DNA binding abilities, suggesting differing mechanisms of action for CMM and ADM (DuVernay *et al.*, 1980).

G. Effects of Anthracyclines on Mitochondrial Function and Energy Metabolism

Although DNA–anthracycline interactions clearly contribute significantly to the mechanism of action of anthracyclines, not all the biological effects of anthracyclines can be directly attributed to nucleic acid synthesis inhibition.

Effects on mitochondrial function have been suggested by several groups (Gosalvez *et al.*, 1974; Iwamoto *et al.*, 1974; Kishi *et al.*, 1976; Andreini *et al.*, 1977; Bertazzoli and Ghione, 1977; Myers *et al.*, 1977; Thayer, 1977). Several mechanisms have been proposed to account for the mitochondrial effects of ADM. These include generation of the superoxide radical (Thayer, 1977), perturbation of the electron transport system (Kishi *et al.*, 1976; Bertazzoli and Ghione, 1977; Bertazzoli *et al.*, 1978), inhibition of the respiratory chain enzymes succinooxidase and NADH-oxidase (Iwamoto *et al.*, 1974), and the inhibition of cytochromes a and a_3 synthesis (Andreini *et al.*, 1977).

It has been postulated that the mitochondrial effects of ADM may be responsible for the cardiotoxicity of this agent. Kishi and co-workers (1976) have demonstrated that ADM inhibits the beef heart mitochondrial enzymes NADH-oxidase and succinooxidase (both enzymes requiring coenzyme Q_{10}) and that several forms of coenzyme Q protect against this inhibition. The role of lipid peroxidation in cardiac toxicity has been reported and its amelioration by α-tocopherol has been suggested (Myers *et al.*, 1976, 1977). Thus although these effects may be responsible in part for the antitumor actions of these compounds, it is becoming evident that the cardiotoxicity of ADM may be largely due to its effects on mitochondrial function and energy metabolism.

H. Antimitotic Effects of Anthracyclines

Silvestrini and co-workers (1970) reported evidence of antimitotic effects of DNM in cultured mouse cells at drug concentrations much too low to affect nucleic acid synthesis. The antimitotic effect was rapid in onset, occurring even when administered within minutes prior to prophase (Silvestrini *et al.*, 1970). This effect was further characterized in a subsequent study (Silvestrini *et al.*, 1973). Kitaura and co-workers (1972) demonstrated similar effects for ADM.

In keeping with a possible effect of the anthracyclines on processes involved with both movement of cellular components and mitosis, Danø (1971, 1972a,b) has suggested that ADM and DNM might interfere with the function of microtubules. This hypothesis is based on the cross-resistance between the anthracyclines and the antimitotic vinca alkaloids seen with tumor cells. Additional support for this hypothesis derives from studies with the DNM analogue *N*-acetyldaunorubicin (DiMarco, 1975b) and the ADM congener AD-32 (Israel *et al.*, 1975; Krishan *et al.*, 1976; Sengupta *et al.*, 1976). The former agent is a weak inhibitor of nucleic acid synthesis but has significant antimitotic activity (DiMarco, 1975b). Furthermore, AD-32 has been reported to be an effective antitumor agent (Israel *et al.*, 1975), but it apparently does not enter the cell nucleus (Krishan *et al.*, 1976) or bind to isolated DNA (Sengupta *et al.*, 1976). Thus the antimitotic effects of these agents may play a role in the antitumor actions of this drug class.

I. Effects of Anthracyclines on the Cell Surface and Cytoplasmic Membrane

Murphree and co-workers (1976) reported essentially complete inhibition of the growth of sarcoma 180 cells in culture by ADM at concentrations that had no effect on the rate of incorporation of [^{3}H]thymidine and [^{3}H]uridine into nucleic acids. Their findings indicated a correspondence in the concentrations of ADM needed for both cytotoxicity and cell surface phenomena. The finding that ADM increased the rate of cellular agglutination by concanavalin A, at low (i.e., 10^{-7} M) drug concentrations, suggested a direct membrane action of ADM (Murphree *et al.*, 1976). Tritton and co-workers (Tritton *et al.*, 1978) and others (Murphree *et al.*, 1977) extended these studies and demonstrated effects on membrane fluidity by ADM. Decreased fluidity was observed in cardiolipin containing lipid bilayers, indicating differential sites of action of ADM. A number of other studies have implicated a direct interaction of anthracyclines with cell membranes (Schioppacassi and Schwartz, 1977; Goldman *et al.*, 1978) and cytoskeleton (Na and Timasheff, 1977). These studies suggest an action of ADM at the membrane level affecting the movement of molecules in the membrane itself.

IV. ANTHRACYCLINE STRUCTURE–ACTIVITY RELATIONSHIPS

The basic chemical structure of the majority of the clinically important anthracycline antitumor antibiotics consists of an aglycone that is a derivative of the basic tetrahydronaphthancene quinone moiety, as shown in Fig. 12. This aglycone is conjugated, via glycosidic linkages, to a glycosidic side chain containing a minimum of one sugar residue, which is usually the amino sugar daunosamine, also shown in Fig. 12. This section will cover some of the many

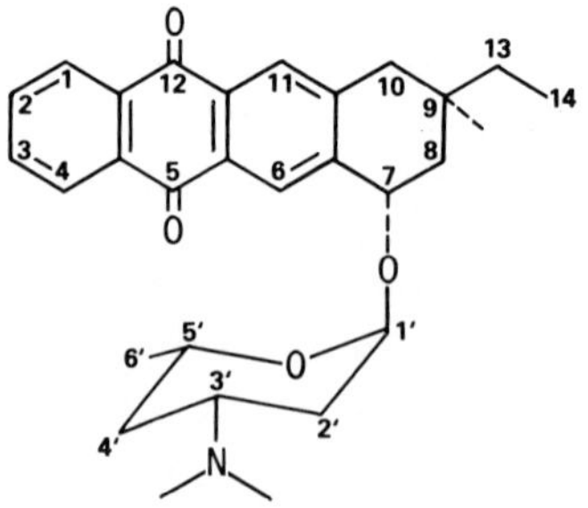

Fig. 12. The basic structure of the anthracycline molecule consisting of an aglycone (tetrahydronaphthacene quinone moiety) conjugated via glycosidic linkages to a side chain containing one or more sugar groups.

structural modification studies, currently under active investigation by several groups, and attempt to correlate the results as derivatives of the basic anthracycline molecule.

A. Modifications at Positions 2 and 3 of the Aglycone

The *in vitro* cytotoxic activities of the 2,3-dimethyl analogues of ADM and DNM were studied by Arcamone and colleagues (1978) and found to be approximately two times more potent than their respective parent compounds. In addition, some increase in *in vivo* effectiveness (longer survival times for drug-treated animals) was also observed against mouse L1210 leukemia. In contrast, the 2,3-dichloro analogue of DNM exhibited significant decreases in *in vitro* cytotoxicity, *in vivo* antitumor potency, and *in vivo* antitumor efficacy against L1210 leukemia.

Thus substitutions at positions 2 and 3 of the anthracycline aglycone is at best correlated with a minimal increase in antitumor activity (as for the dimethyl analogues). Generally, modifications at these positions confer a decrease in antitumor potency and efficacy (Arcamone *et al.*, 1978).

B. Modifications at Positions 1 and 4 of the Aglycone

Substitution of CH_3 groups at positions 1 and 4 of DNM resulted in a two-fold decrease in *in vivo* potency with no change observed for *in vitro* potency, and *in vivo* efficacy, against L1210 leukemia (Arcamone *et al.*, 1978). Substitution of Cl groups at positions 1 and 4 of DNM resulted in a slight increase in *in vitro* potency against HeLa cells and approximately an eightfold decrease in *in vivo* potency against L1210 leukemia. A decrease in *in vivo* effectiveness was also observed (Arcamone *et al.*, 1978).

Thus, similar to the findings of the previous section, substitutions at positions 1 and 4 of the aglycone seem to afford no advantage with regard to enhancing antitumor effects of ADM or DNM (Arcamone *et al.*, 1978). In general, substitutions of chloro groups on positions 1 through 4 confer decreased antitumor effects.

C. Modifications at Position 4 of the Aglycone

The methoxy group (OCH_3) at position 4 of ADM and DNM is not essential for the biochemical and biological effects of these agents (Supino *et al.*, 1977). As indicated in Table V, removal of the OCH_3 groups at position 4 of DNM resulted in a 25- to 100-fold increase in activity *in vitro* as well as *in vivo* (Supino *et al.*, 1977). Similarly, removal of the OCH_3 group from position 4 of ADM resulted in a 65- to 200-fold increase in activity. Similar increases in potencies

TABLE V

In Vitro and in Vivo Antitumor Activities of Adriamycin, Daunomycin, and Their 4-Demethoxyanalogues

Anthracycline	In vitro cytotoxicity,[a] IC_{50} (ng/ml)	In vivo antitumor activity[b]				DNA binding to calf thymus DNA[e]	
		L1210 leukemia		P388 leukemia		K_{app} ($\times 10^6\ M^{-1}$)	N_{app}
		Dose[c] (mg/kg)	MST^d	Dose[c] (mg/kg)	MST^d		
Daunomycin	10.00	2.9	144	4.0	205	3.3 ± 0.8	0.18
4-Demethoxydaunomycin	0.15	1.0	150	0.7	200	2.4 ± 0.3	0.20
Adriamycin	15.00	2.9	141	–	–	–	–
4-Demethoxyadriamycin	0.10	0.5	166	–	–	–	–

[a] Inhibition of colony-forming ability of cultured HeLa cells after 24-hr drug treatment as previously described (Arcamone *et al.*, 1978).

[b] Activity determined as previously reported (Arcamone *et al.*, 1978) employing mouse L1210 and P388 leukemias *in vivo*. Tumor inoculum 10^5 cells i.p. for L1210 leukemia and 10^6 cells i.p. for P388 leukemia.

[c] Represents optimal dose showing no toxicity.

[d] Median survival time expressed as percent of untreated controls.

[e] Results obtained from Zunino *et al.* (1976).

toward the inhibition of the incorporation of [^{3}H]thymidine were also observed (Supino *et al.*, 1977).

Conversion of the OCH$_3$ group of DNM to an OH group, as in CMM (Fig. 9), resulted in increases in potencies (Gause *et al.*, 1974; Crooke, 1977) and a broadening of the antitumor spectrum (Crooke, 1977). In addition, the nature and the degree of the cardiotoxicity changes have been reported to be altered (Buyniski, 1980).

Thus, in contrast to the changes reported previously, removal of the methoxy group from position 4 of ADM and DNM or substitution of a hydroxyl group at this location (e.g., CMM) confers increased antitumor potency and, in the case of CMM, a broadening of antitumor spectrum and some amelioration in the toxicities.

D. Modification at Position 5 of the Aglycone

A significant reduction in a toxic side effect of DNM was reported for its analogue 5-iminodaunomycin by Tong and co-workers (1979a). Structurally, this analogue differs only at position 5 of the aglycone, in which the quinoid carbonyl group is replaced by an imine group (C $=$ N). The results of a comparative study employing ADM, DNM, and 5-iminodaunomycin are summarized in Table VI. Although ADM was superior to the other two agents with respect to antitumor effectiveness and potency against P-388 leukemia, DNM and 5-iminodaunomycin exhibited equivalent antitumor activities. DNM inhibited RNA synthesis at concentrations four times lower than 5-iminodaunomycin. More importantly, 5-iminodaunomycin exhibited a four-fold decrease in cardiotoxicity (Tong *et al.*, 1979a). Thus, although minor changes in the antitumor effects of DNM occurred on modification at position 5, of major importance is the significant reduction in cardiotoxicity.

E. Modification at Positions 4, 7, and 9 of the Aglycone

No therapeutic advantage was afforded by epimerization of the substituents at positions 7 and 9 of 4-demethoxydaunomycin (e.g., 4-demethoxy-7, 9-diepidaunomycin, both α- and β-anomers). Supino and co-workers (1977) reported a loss of activity for these analogues relative to DNM with similar results obtained for ADM and its derivatives. Thus the steric requirements about position 9 and especially position 7 are critical for antitumor activity.

F. Modification at Postion 10 of the Aglycone

Modifications at position 10 of the aglycone pertain mainly to the pyrromycinone and aklavinone families of anthracyclines, although studies on the

TABLE VI

In Vivo and *in Vitro* **Activity of 5-Imino-daunorubicin as Compared with Daunorubicin and Andriamycin**[a]

| | In vivo antitumor activity[b] qd 1–9 | | q4d 5,9,13 | | Cardio-toxicity[c] | IC$_{50}$ values (μM)[d] | |
Anthracycline	Dose (mg/kg)	% T/C	Dose (mg/kg)	% T/C	(mg/kg)	DNA synthesis	RNA synthesis
Adriamycin	1.56	176 ± 72	16.0	120 ± 12	11	1.5	0.7
	0.78	197 ± 26	8.0	159 ± 20			
	0.39	174 ± 14	4.0	146 ± 15			
	0.20	160 ± 7	2.0	130 ± 13			
Daunorubicin	1.56	148 ± 35	16.0	126 ± 12	14	1.0	0.3
	0.78	160 ± 27	8.0	132 ± 4			
	0.39	153 ± 9	4.0	128 ± 12			
	0.20	144 ± 9	2.0	126 ± 15			
5-Imino-	4.0	153 ± 3	24.0	126 ± 3	64	1.6	1.3
daunomycin	2.0	170 ± 15	12.0	116 ± 14			
	1.0	184 ± 11	6.0	124 ± 1			
	0.5	145 ± 8	3.0	130 ± 6			
			1.5	126 ± 8			

[a] Data obtained from Tong *et al.* (1979a).
[b] Activity against mouse P388 leukemia.
[c] Minimum cumulative cardiotoxic dose.
[d] 50% inhibitory concentrations employing cultured L1210 cells.

latter group have not been performed. The structures of these groups of an-thracyclines are shown in Fig. 2, Chapter 8. The ADM–DNM group of com-pounds lacks a substitutent at this position (Fig. 1, Chapter 8).

Initial studies examining the effect of modifications at position 10 of the ag-lycone employed the 10-descarbomethoxy analogues of MCM and RDM, the structures of which are shown in Fig. 2. The importance of the carbomethoxy group (see Fig. 2) at this position with regard to the antitumor activity and the molecular pharmacology of these agents has been previously reported (DuVernay *et al.*, 1979a; DuVernay, 1979) and is summarized in Table VII. This table shows the structure activity relationships obtained regarding the carbomethoxy group at position 10 of the aglycone with regard to DNA binding affinity, nucleolar RNA synthesis inhibitory potency, and antitumor activity both *in vivo* and *in vitro*. The decreased antitumor activity for both MCM and RDM, on removal of the 10-carbomethoxy group and the corresponding loss of nucleolar RNA synthesis inhibitory activity, suggests this latter metabolic process as a subcellular target of the class II (pyrromycinone-based) anthracyclines (DuVer-nay *et al.*, 1979a). The correlation of these findings with DNA binding abilities

TABLE VII

Structure–Activity Relationships of Class II Anthracyclines: The Carbomethoxy Group at Position 10 of the Aglycone

| Anthracycline | K_{app} ($\times$ 10^6 M^{-1})[a] | | | | IC_{50}[a] No-RNA synthesis (μM) | IC_{50}[a] cell survival (μM) | In vivo[b] antitumor activity (mg/kg/inj) |
	M. luteus DNA	Calf thymus DNA	Salmon sperm DNA	Cl. perfr. DNA			
Marcellomycin	5.25	5.03	9.51	6.05	0.01	0.75	0.20
Descarbomethoxy-marcellomycin	1.21	2.14	1.28	1.26	2.56	3.80	4.0
Mimimycin	–	0.33	0.32	–	–	–	51.2[c]
Rudolfomycin	2.02	1.98	3.11	2.44	0.29	0.31	0.20
Descarbomethoxy-rudolfomycin	0.42	1.42	1.54	0.96	9.13	5.0	16.0
Musettamycin	2.32	2.21	1.99	2.96	0.014	–	0.80
Collinemycin	–	0.42	0.59	–	–	–	12.8[c]

[a] Obtained from DuVernay et al. (1979a).

[b] Minimum effective doses (% T/C = 129) against mouse L1210 leukemia. Doses were administered once daily on days 1–5 as previously reported (DuVernay et al., 1979a; DuVernay, 1979).

[c] Doses administered once on day 1.

(DuVernay et al., 1979c) demonstrated the requirements for DNA–drug interactions in the antitumor action of these agents. Furthermore, the correlation of a molecular event with antitumor activity for these anthracyclines has been demonstrated.

Additional modification studies of the 10-carbomethoxy group, in this case MSM and MCM, have been recently reported (DuVernay, 1979). Those modifications involve epimerization of the carbomethoxy group of MSM and MCM yielding CLM and MIMI, respectively, the structures of which are shown in Fig. 3. The activity changes observed were even more marked than those obtained for the 10-descarbomethoxy analogues, as shown in Table VII. Epimerization of the group at position 10 is correlated with a marked decrease in both DNA binding ability and antitumor activity. Thus the carbomethoxy group at position 10 of the class II anthracycline molecule appears to be an important requirement for antitumor activity. Furthermore, the stereospecific environment about this group appears to be critical for optimal antitumor activity.

G. Modifications at Position 13 of the Aglycone

Smith and co-workers (1978) reported on a series of analogues of ADM and DNM that were modified at position 13. Included were the 13-dihydro analogues of DNM and ADM in which the carboxyl group at position 13 was replaced by a

CH_2 group. These analogues were approximately equipotent with DNM and ADM, respectively, toward the inhibition of nucleic acid synthesis while retaining high antitumor activity at potencies comparable to those of their respective parent compounds (Smith *et al.*, 1978) (see Table VIII). In addition, the pyrromycinone-based anthracyclines all contain a methylene group (dihydro derivatives of the carboxyl group) at position 13. These anthracyclines exhibit significant changes in antitumor potency and efficacy from those of ADM and DNM, as will be discussed. The results indicated in Table VIII show that the 13-carboxyl group of ADM and DNM is not intrinsically required for their biological activities. Although the 13-dihydro analogues of ADM and DNM are comparable to their respective parent compounds in terms of potency and effi-

TABLE VIII

In Vitro and *in Vivo* Activities of the 13-Dihydro Analogues of Adriamycin and Daunomycin[a]

Drug	Nucleic acid synthesis inhibition, IC_{50} (μM)[b] DNA	RNA	Antitumor activity in mice P388, qd 1–9 Dose (mg/kg)	T/C[c] (n)	P388, qd 5, 9, 13 Dose (mg/kg)	T/C (n)
Daunomycin	0.66	0.33	1.56	148 ± 35 (8)	16	127 ± 11 (17)
			0.78	167 ± 27 (8)	8	134 ± 6 (17)
			0.39	153 ± 9 (8)	4	131 ± 13 (17)
			0.20	144 ± 9 (8)		
Adriamycin	1.5	0.58	1.56	176 ± 72 (8)	16	130 ± 10 (4)
			0.78	197 ± 26 (8)	8	157 ± 21 (17)
			0.39	174 ± 14 (8)	4	142 ± 14 (17)
			0.20	160 ± 7 (8)	2	133 ± 14 (17)
					1	133 ± 4 (5)
13-Dihydro-daunomycin	1.3	0.84	3.13	160 ± 3 (2)	18.8	140
			1.56	160 ± 9 (2)	9.4	132
			0.78	134 ± 1 (2)	4.7	131
			0.39	140 ± 9 (2)		
13-Dihydro-adriamycin	1.8	1.1	6.25	153	37.5	147
			3.13	164 ± 1 (2)	18.8	147
			1.56	156 ± 2 (2)	9.4	154
			0.78	161 ± 3 (2)	4.7	128
			0.39	140 ± 11 (2)		

[a] Data obtained from Smith *et al.* (1978).

[b] IC_{50}, 50% inhibitory concentrations, determined in cultured L1210 cells as previously reported (Tong *et al.*, 1976).

[c] Ratio of average survival times of treated mice to untreated controls in percent. The average survival time of untreated controls is approximately 11 days. Activity is defined as values of T/C > 125.

cacy, further studies are required to evaluate their toxicities and thus determine if they offer any advantage over their parent compounds.

Substitution of the carboxyl group at position 13 of DNM with a benzyhydrazone function resulted in the analogue rubidazone, which was equal to or slightly superior to DNM in efficacy against P388 leukemia and B16 melanoma *in vivo* (Henry, 1975). In addition, as shown in Table IX, rubidazone was three to six times more potent than DNM. Results obtained with the schedule-sensitive neoplasm L1210 leukemia, *in vivo,* while being less marked, suggested significant antitumor activity for rubidazone (Henry, 1975). The nucleic acid synthesis inhibitory potency of DNM was significantly greater than that of rubidazone (Table IX). Finally, the therapeutic index of rubidazone was about two times greater than that of DNM, reflecting a decrease in toxicity associated with this analogue (Moral *et al.,* 1972). The benzhydrazone derivative of ADM, also indicated in Table IX, showed a decrease in potency and a slight reduction in efficacy against P388 leukemia, as compared to ADM (Henry, 1975). Although the nucleic acid synthesis inhibitory potency was significantly decreased, no further results are available on this analogue.

Finally, a comparison of the structures of the aklavinone- and the pyrromycinone-based anthracyclines with the ADM–DNM group (See Figures 1 and 2, Chapter 8) reveals that the former two groups lack a carboxyl function. Although other structural differences are present, this modification may be an

TABLE IX

The *in Vivo* and *in Vitro* Activities of Analogues of Adriamycin and Daunorubicin Modified at Position 13 of the Aglycone[a]

	In vivo L1210		*In vivo* P388		*In vitro* IC$_{50}$ values (μM)[b]	
Anthracycline	Optimal dose (mg/kg)	ILS[c]	Optimal dose (mg/kg)	ILS[c]	DNA synthesis	RNA synthesis
Adriamycin	1.7	63	1.0	112	0.8	0.9
			0.5	140		
Daunorubicin	1.7	43	0.50	70	0.3	0.3
			0.85	108		
Rubidazone	5.9	27	2	75	2.7	2.0
Adriamycin-13-benzhydrazone	–	–	6	152	6.5	3.0

[a] Results obtained from Henry (1975).

[b] Determined by measuring drug effect on incorporation of labeled precursors into acid-insoluble material, employing cultured L1210 cells (Henry, 1975).

[c] ILS, percentage increased life span.

important determinant of the increased activities exhibited by the pyr-romycinone- and aklavinone-based anthracyclines. Thus modification at position 13 of the anthracycline aglycone may offer important therapeutic advantages by conferring significant increases in antitumor activity while decreasing undesirable side effects.

H. Modifications at Position 14 of the Aglycone

Early studies on the antitumor activity and biological effects of the protype compounds DNM and ADM demonstrated the importance of modifications at position 14 (Henry, 1975). Conversion of the CH_3 group at position 14 of DNM to a CH_2OH group (e.g., ADM) resulted in greater efficacy and a broader spectrum of antitumor activity (Blum and Carter, 1974; Carter, 1975; Henry, 1975). Cleavage of the carbon at position 14 to leave the carboxylic acid group attached to position 9 resulted in a marked decrease in the potency for nucleic acid synthesis inhibition (Tong *et al.*, 1976). This decrease in activity *in vitro* may have been due to decreased cellular uptake because of the more polar character of this analogue. Conversion of this carboxylic acid function to a methyl ester derivative resulted in an analogue that exhibited potencies comparable to those of ADM and DNM toward nucleic acid synthesis inhibition. Both analogues possessed significant antitumor efficacy against P388 leukemia; however, antitumor potencies were substantially decreased relative to ADM and DNM. The ranking of these compounds with regard to antitumor efficacies was ADM > DNM $\simeq$ the 9-COOH analogue > 9-COOCH$_3$ analogue (Tong *et al.*, 1976). The slight *in vivo* superiority of both the 9-COOH and the 9-COOCH$_3$ analogues contrasted with the *in vitro* results. However, since these two analogues differ substantially in polarity, one would suspect that they would be transported and metabolized differently by the host.

A series of anthracycline analogues modified at position 14 were studied, including adriamycin-14-octanoate. Increased antitumor efficacies, relative to ADM, against mouse sarcoma 180 ascites *in vivo* were obtained for several of these analogues while only two analogues, including adriamycin-14-octanoate, retained potencies equivalent to ADM. This latter finding may be accounted for on the basis of a rapid *in vivo* conversion to ADM by mouse serum esterases (Arcamone, 1977). Thus esterification of the 14-hydroxyl group leads to modifications in the distribution characteristics of these analogues, which may offer a therapeutic advantage for these analogues.

I. Modifications at Position 1' of the Sugar

Epimerization of the glycosidic linkage attached at position 1' (e.g., the β-anomer of 7) resulted in a loss of antitumor activity (DiMarco *et al.*, 1976).

J. Modifications at Position 2' of the Sugar

Hydroxylation of the daunosamine sugar at position 2' of DNM resulted in a loss of antitumor activity against L1210 leukemia as well as a significant decrease in nucleic acid synthesis inhibitory potency in *in vitro* cell-free systems (DiMarco *et al.*, 1977).

K. Modifications at Position 4' of the Sugar

Removal of the hydroxyl group from position 4' of the sugar of DNM and ADM resulted in analogues that exhibited no significant change in DNA binding ability or nucleic acid synthesis inhibition (DiMarco *et al.*, 1977). However, 4'-deoxyadriamycin was slightly more potent against L1210 leukemia than ADM and markedly more potent against HeLa cells *in vitro*. Similar changes, though less marked, occurred on removal of the hydroxyl group from DNM (DiMarco *et al.*, 1977).

Epimerization of the hydroxyl group at position 4' of DNM resulted in insignificant changes in *in vivo* and *in vitro* activities. A slight decrease in activity both *in vitro* and *in vivo* occurred on epimerization of the hydroxyl group at position 4' of the sugar side chain of ADM (DiMarco *et al.*, 1977).

The importance of modifications at position 4' of the sugar side chain of the anthracycline molecule, with regard to antitumor activity, is clearly demonstrated in the pyrromycinone-based anthracyclines. Figure 13 shows the structures of the three anthracyclines PYM, MSM, and MCM. These compounds are identical with respect to the PYM portion of the molecule but differ in the

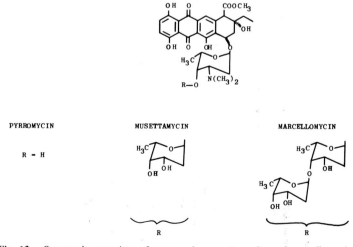

Fig. 13. Structural comparison of pyrromycin, musettamycin, and marcellomycin.

TABLE X

Structure–Activity Relationships of Class II Anthracyclines: The Length of the Glycosidic Side Chain

Anthracycline	Number of sugar groups in side chain	K_{app} ($\times\ 10^6\ M^{-1}$)[a]					IC_{50} (μM)			In vivo[d] antitumor activity (mg/kg)
		Poly(dGdC)-poly(dGdC)	M. luteus DNA	Calf thymus DNA	Cl. perfr. DNA	Poly(dAdT)-Poly(dAdT)	DNA[b] synth.	RNA[b] synth.	No-RNA[c] synth.	
Pyrromycin	1	0.88	0.87	0.98	1.01	1.33	5.7	4.5	6.15	8.0
Musettamycin	2	2.46	2.32	2.21	2.96	6.79	10.0	1.5	0.014	0.8
Marcellomycin	3	4.75	5.25	5.03	6.05	13.23	11.3	1.7	0.009	0.2

[a] Obtained from DuVernay et al. (1979b).
[b] Obtained from Table I.
[c] Obtained from Table II.
[d] Against mouse L1210 leukemia. Doses administered once daily over days 1–5 as previously reported (DuVernay, 1979). Minimal effective doses (% T/C = 129).

number of sugar residues present in the glycosidic side chain. Table X shows the structure activity relationships obtained regarding the length of the glycosidic side chain and correlates the effect of increasing the number sugar residues in the glycosidic side chain with the affinity for binding to DNA, the potency for the inhibition of DNA, whole cellular RNA, nucleolar RNA syntheses, and *in vivo* antitumor potencies (Crooke *et al.*, 1978; DuVernay *et al.*, 1979b; DuVernay, 1979). Using the values obtained for PYM as baseline, the addition of the second sugar group, in this case 2-deoxyfucose to obtain MSM, significantly increases the affinity constants for all DNAs studied and markedly increases the potency for the inhibition of nucleolar RNA synthesis with a simultaneous increase in antitumor activity both *in vivo* and *in vitro*. Addition of the third sugar residue, also 2-deoxyfucose to obtain MCM, significantly increases the DNA binding ability and further increases the nucleolar RNA synthesis inhibitory potency. Thus an increase in the length of the glycosidic side chain is correlated with higher affinities for DNA, greater potency for the inhibition of nucleolar RNA synthesis, and increased antitumor activities both *in vivo* and *in vitro*.

To examine the importance of the sugar composition of the glycosidic side chain, the structures of the three class II anthracyclines MSM, MCM, and RDM were compared, the structures of which are shown in Fig. 14. All three anthracyclines are identical with respect to the MSM portion of the molecule but differ in the terminal sugar residue of the glycosidic side chain. The terminal sugar group of MSM, a disaccharide, is identical to that of MCM, a trisaccharide, whereas that of RDM, a trisaccharide, is rednosamine. The structure activity relationships obtained regarding the terminal sugar residue of the glycosidic side chain are shown in Table XI. This table correlates the change in

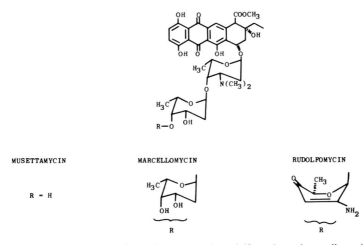

MUSETTAMYCIN   MARCELLOMYCIN   RUDOLFOMYCIN

Fig. 14.   Structural comparison of musettamycin, rudolfomycin, and marcellomycin.

TABLE XI

Structure–Activity Relationships of Class II Anthracyclines: The Terminal Sugar Group of the Glycosidic Side Chain

Anthracycline	Terminal sugar group in side chain	K_{app} ($\times 10^6$ M^{-1})[a]					IC_{50} (μM)			In vivo[d] antitumor activity (mg/kg)
		Poly(dGdC)-poly(dGdC)	M. luteus DNA	Calf thymus DNA	Cl. perfr. DNA	Poly(dAdT)-poly(dAdT)	DNA[b] synth.	RNA[b] synth.	No-RNA[c] synth.	
Musettamycin	2-deoxyfucose	2.46	2.32	2.21	2.96	6.79	10.0	1.50	0.014	0.80
Rudolfomycin	rednosamine	1.74	2.02	1.98	2.44	6.88	69.7	3.65	0.290	0.20
Marcellomycin	2-deoxyfucose	4.74	5.25	5.03	6.05	13.23	11.3	1.70	0.009	0.20

[a] Obtained from DuVernay et al. (1979b).
[b] Obtained from Table I.
[c] Obtained from Table II.
[d] Minimum effective doses (% T/C = 129) against mouse L1210 leukemia. Doses administered once daily over days 1–5 as previously reported (DuVernay, 1979).

the terminal sugar residue with the change in affinities for DNA binding and the nucleolar RNA synthesis inhibitory potencies (Crooke *et al.*, 1978; DuVernay *et al.*, 1979b; DuVernay, 1979). Since all three anthracyclines are identical with regard to the MSM portion of the molecule, the values obtained for this agent can be considered as baseline. Addition of the terminal sugar residue rednosamine did not significantly alter the DNA binding affinities and actually decreased the nucleolar RNA synthesis inhibitory potency by a factor of 20. In contrast, addition of the terminal sugar residue 2-deoxyfucose (e.g., MCM) significantly increased the DNA binding affinities and further increased the potency for the inhibition of nucleolar RNA synthesis. Thus the presence of the terminal sugar residue 2-deoxyfucose was correlated with enhanced DNA binding ability and nucleolar RNA synthesis inhibitory potency.

L. Modifications at Position 6' of the Sugar

Hydroxylation at position 6' of DNM resulted in a marked decrease in nucleic acid synthesis inhibitory potency *in vitro* as well as a loss of antitumor activity. There was also a significant decrease in DNA binding ability. Similar results were obtained for the 4'-epi-6'-hydroxy analogues of DNM and ADM (DiMarco *et al.*, 1977).

M. Modifications of the Amino Group at Position 3' of the Sugar

Tong and co-workers (1979b) reported on the synthesis and some studies on several N-alkylated analogues of ADM and DNM. These analogues are all modified at the three-amino group of the sugar side chain and all the analogues exhibited increased selectivity for the inhibition of whole cellular RNA synthesis. The N',N;-dibenzyl analogue of DNM was reported to have a 10-fold lower cardiotoxic potential, relative to DNM. Of the other analogues studied most exhibited no change in cardiotoxidity relative to parent compounds, whereas N',N'-dimethyladriamycin was nearly two times more cardiotoxic when minimum cumulative cardiotoxic doses were compared (Tong *et al.*, 1979b). Finally, the antitumor activities of these analogues was generally not significantly changed from the parent compounds. Two exceptions include N',N'-demethyldaunomycin, which exhibited greater efficacy and decreased potency relative to DNM, and the N',N'-diethyl analogue of DNM and ADM, which exhibited significant decreases in antitumor potencies with minimal changes in efficacy (Tong *et al.*, 1979b).

V. CONCLUSIONS

Studies on the molecular pharmacology of anthracyclines have provided valuable information regarding structural loci on the anthracycline molecule that may be important in conferring increased activity and decreased toxicities. Further studies are required to obtain agents with better therapuetic indices than those presently available with the existing anthracyclines. The results obtained from structure activity relationship studies indicate that structural loci that are important in governing increased potencies and/or efficacies include positions 4, 9, 10, 13, and 14 of the aglycone, and positions 4' and the 3'-amino group of the sugar side chain. Structural loci that may be important in conferring improved or decreased toxicities include positions 4, 5, 10, 13, and 14 of the aglycone and the 3' amino group of the side chain. Thus relatively minor structural modifications can confer significant changes in the mechanism of action of these compounds, suggesting that, as a class of compounds, the anthracyclines are heterogeneous with respect to mechanisms of action.

REFERENCES

Andreini, G., Beretta, C. M., and Sonzogni, O. (1977). *Pharmacol. Res. Commun.* **9**, 155–164.
Arcamone, F. (1977). *Lloydia* **40**, 45–66.
Arcamone, F., Cassinelli, G., Fantini, G., Grein, A., Orezzi, P., Pol, C., and Spalla, C. (1969). *Biotechnol. Bioeng.* **11**, 1101.
Arcamone, R., Bernardi, L., Patelli, B., Giardino, P., DiMarco, A., Casazza, A. M., Soranzo, C., and Pratesi, G. (1978). *Experientia* **34**, 1255–1256.
Arlandini, E., Vigevani, A., and Arcamone, F. (1977). *Farmaco* **32**, 314–323.
Beerman, T. A., and Goldberg, I. H. (1977). *Biochim. Biophys. Acta* **475**, 281–293.
Bertazzoli, C., and Ghione, M. (1977). *Pharmacol. Res. Commun.* **9**, 235–250.
Bertazzoli, C., Sala, L., Ballerini, L., Watanabe, T., and Folkers, K. (1978). *Res. Commun. Chem. Pathol. Pharmacol.* **15**, 797–800.
Bhuyan, B. K., and Smith, C. G. (1965). *Proc. Natl. Acad. Sci. U.S.A.* **54**, 566–572.
Bhuyan, B. K., and Smith, C. G. (1975). "Nogalamycin," In "Antineoplostie and Immunosuppressive Agents," (eds. A. C. Sartorelli, and D. G. Johns) pp. 623–632, Springer-Verlag, Berlin.
Blum, R. H., and Carter, S. K. (1974). *Ann. Intern. Med.* **80**, 249.
Böhner, R., and Hagen, U. (1977). *Biochim. Biophys. Acta* **479**, 300–310.
Brazhnikova, M. G., Zbarsky, V. B., Ponomarenko, V. T., and Potapova, N. P. (1974). *J. Antibiot.* **27**, 254–259.
Brockmann, H., and Brockmann, H., Jr. (1960). *Naturwissenschaften* **47**, 135.
Brockmann, H., and Lenk, W. (1959). *Chem. Ber.* **92**, 1904–1909.
Brockmann, H., Pia, L. S., and Lenk, W. (1957). *Angew. Chem.* 69: 477.
Buyniski, J. and Hirth, R. S. (1980). In "Anthracyclines: Current Status and New Developments", (S. T. Crooke and S. D. Reich, eds.), pp. 157–170, Academic Press, New York.
Calendi, E., DiMarco, A., Reggiani, M., Scarpinato, B., and Valentini, L. (1965). *Biochim. Biophys. Acta* **103**, 25–49.
Carter, S. K. (1975). *J. Natl. Cancer Inst.* **55**, 1265–1274.
Crook, L. E., Rees, K. R., and Cohen, A. (1972). *Biochem. Pharmacol.* **21**, 281–286.
Crooke, S. T. (1977). *J. Med.* **8**, 295–316.
Crooke, S. T., DuVernay, V. H., Galvan, L., and Prestayko, A. W. (1978). *Mol. Pharmacol.* **14**, 290–298.
Danø, K. (1971). *Cancer Chemother. Rep.* **55**, 133–141.

Danø, K. (1972a). *Cancer Chemother. Rep.* **56,** 321-326.

Danø, K. (1972b). *Cancer Chemother. Rep.* **56,** 701-708.

Danø, K., Frederiksen, S., and Hellung-Larsen, P. (1972). *Cancer Res.* **32,** 1307-1314.

Daskal, Y. (1979). In "Effects of Drugs on the Cell Nucleus," (H. Busch, S. T. Crooke, and Y. Daskal, eds.) vol. 1, pp. 107-125, Academic Press, New York.

Daskal, Y., Woodard, C., Crooke, S. T., and Busch, H. (1978). *Cancer Res.* **38,** 467-473.

DiMarco, A. (1975a). *In* "Handbook of Experimental Pharmacology" (A. C. Sartorelli and D. G. Johns, eds.), Vol. 38/2, pp. 593-614. Springer-Verlag, Berlin and New York.

DiMarco, A. (1975b). *Cancer Chemother. Rep.* **59,** (Part 6) 91.

DiMarco, A., Gaetani, V., Orezzi, P., Scarpinato, B., Silvestrini, R., Soldati, M., Dasdia, T., and Valenti, L. (1964). *Nature (London)* **201,** 706.

DiMarco, A., Silvestrini, R., Dasdia, T., and DiMarco, S. (1965a). *Riv. Ital. Istochim.* **11,** 211.

DiMarco, A., Silvestrini, R., DiMarco, S., and Dasdia, T. (1965b). *J. Cell Biol.* **27,** 545-550.

DiMarco, A., Gaetani, M., and Scarpinato, B. (1969). *Cancer Chemother. Rep.* **53,** 33-37.

DiMarco, A., Arcamone, F., and Zunino, F. (1975). *In* "Antibiotics II—Mechanism of Action of Antimicrobial and Antitumor Agents" (J. W. Corcoran and F. E. Hahn, eds.), pp. 101-128. Springer-Verlag, Berlin and New York.

DiMarco, A., Casazza, A. M., Gambetta, R., Supino, R., and Zunino, F. (1976). *Cancer Res.* **36,** 1962-1966.

DiMarco, A., Casazza, A. M., Dasdia, T., Necco, A., Pratesi, G., Rivolta, P., Velcich, A., Zaccara, A., and Zunino, F. (1977). *Chem.-Biol. Interact.* **19,** 291-302.

Doyle, T. W., Grulich, R. E., Nettleton, D. E., and Essery, J. M. (1978). *Proc. 61st Can. Chem. Conf. Exhib., Winnipeg, Manit.*

Doyle, T. W., Nettleton, D. E., Grulich, R. E., Balitz, D. M., Johnson, J. L., and Vulcano, A. L. (1979). *J. Am. Chem. Soc.* **101:**7041-7049.

DuVernay, V. H. (1979). Ph.D. Thesis, Baylor Coll. of Med., Houston, Texas.

DuVernay, V. H., Essery, J. M., Doyle, T. W., Bradner, W. T., and Crooke, S. T. (1979a). *Mol. Pharmacol.* **15,** 341-356.

DuVernay, V. H., Pachter, J. A., and Crooke, S. T. (1979b). Biochemistry **18,** 4024-4030.

DuVernay, V. H., Pachter, J. A., and Crooke, S. T. (1979c). *Mol. Pharmacol.* **16,** 623-632.

DuVernay, V. H., Pachter, J. A., and Crooke, S. T. (1980). *Cancer Res.* **40,** 387-394.

Ellen, K. A. O., and Rhode, S. L. (1970). *Biochim. Biophys. Acta* **209,** 415.

Essery, J. M., and Doyle, T. W. (1979). *J. Antibiot.* **32,** 247-250.

Facchinetti, T., Montovani, A., Cantoni, L., Cantoni, R., and Salmona, M. (1978). *Chem.-Biol. Interact.* **20,** 97-102.

Gabbay, E. J., Grier, D., Fingele, R., Reiner, R., Pearce, S. W., and Wilson, W. D. (1976). *Biochemistry* **15,** 2062-2069.

Gause, G. F., Brazhnikova, M. G., and Shorin, V. A. (1974). *Cancer Chemother. Rep., Part 2* **58,** 255-256.

Gellert, M., Smith, C. E., Neville, D., and Felsenfeld, G. (1965). *J. Mol. Biol.* **11,** 445-457.

Goldman, R., Fachinetti, T., Bach, D., Raz, A., and Shinitzky, M. (1978). *Biochim. Biophys. Acta* **512,** 254-269.

Goodman, M. F., Bessman, M. J., and Bachur, N. R. (1974). *Proc. Natl. Acad. Sci. U.S.A.* **71,** 1193-1196.

Gosalvez, M., Blanco, M., Hunter, J., Miko, M., and Chance, B. (1974). *Eur. J. Cancer* **10,** 567-574.

Gottlieb, J. A., and Hill, C. S. (1974). *N. Engl. J. Med.* **290,** 193-197.

Henry, D. W. (1975). *Cancer Chemother., Div. Med. Chem. Symp., Meet. Am. Chem. Soc., 169th, Washington, D.C.* pp. 15-57.

Hittlema, W. N., and Rao, P. N. (1975). *Cancer Res.* **35,** 3027-3035.

Hyman, R. W., and Davidson, N. (1971). *Biochim. Biophys. Acta* **228,** 38–48.
Isetta, A. M., Initini, C., and Soldat, M. (1971). *Experientia* **27,** 202–204.
Israel, M., Modes, E. J., and Frei, E., III (1975). *Cancer Res.* **35,** 1365–1368.
Iwamoto, Y., Hansen, I. L., Porter, T. H., and Folkers, K. (1974). *Biochem. Biophys. Res. Commun.* **58,** 633–638.
Kann, H. H., and Kohn, K. W. (1972). *Mol. Pharmacol.* **8,** 551–560.
Kishi, T., Watnabe, T., and Folkers, K. (1976). *Proc. Natl. Acad. Sci. U.S.A.* **73,** 4653–4656.
Kitaura, K., Imai, R., Ishihara, Y., Yanai, H., and Takahira, H. (1972). *J. Antibiot.* **25,** 509–514.
Krishan, A., Israel, M., Modest, E. J., and Frei, E., III (1976). *Cancer Res.* **36,** 2114–2116.
Krishan, A., Ganapathi, R. N., and Israel, M. (1978). *Cancer Res.* **38,** 3656–3662.
Lee, Y. C., and Byfield, J. E. (1976). *J. Natl. Cancer Inst.* **57,** 221–224.
Lefrak, E. A., Pitha, J., Rosenheim, S., and Gottlieb, J. (1973). *Cancer (Philadelphia)* **32,** 302–314.
Lerman, L. S. (1961). *J. Mol. Biol.* **3,** 18–30.
Litchfield, J. T., Jr., and Wilcoxon, F. (1949). *J. Pharmacol. Exp. Ther.* **96,** 99–113.
Lown, J. W., Sim, S. K., Majundar, K. C., and Chang, R. Y. (1977). *Biochem. Biophys. Res. Commun.* **76,** 705–710.
Massimo, L., Dagna-Bricarelli, F., and Cherchi, M. G. (1971). *In* "International Symposium on Adriamycin (S. K. Carter, A. DiMarco, M. Ghione, eds.), pp. 35–46. Springer-Verlag, Berlin and New York.
Meriwether, W. D., and Bachur, N. R. (1972). *Cancer Res.* **32,** 1137–1142.
Merski, J., Daskal, Y., Crooke, S. T., and Busch, H. (1979). *Cancer Res.* **39,** 1239–1244.
Momparler, R. L., Karon, M., Siegel, S. E., and Avila, F. (1976). *Cancer Res.* **36,** 2891–2895.
Mong, S., DuVernay, V. H., Strong, J. E. and Crooke, S. T. (1980). *Mol. Pharmacol.* **17:**100–105.
Moral, R., Ponsinet, G., and Jolles, G. (1972). *C. R. Acad. Sci., Ser. D* **275,** 301–304.
Murphree, S. A., Cunningham, L. S., Hwang, K. M., and Sartorelli, A. C. (1976). *Biochem. Pharmacol.* **25,** 1227–1231.
Murphree, S. A., Tritton, T. R., and Sartorelli, A. C. (1977). *Fed. Proc.* **36,** 303.
Myers, C. E., McGuire, W., and Young, R. (1976). *Cancer Treat. Rep.* **60,** 961–962.
Myers, C. E., McGuire, W. P., Liss, R. H., Ifrim, I., Grotzinger, K., and Young, R. C. (1977). *Science* **197,** 165–167.
Na, G., and Timasheff, S. N. (1977). *Arch. Biochem. Biophys.* **182,** 147–154.
Nettleton, D. E., Bradner, W. T., Bush, J. A., Coon, A. B., Mosely, J. S., Myllymaki, R. W., O'Herron, F. A., Schrieber, R. H., and Vulcano, A. L. (1977). *J. Antibiot.* **30,** 525–529.
Oki, T. (1977). *J. Antibiot.* **30,** Suppl., S70–S84.
Oki, T., Matsuzawa, Y., Yoshimoto, A., Numata, K., Kitamura, I., Hori, S., Takamatsu, A., Umezawa, H., Ishizuka, M., Naganawa, H., Suda, H., Hamada, M., and Takeuchi, T. (1975). *J. Antibiot.* **28,** 830–834.
Parker, L., M., Hirst, M., and Israel, M. (1978). *Cancer Treat. Rep.* **62,** 119–127.
Pater, M. M., and Mak, S. (1974). *Nature (London)* **250,** 788.
Perry, R. R. (1963). *Exp. Cell Res.* **29,** 400.
Pigram, W. J., Fuller, W., and Hamilton, L. D. (1972). *Nature (London), New Biol.* **235,** 17–19.
Pratesi, G., Casazza, A. M., and DiMarco, A. (1978). *Cancer Treat. Rep.* **62,** 105–110.
Reuser, R. (1975). *Biochim. Biophys. Acta* **383,** 266–273.
Revet, B. M. J., Schmir, M., and Viongrad, J. (1971). *Nature (London), New Biol.* **229,** 10–13.
Rusconi, A., and Calendi, E. (1966). *Biochim. Biophys. Acta* **119,** 413.
Schurig, J., Bradner, W. T., Huftalen, J. B., and Doyle, T. W. (1980). In "Anthracyclines: Current Status and New Developments," (S. T. Crooke and S. D. Reich, eds.), pp. 141–149, Academic Press, New York.
Schwartz, H. S. (1975). *Res. Commun. Chem. Pathol. Pharmacol.* **10,** 51–64.

Sengupta, S. K., Seshadri, R., Modest, E. J., and Israel, M. (1976). *Proc. Am. Assoc. Cancer Res.* **17**, 109.

Silvestrini, R., DiMarco, A., and Dasdia, T. (1970). *Cancer Res.* **30**, 966.

Silvestrini, R., Lenaz, L., Difronzo, G., and Sanfilippo, O. (1973). *Cancer Res.* **33**, 2954–2958.

Smith, T. H., Fujiwara, A. N., and Henry, D. W. (1978). *J. Med. Chem.* **21**, 280–283.

Snyder, A. L., Kann, H. E., and Kohn, K. W. (1971). *J. Mol. Biol.* **58**, 555–565.

Strong, J. E., and Crooke, S. T. (1978). *Cancer Res.* **38**, 3322–3326.

Supino, R., Necco, A., Dasdia, T., Casazza, A. M., and DiMarco, A. (1977). *Cancer Res.* **37**, 4523–4528.

Tatsumi, K., Nakamura, T., and Wakisaka, G. (1974). *Gann* **65**, 237–247.

Thayer, W. S. (1977). *Chem.-Biol. Interact.* **19**, 265–278.

Tong, G. L., Lee, W. W., Black, D. R., and Henry, D. W. (1976). *J. Med. Chem.* **19**, 395–398.

Tong, G. L., Henry, D. W., and Acton, E. M. (1979a). *J. Med. Chem.* **22**, 36–39.

Tong, G. L., Yu, H. Y., Smith, T. H., and Henry D. W. (1979b). *J. Med. Chem.* **22**, 912–918.

Tritton, T. R., Murphree, S. A., and Sartorelli, A. C. (1978). *Biochem. Biophys. Res. Commun.* **84**, 802–805.

Tsou, K. C., and Yip, K. F. (1976). *Cancer Res.* **36**, 3367–3373.

Unuma, T., and Busch, H. (1967). *Cancer Res.* **27**, 1232–1242.

Vecchi, A., Cairo, M., Mantovani, A., Sironi, M., and Sprenfico, F. (1978). *Cancer Treat. Rep.* **62**, 111–117.

Wang, J. J., Chervinshy, D. S., and Rosen, J. M. (1972). *Cancer Res.* **32**, 511–515.

Ward, D. C., Reich, E., and Goldberg, I. H. (1965). *Science* **149**, 1259–1263.

Waring, M. (1970). *J. Mol. Biol.* **54**, 247–279.

Wilkinson, P. M., Israel, M., Pegg, W. J., and Frei, E., III (1979). *Cancer Chemother. Pharmacol.* **2**, 121–125.

Zunio, F., Gambetta, R., DiMarco, A., and Zaccara, A. (1972). *Biochim. Biophys. Acta* **277**, 489–498.

Zunio, F., Romolo, G., DiMarco, A., Luoni, G., and Zaccara, A. (1976). *Biochem. Biophys. Res. Commun.* **69**, 744–750.

Zunio, F., Gambetta, R., DiMarco, A., Velcich, A., and Zaccara, A. (1977). *Biochim. Biophys. Acta* **476**, 38–46.

15
VINCA ALKALOIDS: MOLECULAR AND CLINICAL PHARMACOLOGY
Richard A. Bender

I. INTRODUCTION

The common periwinkle plant, *Vinca rosea,* is an ever-blooming herb that is widely cultivated in ornamental gardens throughout the world. In the natural state, pink and white varieties are found, as illustrated in Fig. 1. This plant has found numerous uses in indigenous medicine throughout the world. It has been used to control hemorrhage and scurvy, as a mouthwash for toothaches, and in the healing and cleansing of chronic wounds. Moreover, it has been used to treat diabetic ulcer and as an oral hypoglycemic agent (Johnson *et al.,* 1963). Pioneering work at Lilly Research Laboratories in the early 1960s failed to confirm its hypoglycemic activity but did demonstrate the effect of a particular extract of the periwinkle plant on the bone marrow of experimental animals. More detailed investigation led to the preparation of a class of alkaloid substances that had antileukemic activity in mice. These alkaloids were vincristine (VCR),

CANCER AND CHEMOTHERAPY, VOL. III

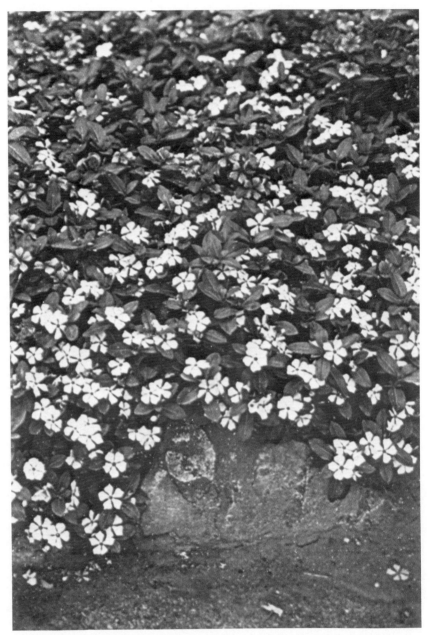

Fig. 1.   Photograph of white and pink *(Vinca rosea linn)* periwinkle plants.

vinblastine (VBL), vinleurosine, and vinrosidine. The greater potency of VCR and VLB against murine tumors, particularly P1534, occasioned their development for clinical use (Johnson *et al.*, 1963). The remainder of this chapter deals with their clinical and molecular pharmacology.

II. MOLECULAR STRUCTURE

Both VCR and VLB were extensively investigated using several structural probes and found to be dimeric substances consisting of two structurally similar multiringed compounds, vindoline and catharanthine, linked together by a carbon–carbon bridge. Curiously, neither vindoline nor catharanthine have any antitumor activity by themselves. The chemical formula for VCR is $C_{46}H_{54}N_4O_{10}$ and that for VLB is $C_{46}H_{56}N_4O_9$. Their close structural similarity is further emphasized by comparison of their molecular structures as depicted in Fig. 2A.

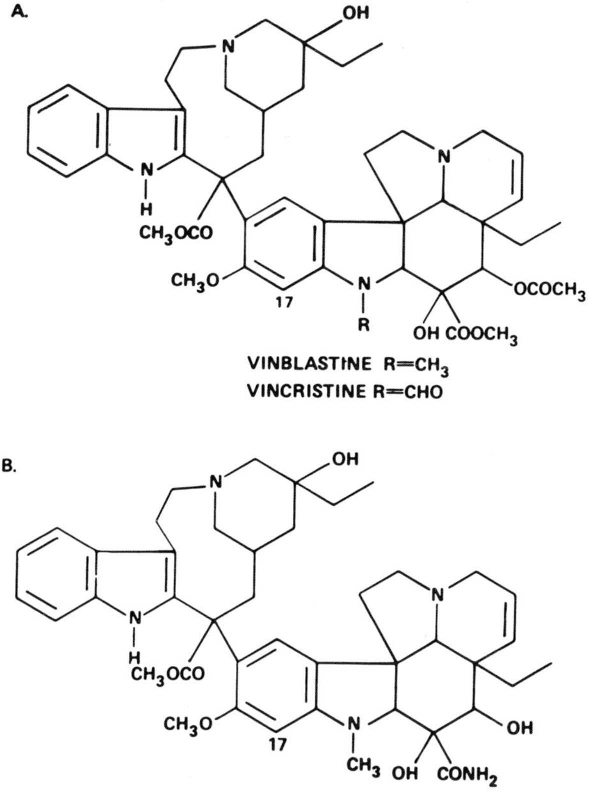

VINBLASTINE R=CH₃
VINCRISTINE R=CHO

Fig. 2. Molecular structure of vincristine, vinblastine (A), and vindesine (B).

VLB has a methyl group instead of the formyl group found on VCR. A new structural analogue, vindesine, currently under intensive investigation is depicted in Fig. 2B. The similarity of the molecular structures of these compounds is in striking contrast to their varied clinical spectrum of antitumor activity and toxicity.

III. MOLECULAR PHARMACOLOGY

A. Mechanism of Cellular Entry

Most antitumor agents must enter the cell and interact with an intracellular target to be effective. Some substances diffuse through the cell membrane passively; others do so in association with a carrier protein. A number of compounds require an expenditure of energy to traverse the cell membrane, so-called active transport. This appears to be the case with the vinca alkaloids. Bleyer *et al.* (1975) have provided evidence for carrier-mediated transport of VCR in L1210 and P388 murine leukemia cell lines. They found a Michaelis constant (K_m) for transport of 9.2 μM, with energy dependence, a Q_{10} of 6.3 and marked inhibition of cellular entry by the structural congener VLB. These data are strongly in favor of both carrier mediation and energy dependence for VCR transport in murine cell lines. Intracellular VCR appeared to be present in at least two distinct fractions: One fraction was irreversibly bound, presumably to the protein, tubulin, as will be discussed later, and a second fraction was exchangeable (VCR_{ex}) and free to exit the cell when resuspended in VCR-free media. We have postulated the existence of a third fraction, VCR bound to nontubulin proteins, the nature and details of which remain the subject of speculation. The presumed or proven role that each of these intracellular fractions plays in VCR's antitumor effect will be discussed in Sections III,B and III,C. A schematic representation of the transmembrane movement of VCR is found in Fig. 3.

Although study of the membrane transport of VLB remains to be performed, the close structural similarities of VCR and VLB and VLB's apparent specificity for the same membrane carrier site suggest that VLB too enters mammalian cells by an energy-dependent, carrier-mediated route. Further investigation of vinca alkaloid transport, particularly in resistant and nonresistant tumor cell lines, remains an important area of study. In addition, the existence of a putative "heterocyclic carrier" common to the vinca alkaloids—actinomycins, bleomycins, and anthracyclines—remains to be confirmed.

B. Interaction with Tubulin

Tubulin is the basic protein subunit of microtubules. Microtubules are abundant in eukaryotic cells, where they are associated with a number of essential functions, which include maintenance of cell shape, mitosis, meiosis, secretion,

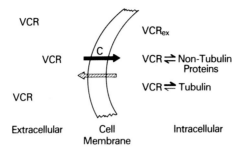

Fig. 3. Schematic representation of putative mechanism for vinca alkaloid transport (notably vincristine). The solid arrow and letter C depict an influx carrier and the dashed arrow an efflux mechanism that may or may not involve a carrier. Intracellular vincristine may exist bound to tubulin or nontubulin proteins or "free" in the intracellular volume as VCR_{ex}.

and axonal transport (Olmsted and Borisy, 1973). Many of the unique aspects of microtubules arise from the ability of tubulin to polymerize and depolymerize into smaller and larger units. Detailed study of tubulin polymerization suggests that it is a highly organized process having both pattern and direction (Tucker, 1977). Tubulin itself is a complex protein compound of α and β subunits, each having a molecular weight of about 55,000 (Luduena *et al.*, 1977). The recognition that VLB caused dissolution of microtubules *in vivo* (Bensch and Malawista, 1969) and induced tubulin-rich crystals intracellularly (Bryan, 1972) suggested that a primary site for the vinca alkaloid's cellular effect was tubulin. Subsequent investigations by Owellen *et al.* (1972, 1976) revealed that VCR and VLB bound to tubulin rapidly and with high affinity and were characterized by binding constants of 8.0×10^6 and 6.0×10^6 liters/mole, respectively. However, other investigators found a binding constant of 2×10^4 liters/mole using tubulin isolated from a different source, suggesting that there may be species differences in tubulin proteins (Lee *et al.*, 1975). Such speculation awaits additional laboratory confirmation. Interestingly, the stoichiometry and free-energy requirements for VCR and VLB binding to tubulin appear to be identical (Lee *et al.*, 1975).

Tubulin binding is a property shared by two other classes of antitumor agents, the ansa macrolides (maytansine) and the epipodophyllotoxins (VP-16 and VM-26). Indeed, it appears that VCR and maytansine may share a common tubulin binding site (Mandelbaum-Shavit *et al.*, 1976; Cortese *et al.*, 1977). The interaction of three classes of antineoplastic drugs with tubulin lends credence to the basic role of tubulin in cellular function and emphasizes its importance as an intracellular target of antineoplastic agents.

C. Cellular Action of the Vinca Alkaloids

The antitumor effect of VCR and VLB has been investigated from several aspects. The work of Creasey *et al.* (Creasey and Markiw, 1964, 1965; Creasey,

1968) originated from the concept that the effect of vinca alkaloids on mitosis arose from their effect on nucleic acid metabolism. He demonstrated that VLB concentrations of 0.2 mM inhibited uridine incorporation into RNA and, to a lesser extent, thymidine incorporation into DNA. In addition, VCR and VLB were found to inhibit the entry of glutamic acid into murine tumor cells. However, as will be discussed, the concentrations of VCR and VLB achieved *in vivo* are about 1000 times lower than those studied by Creasey *et al.*, suggesting that other mechanisms must be operative *in vivo*. It is of interest that recent studies by Peterson *et al.* (1976) on rat brain synaptosomes do confirm that micromolar concentrations of VLB may inhibit amino acid transport *in vitro*. Thus inhibition of transport of certain essential cellular substrates may be one mechanism of vinca action.

The known binding of VCR and VLB to microtubular protein prompted *in vitro* study of the effect of the vincas on tubulin polymerization. Owellen *et al.* (1976) demonstrated that tubulin polymerization was inhibited by VCR and VLB to a similar degree but that considerably higher concentrations of the separate vindoline and catharanthine portions of the dimeric molecule were required, consistent with their lack of cytotoxicity *in vivo* and *in vitro* (Johnson *et al.*, 1963). Inhibition of tubulin polymerization into microtubules, with subsequent arrest of cells in metaphase, does not require that cells be exposed to VCR or VLB only during mitosis or M phase. In fact, studies by Madoc-Jones and Mauro (1968) and by Jellinghaus *et al.* (1977) suggest that VCR can damage a cell during any phase of the cell cycle but that the effect may not be seen until the cell enters mitosis and is arrested in metaphase. Thus, although VCR and VLB appear to be phase-apecific with respect to their antitumor effect, all cycling cells are at risk for vinca-induced cytotoxicity because of VCR's and VLB's persistence intracellularly. An extension of these observations examines the reversibility of the mitotic arrest of cells exposed to vinca alkaloids. Bruchovsky *et al.* (1965) and Madoc-Jones and Mauro (1968) reported a lack of reversibility of the mitotic arrest of cells exposed to the vinca alkaloids; however, whether mitotic arrest is translated into a subsequent loss of cell viability is not clear. Tucker *et al.* (1977) demonstrated spindle dissolution in 50% of Chinese hamster fibroblasts exposed briefly to VLB without subsequent cell death as determined by the cells' continued ability to form colonies. These results are consistent with earlier reports of the reversibility of vinca alkaloid-induced mitotic arrest following resuspension of cells in fresh media (Krishan, 1968), although cellular recovery may not be complete (Journey *et al.*, 1968). Moreover, they serve to highlight the lack of clarity regarding the antitumor action(s) of the vinca alkaloids.

Cytotoxic concentrations of VCR and VLB have been investigated using soft agar cloning techniques (Chu and Fisher, 1968; Jackson and Bender, 1978). These studies have demonstrated that maintained VCR concentrations of 4 × 10^{-8} M are 100% lethal to dividing murine leukemia cells and that concentrations of $\sim 1 \times 10^{-8}$ M produced a 50% kill (Jackson and Bender, 1978). Using a murine bioassay technique, Wilkoff *et al.* (1968) calculated a minimum effective VCR concentration of between 1.2×10^{-8} M and 1.2×10^{-9} M in L1210 leukemia cells. Investigation of the cytotoxic threshold in human tissues has focused on a lymphoblastoid cell line, CEM. Constant *in vitro* exposure of CEM cells to 1×10^{-8} M VCR revealed this to be a maximally effective concentration in inhibiting cell proliferation (Jackson and Bender, 1978). Interestingly, Schrek (1974) noted a difference in the *in vitro* VCR concentration needed to produce morphologic changes in normal lymphocytes and those of chronic lymphocytic leukemia. Following a 7-day exposure, 1.2×10^{-5} M and 9.7×10^{-7} M were found to be minimal effective concentrations in these two cell types, respectively. This differential sensitivity may help explain VCR's effectiveness in the treatment of acute and chronic lymphocytic leukemia with relative sparing of normal lymphocytes. The clinical relevance of these experimentally derived *in vitro* cytotoxic concentrations will be clarified in the following section on clinical pharmacology.

IV. CLINICAL PHARMACOLOGY

A. Vincristine

Investigation of the human pharmacology of the vinca alkaloids has been greatly assisted by the use of tritiated radiochemicals (Owellen and Donigian, 1972) and, more recently, by a radioimmunoassay (Owellen *et al.*, 1977a). Bender *et al.* (1977) studied four patients with malignant lymphoma using radioactively labeled VCR that had been purified by high-pressure liquid chromatography (HPLC). Each patient received a standard clinical dose of 2 mg and the disappearance of blood radioactivity was measured. A peak value of 3.6×10^{-7} M was reached at 2.5 min with a triphasic decay and thereafter with half-lives of 0.85, 7.4, and 164 min (see Fig. 4). Owellen *et al.* (1977a). was able to identify similar half-lives of 3.4 and 155 min. Extensive binding of VCR to formed blood elements was noted, with greater than 50% of the radiolabel bound 20 min after injection. Owellen and Hartke (1975) had previously determined that binding to blood elements occurred in order: plasma > platelets > red blood cells > white blood cells. Their extensive binding to blood platelets may explain their role, particularly VCR, in the management of idiopathic thrombocytopenia purpura, a disorder of blood platelets.

The extensive tissue binding of VCR may help explain some unique features of its excretion. Over a 72-hr period of study, 12% of the radioactivity was excreted in the urine, of which one-half was metabolites and/or decomposition products. Approximately 69% was excreted in the feces, with about 40% as metabolites

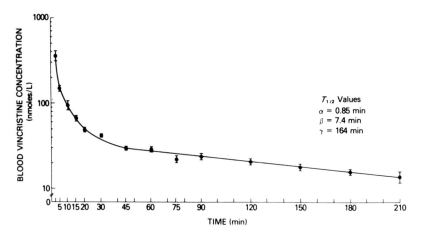

Fig. 4. The blood disappearance curve of tritiated vincristine in man. The $t_{\frac{1}{2}}$ values are derived by linear regression analysis. Correction for metabolism and/or decomposition is not included in the concentration measurements. (From Bender *et al.*, 1977.)

and/or decomposition products (Bender *et al.*, 1977). Resolution of parent drug from metabolites and/or decomposition products was carried out using HPLC techniques. The high percentage of radioactivity excreted in the feces of these patients and previous reports of substantial biliary excretion in animals (Castle *et al.*, 1976; El Dareer *et al.*, 1977) suggested the biliary route to be the principal route of elimination in man. This was confirmed by Jackson *et al.* (1978) employing intravenously administered tritiated VCR in a patient with a choledochal T tube. Following a total dose of 0.5 mg, VCR and its metabolic and/or decomposition products were rapidly concentrated in the bile. The highest biliary concentration (6×10^{-7} M) occurred 2–4 hr following injection and was more than 100 times higher than the concentration recorded in the simultaneous plasma sample (see Fig. 5). Following that, the plasma and biliary concentrations declined with similar half-lives with the biliary VCR concentration about 20 times higher than that in the plasma at the 72-hr time point. Biliary excretion was cumulative over this time interval with 49.6% of the injected radiolabel present in the bile by 72 hr (see Fig. 6). Curiously, only 4.2% of the radiolabel was recovered in the feces, in contrast to the earlier study by Bender *et al.* (1977), where 69% of the administered dose was excreted in the feces. However, as no biliary samples were obtained in the latter study, the biliary contribution to fecal excretion likely explains the difference and validates the notion that biliary excretion is the principal route in man. Products of VCR metabolism and/or decomposition rapidly appeared in the bile and only 46.5% of the drug was in the parent form by the 2-hr collection, as determined by HPLC analysis. However, while hepatic metabolism appears to be implicated, the origin of the radioactive

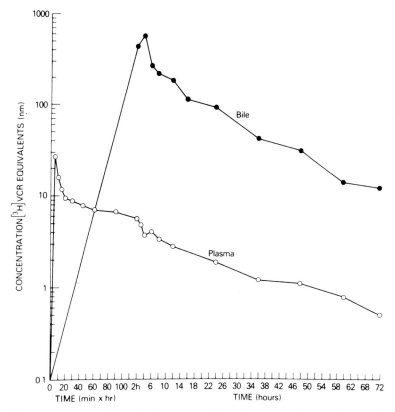

Fig. 5.   Concentration of tritiated vincristine and its metabolic and/or decomposition products in the plasma and bile at various time points in man. (From Jackson *et al.*, 1978.)

species appearing in the bile remains unclear as the parent drug was found to decompose when incubated in physiologic buffer at 37° (Jackson *et al.*, 1978).

B. Vinblastine

The pharmacokinetics of VLB in man were originally described by Owellen *et al.* (1975) using a radioactively labeled drug. They noted that the clearance of radioactivity from the blood was biphasic with half-lives of 4.5 and 190 min, very similar to those described for VCR. However, more recent work using a radioimmunoassay to determine VLB concentrations noted a triphasic blood decay with α and β half-lives of 3.9 and 53 min, respectively, and a long terminal half-life of about 20 hr (Owellen *et al.*, 1977b). A representative decay curve is seen in Fig. 7. It may be seen that peak VLB concentrations are in the

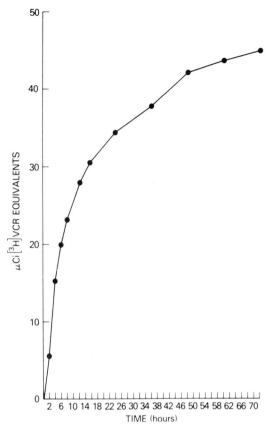

Fig. 6. Cumulative biliary excretion of tritiated vincristine and its metabolic and/or decomposition products during a 72-hr period of study following intravenous injection of 158 μCi of tritiated drug. Samples were collected at various time points from a T tube located in the common bile duct of a single patient. (From Jackson *et al.*, 1978.)

range of 300–400 n*M*/liter. As was the case with VCR, extensive binding to blood components occurred rapidly, with plasma and platelets binding more avidly than white cells and red cells.

Excretion of radioactivity in the urine and feces over the 3-day period of study was 13.6% and 9.9% respectively. Although the urinary excretion of VCR and that of VLB are similar, the disparity between the fecal excretion (69% vs. 9.9%) is puzzling. Although it seems clear that both drugs are retained by the tissues to some degree and therefore do not appear in the urine or feces, a sevenfold difference in tissue retention between the two alkaloids seems unlikely. The identification of metabolites was carried out by thin-layer chromatography, a technique with limited resolution when compared to HPLC. Only two major

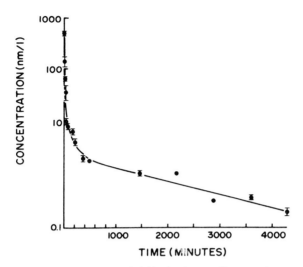

Fig. 7.   The blood disappearance curve of vinblastine in man. Concentrations were measured at various time points using a radioimmunoassay. (From Owellen *et al.*, 1977b.)

species were identified in specimens of urine and feces. One species co-migrated with VLB and appeared to be the parent drug. The second species was identified as deacetylvinblastine or vindesine (see Fig. 2B). Interestingly, vindesine is a more potent cytotoxic agent than VLB in experimental tumors and is currently undergoing phase II clinical testing. Earlier work by Owellen and Hartke (1975) using tritiated VLB suggested more extensive fecal excretion and metabolism. However, metabolism of the tritiated VLB to vindesine and tritiated acetic acid and acetate derivatives of the parent compound is felt to explain the differences between the results obtained using the radiochemical and radioimmunoassay (Owellen *et al.*, 1977b).

C. Drug Interactions

The interactions of VCR and VLB with other drugs are of interest although their clinical significance remains to be defined. Low concentrations (0.005 mg/ml) of several amino acids—namely, glutamic acid, aspartic acid, ornithine, citrulline, and arginine—completely reverse the cytotoxic effect of VLB in tissue culture (Johnson *et al.*, 1960). This observation may have clinical relevance for the patient receiving hyperalimentation. VCR has been shown to augment methotrexate uptake by human acute myeloblastic leukemia cells *in vitro* at a clinically achievable VCR concentration of 0.1 μM (Bender *et al.*, 1975). However, more recent work on human lymphoblastoid cells in tissue culture demonstrates no augmentation of methotrexate uptake at identical VCR concentrations

(Warren *et al.*, 1977). This disparity raises questions regarding individual tumor thresholds for this effect and minimizes its clinical utility. Moreover, recent *in vivo* studies using the L1210 murine leukemia model demonstrate that in a tumor sensitive to methotrexate in which VCR augments methotrexate uptake, therapeutic synergism of methotrexate and VCR is not found at methotrexate concentrations comparable to those achieved clinically in "high-dose" protocols (Bender *et al.*, 1978). Whereas VLB has also been shown to augment methotrexate uptake *in vitro* (Zager *et al.*, 1973), similarly detailed *in vivo* studies or studies employing human tissues remain to be performed.

V. CONCLUSION

The vinca alkaloids demonstrate that drugs that interact with tubulin may have potent cytotoxic effects. Although they have similar mechanisms of action, pharmacokinetic differences have been observed. That analogues with similar properties can have different therapeutic effects and toxicities is evidenced by the vinca alkaloids.

ACKNOWLEDGMENTS

The author would like to acknowledge the stimulation and assistance of Don V. Jackson, Jr., M. D., and Arlene P. Nichols, M. S., in the conduct of some of the studies cited in this chapter.

REFERENCES

Bender, R. A., Bleyer, W. A., Frisby, S. A., and Oliverio, V. T. (1975). *Cancer Res.* **35,** 1305–1308.
Bender, R. A., Castle, M. C., Margileth, D. A., and Oliverio, V. T. (1977). *Clin. Pharmacol. Ther.* **22,** 430–438.
Bender, R. A., Nichols, A. P., Norton, L., and Simon, R. M. (1978). *Cancer Treat. Rep.* **62,** 997–1003.
Bensch, K. G., and Malawista, S. E. (1969). *J. Cell Biol.* **40,** 95–107.
Bleyer, W. A., Frisby, S. A., and Oliverio, V. T. (1975). *Biochem. Pharmacol.* **24,** 633–639.
Bruchovsky, N., Owen, A. A., Becker, A. J., and Till, J. E. (1965). *Cancer Res.* **25,** 1232–1237.
Bryan, J. (1972). *J. Mol. Biol.* **66,** 157–168.
Castle, M. C., Margileth, D. A., and Oliverio, V. T. (1976). *Cancer Res.* **36,** 3684–3689.
Chu, M. Y., and Fisher, G. A. (1968). *Biochem. Pharmacol.* **17,** 753–767.
Cortese, F., Bhattacharyya, B., and Wolff, J. (1977). *J. Biol. Chem.* **252,** 1134–1140.
Creasey, W. A. (1968). *Cancer Chemother. Rep.* **52,** 501–507.
Creasey, W. A., and Markiw, M. E. (1964). *Biochem. Pharmacol.* **13,** 135–142.
Creasey, W. A., and Markiw, M. E. (1965). *Biochim. Biophys. Acta* **103,** 635–645.

El Dareer, S. M., White, V. M., Chen, F. P., Mellett, L. B., and Hill, D. L. (1977). *Cancer Treat. Rep.* **61,** 1269-1277.

Jackson, D. V., and Bender, R. A. (1978). *Cancer Res.* **39,** 4346-4349.

Jackson, D. V., Castle, M. C., and Bender, R. A. (1978). *Clin. Pharmacol. Ther.* **24,** 101-107.

Jellinghaus, W., Schultze, B., and Maurer, W. (1977). *Cell Tissue Kinet.* **10,** 147-156.

Johnson, I. S., Wright, H. F., Svoboda, G. H., and Vlantis, J. (1960). *Cancer Res.* **20,** 1016-1022.

Johnson, I. S., Armstrong, J. G., Gorman, M., and Burnett, J. P. (1963). *Cancer Res.* **23,** 1390-1427.

Journey, L. J., Burdman, J., and George, P. (1968). *Cancer Chemother. Rep.* **52,** 509-516.

Krishan, A. (1968). *J. Natl. Cancer Inst.* **41,** 581-595.

Lee, J. C., Harrison, D., and Timasheff, S. N. (1975). *J. Biol. Chem.* **250,** 9276-9282.

Luduena, R. F., Shooter, E. M., and Wilson, L. (1977). *J. Biol. Chem.* **252,** 7006-7014.

Madoc-Jones, H., and Mauro, F. (1968). *J. Cell. Physiol.* **72,** 185-196.

Mandelbaum-Shavit, F., Wolpert-DeFilippes, M. K., and Johns, D. G. (1976). *Biochem. Biophys. Res. Commun.* **72,** 47-54.

Olmsted, J. B., and Borisy, G. G. (1973). *Annu. Rev. Biochem.* **42,** 507-540.

Owellen, R. J., and Donigian, D. W. (1972). *J. Med. Chem.* **15,** 894-898.

Owellen, R. J., and Hartke, C. A. (1975). *Cancer Res.* **35,** 975-980.

Owellen, R. J., Owens, A. H., and Donigian, D. W. (1972). *Biochem. Biophys. Res. Commun.* **47,** 685-691.

Owellen, R. J., Hartke, C. A., Dickerson, R. M., and Hains, F. O. (1976). *Cancer Res.* **36,** 1499-1502.

Owellen, R. J., Root, M. A., and Hains, F. O. (1977a). *Cancer Res.* **37,** 2603-2607.

Owellen, R. J., Hartke, C. A., and Hains, F. O. (1977b). *Cancer Res.* **37,** 2597-2602.

Peterson, N. A., Raghupahty, E., and Estey, S. T. (1976). *Biochem. Pharmacol.* **25,** 1389-1395.

Schrek, R. (1974). *Am. J. Clin. Pathol.* **62,** 1-7.

Tucker, J. B. (1977). *Nature (London)* **266,** 22-26.

Tucker, R. W., Owellen, R. J., and Harris, S. B. (1977). *Cancer Res.* **37,** 4346-4351.

Warren, R. D., Nichols, A. P., and Bender, R. A. (1977). *Cancer Res.* **37,** 2933-2997.

Wilkoff, L. J., Dulmadge, E. A., and Dixon, G. J. (1968). *Proc. Soc. Exp. Biol. Med.* **127,** 472-478.

Zager, R. F., Frisby, S. A., and Oliverio, V. T. (1973). *Cancer Res.* **33,** 1670-1676.

16

MOLECULAR PHARMACOLOGY OF ALKYLATING AGENTS
Michael Colvin

I. INTRODUCTION

The alkylating agents are a group of drugs that have the common property that their biological effects are mediated through the covalent bonding of alkyl groups of the drug to biological molecules. Historically the alkylating agents have been very important because the nitrogen mustard alkylating agents were the first chemical agents to demonstrate significant antitumor effect in experimental animals and man. The use of these compounds as antitumor agents grew out of the observation that the sulfur mustard used as a war gas in World War I produced not only the intended irritant effect on the lungs and membranes but also

CANCER AND CHEMOTHERAPY, VOL. III
Copyright © 1981 by Academic Press, Inc.
All rights of reproduction in any form reserved.
ISBN 0-12-197803-6

hematopoietic aplasia and lymphoid depletion. Although sulfur mustard was too reactive and toxic for [Fig. 1] clinical administration, the related nitrogen mustards were demonstrated to produce regression of lymphoid tumors in rodents and were tested for activity against lymphoid neoplasias in man (Gilman, 1963). The clinical trials demonstrated that significant regressions of these tumors could be produced, but the tumors recurred and were then drug resistant. These studies stimulated a search for further chemical agents capable of producing tumor regression, and this was the beginning of the present era of cancer chemotherapy.

II. CHEMISTRY OF THE ALKYLATING REACTIONS

Although alkylation reactions constitute one of the major classes of chemical reactions, only those alkylating agents that are stable and alkylate under biological conditions are important as drugs. A diverse group of structures can serve as biological alkylating agents through a variety of mechanisms.

Alkylating agents have traditionally been classified as to whether they undergo $S_N 1$ (first-order) or $S_N 2$ (second-order) reactions. These are kinetic terms reflecting whether the rate of the reactions is dependent on the concentration of the alkylating agent only ($S_N 1$) or on the concentration of both the alkylating agent and the substrate ($S_N 2$).

Mechanistically, the $S_N 1$ reactions (see Fig. 2) represent those in which a very reactive intermediate such as a carbonium ion ($R_1 I$) is formed and reacts very rapidly with the electron-rich substrate, such as an amino group. In such reactions the rate r_1 is much slower than the rate r_2 and thus the overall rate of the reaction is determined by the concentration of $R_1 X$ alone. Mechanistically, the $S_N 2$ reaction (Fig. 3) represents a direct displacement reaction between the substrate and the original alkylating agent. The rate of these reactions will be dependent on the concentration of both the original alkylating agent and the substrate.

The terms $S_N 1$ and $S_N 2$ are usually used to refer to the mechanism of the alkylation reaction rather than the kinetics. In the past such mechanisms were often inferred from kinetic studies. Using modern chemical techniques it is

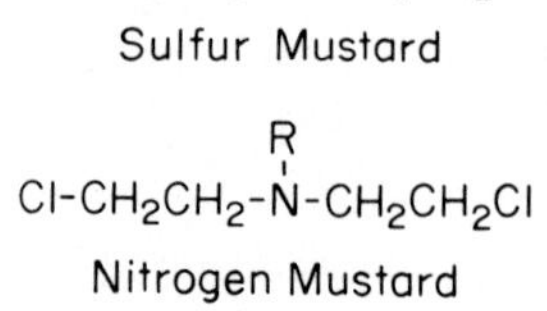

$$Cl-CH_2CH_2-S-CH_2CH_2Cl$$

Sulfur Mustard

$$\overset{R}{\underset{|}{Cl-CH_2CH_2-N-CH_2CH_2Cl}}$$

Nitrogen Mustard

Fig. 1. Structures of sulfur mustard and nitrogen mustard.

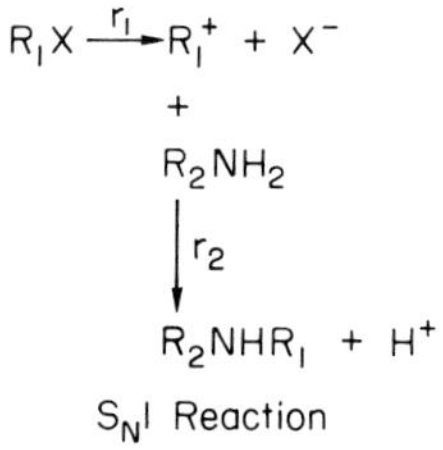

$$R_1X \xrightarrow{r_1} R_1^+ + X^-$$
$$+$$
$$R_2NH_2$$
$$\downarrow r_2$$
$$R_2NHR_1 + H^+$$
$$S_N1 \text{ Reaction}$$

Fig. 2. S_N1 reaction (first order).

increasingly possible to define the exact chemical intermediates and the mechanisms involved in the reactions of the alkylating agents. Such knowledge is important because the intermediates and mechanisms involved may define the target of the alkylation reaction. For example, the evidence now indicates that very reactive intermediates using an S_N1 mechanism are more likely to alkylate the O atoms of nucleotides and the phosphate groups of DNA.

III. CLINICALLY EFFECTIVE ALKYLATING AGENTS

The types of alkylating compounds that have proved to be useful in the clinical therapy of tumors are listed in Table I. Some of these compounds, such as the nitrosoureas and triazenes, were not known to be alkylating agents when they were first developed but were found to be alkylating agents subsequently.

A. Nitrogen Mustards

The first nitrogen mustard derivative to be used extensively clinically was mechlorethamine, shown in Fig. 4. This agent has been shown to alkylate through the aziridine intermediate as illustrated in Fig. 5. The lone pair of electrons in the nitrogen atom provides an electron-rich target for the electrophilic β carbon atom to produce the aziridine intermediate. Although mechlorethamine demonstrated good activity against lymphomas, the therapeutic index of the agent is low, both in experimental animal systems and in clinical use. Furthermore, the extreme reactivity of this agent makes it somewhat dif-

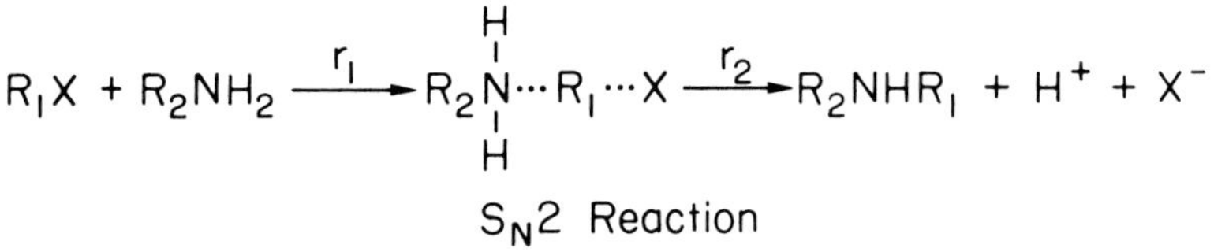

$$R_1X + R_2NH_2 \xrightarrow{r_1} R_2\overset{\displaystyle H}{\underset{\displaystyle H}{N}}\cdots R_1 \cdots X \xrightarrow{r_2} R_2NHR_1 + H^+ + X^-$$

$$S_N2 \text{ Reaction}$$

Fig. 3. S_N2 reaction (second order).

TABLE I

Therapeutically Useful Alkylating Agents

1. Nitrogen Mustards
2. Aziridines
3. Alkyl Alkane Sulfonates
4. Nitrosoureas
5. Triazene Derivatives
6. Epoxides

ficult to administer, in that it cannot be given orally and the drug produces severe vesication if extravasated into tissues. In efforts to develop more effective nitrogen mustards thousands of compounds have been synthesized in which the methyl group is replaced by other chemical groups. Of this number of compounds only three are presently in widespread clinical use. These are chlorambucil, phenylalanine mustard, and cyclophosphamide. The structure of chlorambucil is shown in Fig. 6. In this compound the electron withdrawing properties of the benzene ring produce a less reactive nitrogen mustard. Chlorambucil can be administered by mouth and appears to have a higher therapeutic index than mechlorethamine in clinical use. Phenylalanine mustard is similar in structure to chlorambucil in that the bischloroethylamine group is substituted into the para position of the benzene ring of the amino acid phenylalanine. The chemical and clinical properties of these molecules appear to be similar.

The most widely used alkylating agent is cyclophosphamide (Fig. 7). This compound is interesting in that the parent molecule is not an active alkylating agent, but an alkylating agent, phosphoramide mustard, is produced by metabolism of the parent compound by the hepatic microsomes (Brock and Hohorst, 1963; Colvin *et al.*, 1973; Connors *et al.*, 1974). This compound has been demonstrated to alkylate through an aziridine intermediate (Colvin *et al.*, 1976), as shown in Fig. 5. Cyclophosphamide has been demonstrated to have clinically significant activity against a wide range of tumors and is discussed in detail in another volume of this series.

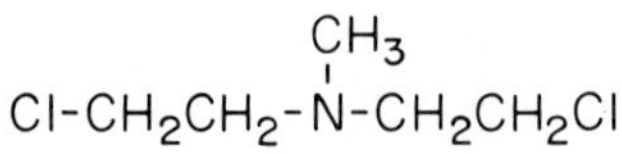

$$\overset{\displaystyle CH_3}{\underset{\displaystyle |}{Cl-CH_2CH_2-N-CH_2CH_2Cl}}$$

Mechlorethamine

Fig. 4.   Structure of mechlorethamine.

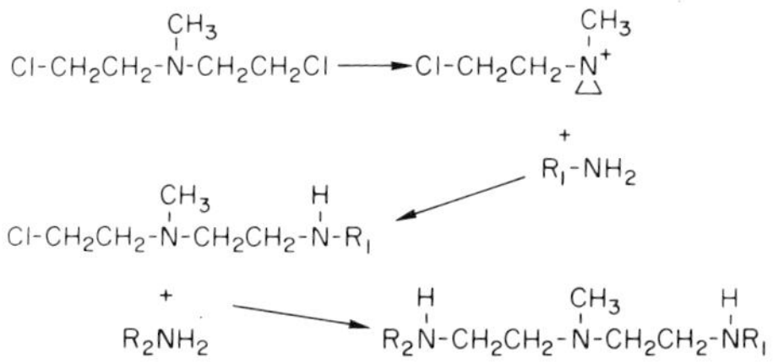

$$Cl\text{-}CH_2CH_2\text{-}\overset{\overset{\displaystyle CH_3}{|}}{N}\text{-}CH_2CH_2Cl \longrightarrow Cl\text{-}CH_2CH_2\text{-}\overset{\overset{\displaystyle CH_3}{|}}{\underset{\underset{\displaystyle \triangle}{}}{N^+}}$$

$$\overset{+}{R_I\text{-}NH_2}$$

$$Cl\text{-}CH_2CH_2\text{-}\overset{\overset{\displaystyle CH_3}{|}}{N}\text{-}CH_2CH_2\text{-}\overset{\overset{\displaystyle H}{|}}{N}\text{-}R_I$$

$$\overset{+}{R_2NH_2} \longrightarrow R_2\overset{\overset{\displaystyle H}{|}}{N}\text{-}CH_2CH_2\text{-}\overset{\overset{\displaystyle CH_3}{|}}{N}\text{-}CH_2CH_2\text{-}\overset{\overset{\displaystyle H}{|}}{N}R_I$$

Fig. 5. Alkylation mechanism of the nitrogen mustard mechlorethamine via the aziridine intermediate.

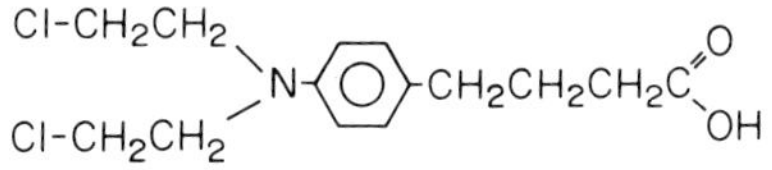

$$\begin{array}{c} Cl\text{-}CH_2CH_2 \\ Cl\text{-}CH_2CH_2 \end{array}\!\!N\!\!-\!\!\langle O \rangle\!\!-\!\!CH_2CH_2CH_2C\!\!\begin{array}{c} {}^{\displaystyle O} \\ {}_{\displaystyle OH} \end{array}$$

Chlorambucil

Fig. 6. Structure of chlorambucil.

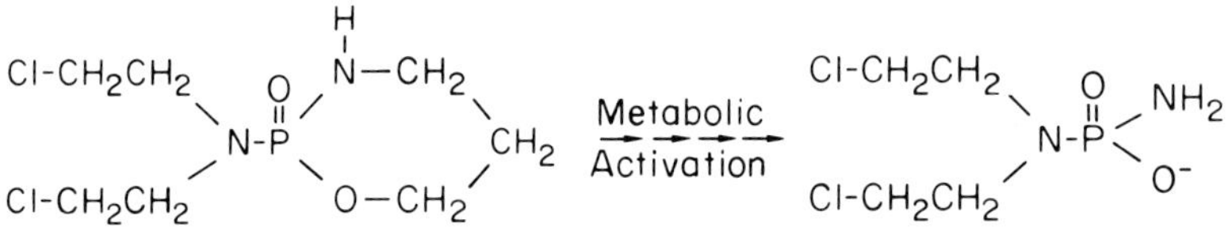

$$\begin{array}{c} Cl\text{-}CH_2CH_2 \\ \\ Cl\text{-}CH_2CH_2 \end{array}\!\!N\text{-}P\!\!\begin{array}{c} \overset{H}{\underset{}{N}}\!\!-\!\!CH_2 \\ \\ O\!\!-\!\!CH_2 \end{array}\!\!\begin{array}{c} \\ CH_2 \\ \end{array}$$
$$\xrightarrow[\text{Activation}]{\text{Metabolic}}$$
$$\begin{array}{c} Cl\text{-}CH_2CH_2 \\ \\ Cl\text{-}CH_2CH_2 \end{array}\!\!N\text{-}P\!\!\begin{array}{c} \overset{O}{}\;NH_2 \\ \\ O^- \end{array}$$

Cyclophosphamide   Phosphoramide
                                              Mustard

Fig. 7. Metabolism of cyclophosphamide to phosphoramide mustard.

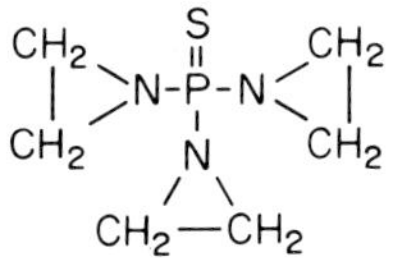

$$\begin{array}{c} CH_2 \\ | \\ CH_2 \end{array}\!\!\!\begin{array}{c} \\ N\text{-}\overset{\overset{\displaystyle S}{\|}}{P}\text{-}N \\ | \\ N \end{array}\!\!\!\begin{array}{c} CH_2 \\ | \\ CH_2 \end{array}$$
$$\begin{array}{c} / \;\;\; \backslash \\ CH_2\!\!-\!\!CH_2 \end{array}$$

Thio-TEPA
(*N,N',N''* - Triethylene Thiophosphoramide)

Fig. 8. Structure of thio-TEPA (*N,N,'N''*-triethylene thiophosphoramide).

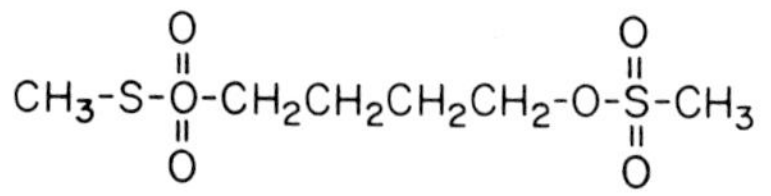

$$CH_3-S-O-CH_2CH_2CH_2CH_2-O-S-CH_3$$

Busulfan

Fig. 9.   Structure of busulfan.

B. Aziridines

Compounds bearing unchanged aziridine groups, such as thio-TEPA (N,N',N''-triethylene thiophosphoramide, Fig. 8), have been used clinically. Although the mechanism of alkylation of these compounds has not been extensively investigated, it is presumed these agents alkylate by opening of the aziridine ring as shown for the nitrogen mustards. Mitomycin C, a natural product that appears to exert its actions through alkylation (Szybalski and Iyer, 1964), bears an aziridine group that is probably involved in alkylation by the molecule. This compound is discussed in detail in a later section.

C. Alkyl Alkane Sulfonates

The only member of this group of compounds in common clinical use is busulfan, shown in Fig. 9. This agent alkylates through an S_N2 attack of the nucleophilic substrate on the molecule as shown in Fig. 10. Although this drug has shown useful clinical activity only in chronic myelocytic leukemia, it is the agent of choice in this disease. The drug is also of considerable experimental interest because of its profound toxic effect on hematopoietic stem cells (Fried *et al.*, 1977) but relative lack of effect on lymphocytic cells. The pharmacological basis for these properties is unknown.

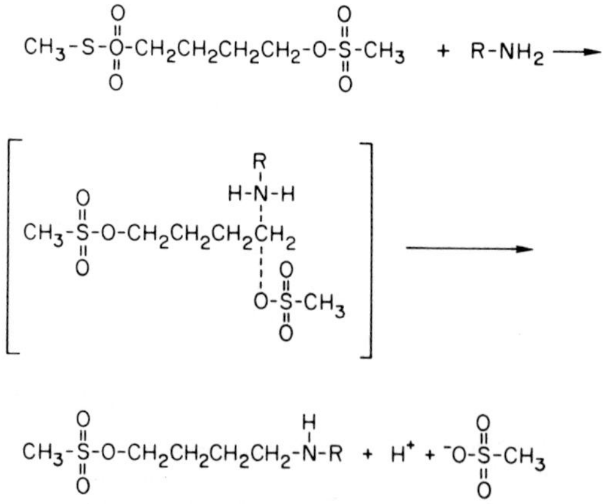

$$CH_3-S-O-CH_2CH_2CH_2CH_2-O-S-CH_3 \; + \; R-NH_2 \longrightarrow$$

$$\left[CH_3-S-O-CH_2CH_2CH_2CH_2 \begin{array}{c} R \\ H-N-H \\ \vdots \\ O \\ \| \\ O-S-CH_3 \\ \| \\ O \end{array} \right] \longrightarrow$$

$$CH_3-S-O-CH_2CH_2CH_2CH_2-N-R \; + \; H^+ + \; ^-O-S-CH_3$$

Fig. 10.   Alkylation mechanism of alkane sufonates.

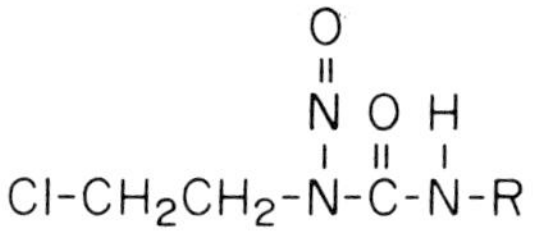

$$
\begin{array}{c}
\text{O} \\
\parallel \\
\text{N}\quad\text{O}\quad\text{H} \\
\mid\quad\parallel\quad\mid \\
\text{Cl-CH}_2\text{CH}_2\text{-N-C-N-R}
\end{array}
$$

Fig. 11.   General structure of the nitrosoureas.

D. Nitrosoureas

The nitrosoureas, a general structure for which is shown in Fig. 11, are a group of compounds introduced into cancer chemotherapy in the early 1960s (DeVita *et al.*, 1965). These agents are distinctive in that they cross the blood–brain barrier readily (Schabel *et al.*, 1965) and exhibit an unusual delayed hematologic toxicity in man (Lessner, 1968).

Because of the structural similarities to the nitrogen mustards it was presumed that these compounds were active as alkylating agents. In the last few years evidence that this drug is an alkylating agent has been provided with the demonstration that the nitrosoureas alkylate nucleic acids and nucleotides (Cheng *et al.*, 1972; Kramer *et al.*, 1974) and the elucidation of the degradation pathway of this agent under physiologic conditions. As shown in Fig. 12, the nitrosoureas decompose under physiologic conditions to form an alkylating chloroethyl diazonium intermediate. Alkylation of a nitrogen in cytosine or guanosine by the chloroethyl group will produce a chloroethyl amino group capable of a second alkylation process (Kramer *et al.*, 1974; Ludlum *et al.*, 1975). Data from Kohn (1977) showing that BCNU produces DNA–DNA cross-links suggests that such a chloroethyl group inserted onto one strand of DNA can alkylate a base on the complementary strand to produce an interstrand cross-link.

E. Triazene Derivatives

Shealy and colleagues (1961; Shealy, 1970) synthesized a series of analogues of 5-aminoimidazole-4-carboxamide (AIC), an intermediate in purine ribonuc-

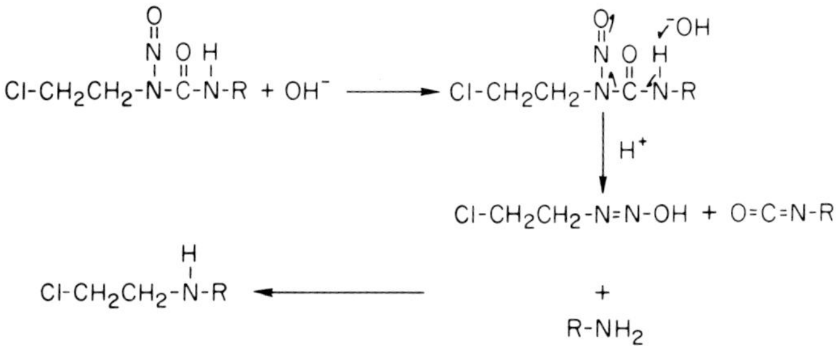

$$
\begin{array}{ccc}
\begin{array}{c}\text{O}\\\parallel\\\text{N}\;\text{O}\;\text{H}\\\mid\;\parallel\;\mid\\\text{Cl-CH}_2\text{CH}_2\text{-N-C-N-R}\end{array} + \text{OH}^- &\longrightarrow& \begin{array}{c}\text{O}\quad\nearrow\!\text{OH}\\\parallel\\\text{N}\;\text{O}\;\text{H}\\\mid\;\parallel\;\mid\\\text{Cl-CH}_2\text{CH}_2\text{-N-C-N-R}\end{array}
\end{array}
$$

$$\Big\downarrow \text{H}^+$$

$$\text{Cl-CH}_2\text{CH}_2\text{-N=N-OH} + \text{O=C=N-R}$$

$$
\begin{array}{c}
\text{H}\\
\mid\\
\text{Cl-CH}_2\text{CH}_2\text{-N-R}
\end{array}
\quad\longleftarrow\quad
\begin{array}{c}
+\\
\text{R-NH}_2
\end{array}
$$

Fig. 12.   Mechanism of decomposition and alkylation of the chloroethylnitrosoureas.

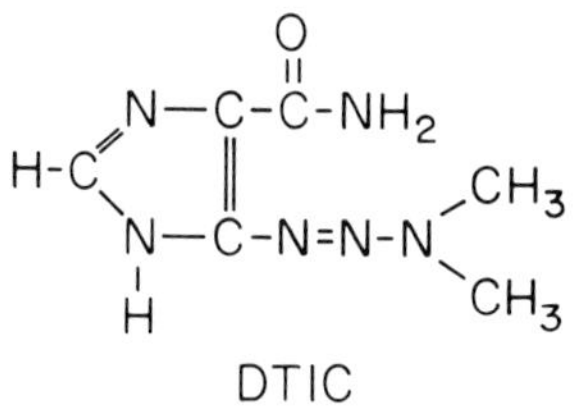

DTIC

Fig. 13.   Structure of DTIC (5-[3,3-dimethyl-1-triazeno]-imidazole-4-carboxamide).

leotide synthesis, and demonstrated antitumor activity of these compounds against rodent tumors. One of these compounds, 5-(3,3-dimethyl-1-triazeno)-imidazole-4-carboxamide (DTIC, Fig. 13), has subsequently been introduced into clinical use. This drug is the most effective single agent for the treatment of malignant melanoma (Luce *et al.*, 1970).

The initial rationale for the activity of these compounds was as inhibitors of purine synthesis. However, subsequent work has indicated that the compound is active as a monofunctional alkylating agent (Bono, 1976; Loo *et al.*, 1976; Skibba *et al.*, 1970) after enzymatic hydroxylation as shown in Fig. 14 (Skibba *et al.*, 1970).

Procarbazine, a hydrazine derivative widely used in the treatment of Hodgkin's disease, may also serve as a methylating agent after enzymatic hydroxylation (Horváth and Institóris, 1967), but it is not established that this is the primary mechanism of action of procarbazine.

F. Epoxides

Epoxides, such as dianhydrogalactitol (Fig. 15), are biological alkylating agents (Sebestyén *et al.*, 1972) that show activity against a large number of

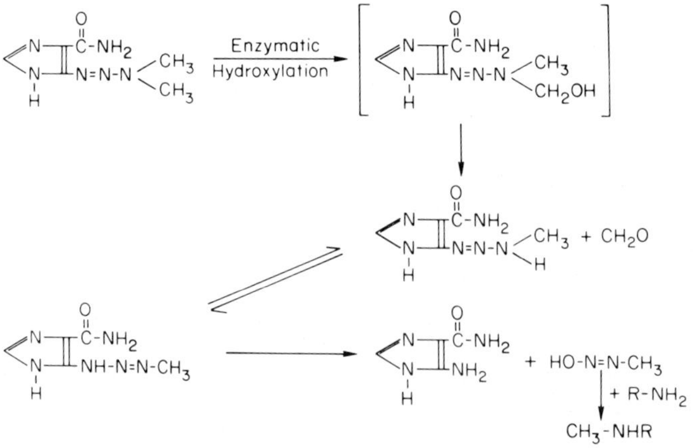

Fig. 14.   Enzymatic hydroxylation of DTIC.

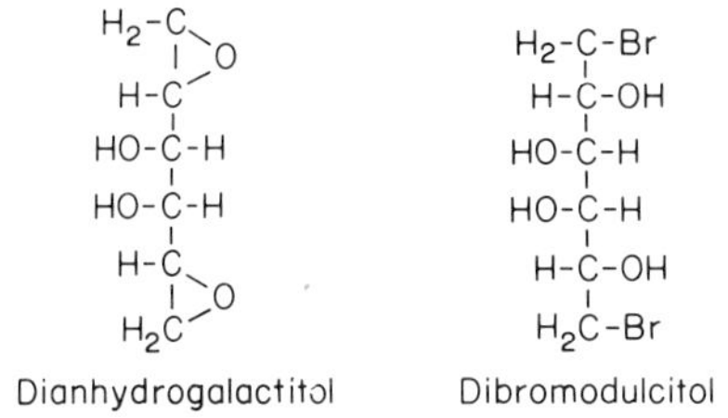

```
    H₂-C                              H₂-C-Br
     |    O                            |
    H-C                               H-C-OH
     |                                 |
  HO-C-H                            HO-C-H
     |                                 |
  HO-C-H                            HO-C-H
     |                                 |
    H-C                               H-C-OH
     |    O                            |
    H₂C                               H₂C-Br

  Dianhydrogalactitol              Dibromodulcitol
```

Fig. 15.   Structures of dianhydrogalactitol and dibromodulcitol.

animal tumors and show clinical activity (Haas *et al.*, 1976). These compounds are chemically similar to ethylenimines and presumably alkylate in a similar fashion. Brominated polyhydroxy compounds such as dibromodulcitol (Fig. 15) can be shown to produce the corresponding diepoxides, which may be responsible for the antitumor activity of the brominated compounds (Horváth and Institóris, 1967).

IV. REACTIONS WITH BIOLOGICAL MOLECULES

A. Biological Targets of Alkylation

Since the alkylating agents are nonspecific electrophilic reagents, there are a variety of targets in the biological milieu with which these reagents will react. Such electron-rich sites are listed in Table II and are present both in small molecules, such as amino acids and nucleotides, and in protein and nucleic acid macromolecules. When radioactive alkylating agents are administered to animals, extensive binding of the radioactivity to both proteins and nucleic acids is observed (Warwick, 1963; Wheeler, 1962). Thus a variety of alkylations of biological molecules is potentially responsible for the biological effect of alkylating agents. However, for the reasons cited in Table III, deoxyribonucleic acid (DNA) is a likely candidate for the site of critical damage to the cell. First, virtually all cytotoxic alkylating agents are also mutagenic and teratogenic, indicating that they damage the genetic material of the cell. Second, of the critical

TABLE II

Targets of Alkylation in Cells

Nucleophilic sites on:
1. Proteins (S, N atoms)
2. Nucleic acids (O, N atoms, PO_4 groups)
3. Amino acids and nucleotides (S, N, O atoms, PO_4 groups)

TABLE III

Reasons for Implicating DNA as a Primary Target of Alkylating Agents

1. Alkylating agents are mutagenic, teratogenic, and carcinogenic, as well as cytotoxic
2. Fewer copies of DNA in cell, as compared to RNA, proteins, and low molecular weight compounds
3. One mechanism of resistance to alklyating agents appears to be capability to repair alkylation lesions in DNA
4. Bifunctional alkylating agents, capable of crosslinking DNA, are in general more effective antitumor agents than monofunctional analogues

molecules in the cell, the most limited in number and the ones whose functions are amplified the most are the DNA strands. Thus damage to the DNA may be amplified through altered transcription of RNA and subsequent translation of RNA into protein. Third, one mechanism of resistance of both eucaryotic cells and bacteria to alkylating agents appears to be the capability to repair alkylation lesions in DNA. Finally, of the clinically useful alkylating agents, by far the largest number are bifunctional, with the ability to cross-link DNA, as will be discussed later. Increasing the functionality of the agents to greater than two does not increase the antitumor activity of the agents. These somewhat intuitive speculations are supported by an increasing amount of experimental evidence on the occurrence and significance of alkylation damage to DNA.

B. Nucleic Acid Targets for Alkylation

The two components of the DNA that can be alkylated are the sugar-phosphate backbone and the bases. The negatively charged phosphates are likely candidates for alkylation. Bannon and Verly (1972) have established that such alkylation does occur. Although phosphate alkylation has been demonstrated to produce strand breaks, Verly (1974) has postulated that phosphate ester formation by ethyl methanesulfonate is not responsible for toxicity. Toxicity from phosphate alkylation would be even less likely for the antitumor alkylating agents, which alkylate phosphate groups less than the S_N1 reagent ethyl methanesulfonate.

Certain sites on the nuclei acid bases are especially susceptible to alkylation. These sites are the 7 nitrogen of guanine, the 1 and 3 nitrogens of adenine, and the 3 nitrogen of cytosine. Of these sites the most reactive and quantitatively important alkylation site is the 7 nitrogen of guanine. The evidence at present indicates that alkylation of the 7 nitrogen is important in the antitumor effect of the antitumor agents, whereas the minor sites of alkylation, especially the 6 oxygen (Loveless, 1969; Gerchman and Ludlum, 1973) and extracyclic amino group of guanine (Weinstein *et al.*, 1976), may be critical for alkylation carcinogenesis.

C. Molecular Consequences of Nucleic Acid Alkylation

The potential molecular consequences of the alkylation by mechlorethamine of the 7 nitrogen of deoxyguanylic acid in DNA is shown in Fig. 16. The remaining chloroethyl group in the nitrogen mustard may react with a deoxyguanylic acid residue in the complementary DNA strand to produce an intermolecular cross-link, with such a residue in the same DNA strand to produce an intramolecular cross-link, or, as recently described, with a group in a protein to produce a DNA-protein cross-link. Since the alkylation of the 7 nitrogen atom introduces a positive charge into the imidazole portion of the deoxyguanylic acid molecule, a degree of instability of the molecule is introduced and scission of the glycosidic bond (Lawley and Brookes, 1957) may occur to release the guanine residue from the DNA chain to produce an apurinic site in the DNA. Alternatively, the

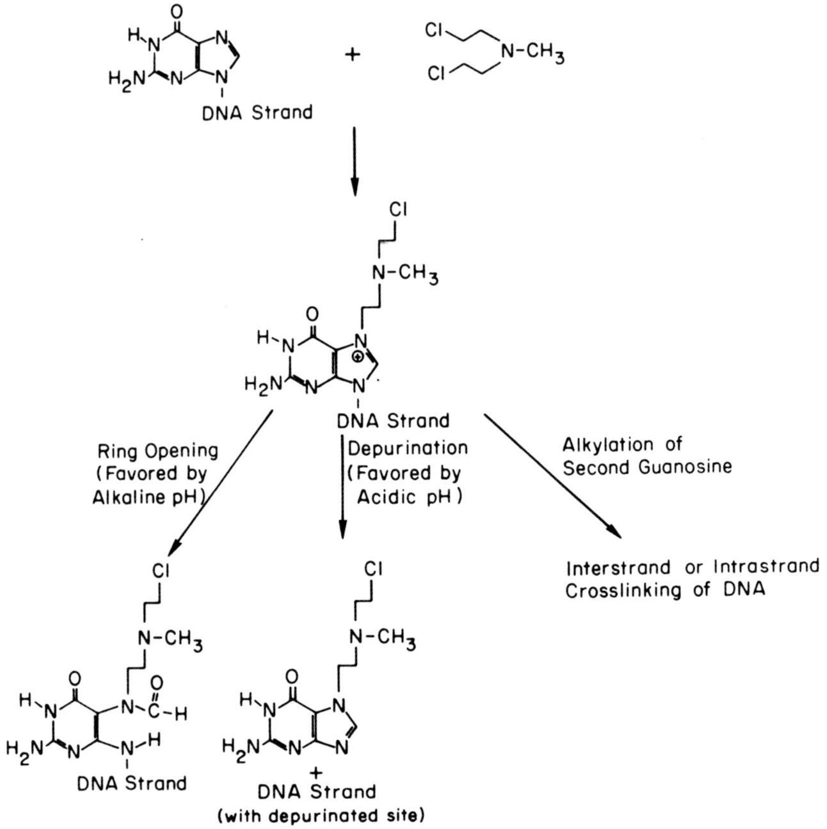

Fig. 16. Molecular consequences of nucleic acid alkylation by mechlorethamine.

imidazole portion of the molecule may open (Lawley and Brookes, 1957), as illustrated in Fig. 16.

Since bifunctional agents are in general cytotoxic at lower concentrations than the analogous monofunctional agents and most of the clinically useful alkylating agents are bifunctional, it seems likely that the cross-linking reaction, and in particular the interstrand cross-link, is important to the antitumor effects of the alkylating agents. However, since most of the alkylations produced by even the bifunctional agents are monofunctional, the effects of the monofunctional alkylations and their potential contributions to both the therapeutic and toxic effects of the agents must be considered. In addition, some clinically effective alkylating agents, such as DTIC, appear to be monofunctional.

Although apurinic sites in the DNA will lead to spontaneous hydrolysis of an adjacent phosphodiester bond, this process is slow and probably not of biological importance (Verly, 1974). However, endonucleases that will produce single-strand breaks at apurinic sites have now been described (Verly, 1974) and are probably responsible for single-strand breaks that are produced by monofunctional agents and for the toxic and therapeutic effects of the monofunctional agents. Although it has been demonstrated that the presence of apurinic sites may produce cross-links, the frequency is such that it is unlikely that these cross-links are responsible for the antitumor activity of monofunctional agents (Burnatte and Verly, 1972). The effect of the ring opening of deoxyguanosine on the functioning of the DNA molecule is unknown, but since the glycosidic bond remains stable the alkylated ring opened deoxyguanosine moiety should be able to participate in cross-linking reactions.

Both cross-links and monofunctional alkylations can be excised from DNA strands, and the role of these repair mechanisms in the differential sensitivity of normal and tumor cells and in the development of drug resistance by tumor cells has been examined extensively (Roberts et al., 1971; Reid and Walker, 1969; Yin et al., 1973). Although it is an attractive hypothesis that normal cells can repair alkylation damage more readily than malignant cells and thus are less susceptible to the effects of alkylating agents, convincing evidence to support this hypothesis has yet to be demonstrated.

A recent advance in the study of the alkylating agents has been the development by Kohn and Grimek-Ewig (1973) of the alkaline elution technique of studying DNA cross-linking. This technique allows cross-linking to be precisely studied in cells after the in vivo administration of therapeutic levels of alkylating agents. These studies have reinforced the importance of DNA cross-links in the mechanism of action of the therapeutic alkylating agents.

Several studies have indicated that, in addition to DNA–DNA cross-links, the alkylating agents can link DNA to protein (Rutman et al., 1961; Klatt et al., 1969). Kohn and colleagues have recently presented evidence that this linkage of

DNA to protein is due to N-7 guanine–protein cross-links, analogous in the guanosine portion of the cross-links to the N-7 guanosine links described earlier (Thomas *et al.*, 1978). These workers have indicated that with mechlorethamine there are several DNA–protein cross-links for each DNA–DNA cross-link. The relative roles of these two types of cross-links in the actions of the alkylating agents have not yet been definitely established, although the DNA–DNA cross-links appear to be more cytotoxic.

D. Functional Effects of Alkylation

Many reports have demonstrated that alkylating agents produce a greater inhibition of DNA synthesis than of RNA or protein synthesis (Warwick, 1963; Wheeler, 1962). An example of this effect is shown in Fig. 17, in which the relative effects of cyclophosphamide metabolites on macromolecular synthesis in murine leukemia cells *in vitro* are demonstrated. Although there are conflicting reports (Rudden and Johnson, 1968; Tomisek *et al.*, 1966; Wheeler and Alexander, 1964), the evidence favors the hypothesis that the inhibition of synthesis is due to damage to the nucleic acid template rather than to inactivation of polymerase enzymes. However, it has been demonstrated in two reports (Chmielewicz *et al.*, 1967; Rudden and Johnson, 1968) that the DNA polymerase template activity of DNA is more sensitve to nitrogen mustard than the RNA polymerase template activity of DNA. These observations indicate that the inhibition of DNA synthesis by alkylating agents may be a complex phenomenon.

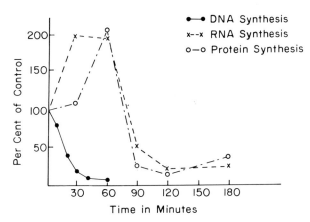

Fig. 17. Effects of cyclophosphamide metabolites on macromolecular synthesis.

E. Transport into Cells

The mechanisms by which alkylating agents enter cells have not been extensively investigated, but several important observations have been made. Goldenberg and colleagues (1971) have shown that the polar compound mechlorethamine enters murine lymphoblasts via an active transport system that also transports choline. Furthermore, these investigators have demonstrated that the entrance of mechlorethamine into cells can be potentiated by pharmacological maneuvers (Goldenberg, 1974).

Goldenberg and his co-workers have also demonstrated that phenylalanine mustard is actively transported into tumor cells (Goldenberg et al., 1977). Additional observations by Vistica and Rabinovitz (Vistica et al., 1977) have indicated that this compound is utilizing a neutral amino acid transport system and that the cytotoxicity of the agent can be inhibited by the presence in the medium of neutral amino acids such as leucine.

BCNU, however, has now been demonstrated by Goldenberg and colleagues to enter cells by passive diffusion (Begleiter et al., 1977). This result is not unexpected from the nonpolar nature of the nitrosoureas and their ready penetration into the central nervous system (Schabel et al., 1965).

A great deal of effort has been expended in attempting to develop alkylating agents that will target to specific tissues or selectively enter tumor cells. Such efforts have not been very successful, but these efforts have not been based on a knowledge of specific transport systems. It seems probable that future efforts based more directly on a knowledge of how the present agents enter cells will be more successful.

F. Cellular Resistance to Alkylating Agents

As with most antitumor agents, the failure of alkylating agent therapy is usually due to the emergence of drug-resistant tumor cells. Several investigators have shown that some resistant cells may show decreased uptake of the alkylating agent (Chun et al., 1969; Goldenberg, 1975), and this mechanism would appear to be an important way in which drug resistance develops. However, some studies that have compared sensitive and resistant cells have demonstrated an enhanced ability of drug-resistant cells to repair the nucleic acid damage inflicted by alkylating agents (Yin et al., 1973). These two types of resistance may explain a phenomenon observed in both animal testing and the clinical use of the alkylating agents. This phenomenon is that tumors resistant to a specific alkylating agent will often show at least some degree of cross-resistance to other alkylating agents. However, this cross-resistance is not complete and tumors resistant to one alkylating agent may show a good response to a different alkylating agent. These results could be explained if transport mechanisms are responsible for the agent-specific resistance and enhanced repair of alkylation damage is responsible for the general cross-resistance to alkylating agents.

V. DISCUSSION

In conclusion, the alkylating agents were the first effective chemical agents used in the therapy of cancer and remain an important component of antitumor therapy. Although the pharmacology of these agents has been difficult to study because they are small, very reactive molecules, in recent years a great deal has been learned about the pharmacology and mechanism of action of these agents. With the enlargement of this knowledge it seems likely that more effective and selective alkylating agents will be developed.

REFERENCES

Bannon, P., and Verly, W. (1972). *Eur. J. Biochem.* **31**, 103–111.
Begleiter, A., Lam, Y.-Y. P., and Goldenberg, G. J. (1977). *Cancer Res.* **37**, 1022–1031.
Bono, V. H., J. (1976). *Cancer Treat. Rep.* **60**, 141–148.
Brock, N., and Hohorst, H.-J. (1963). *Arzneim.-Forsch.* **13**, 1021–1031.
Burnatte, J., and Verly, W. G. (1972). *Biochim. Biophys. Acta* **262**, 449–452.
Cheng, C. J., Fujimura, S., Grunberger, D., and Weinstein, I. B. (1972). *Cancer Res.* **32**, 22–27.
Chmielewicz, Z. F., Fiel, R. J., Bardos, J. J., and Ambrus, J. L. (1967). *Cancer Res.* **27**, 1248–1257.
Chun, E. H. L., Gonzales, L., Lewis, S. F., Jones, J., and Rutman, R. J. (1969). *Cancer Res.* **29**, 1184–1194.
Colvin, M., Padgett, C. A., and Fenselau, C. (1973). *Cancer Res.* **33**, 915–918.
Colvin, M., Brundrett, R. B., Kan, M.-N. N., Jardine, I., and Fenselau, C. (1976). *Cancer Res.* **36**, 1121–1126.
Connors, T. A., Cox, P. J., Farmer, P. B., Foster, A. B., and Jarman, M. (1974). *Biochem. Pharmacol.* **23**, 115–129.
DeVita, V., Carbone, P., Owens, A., Gold, G. C., Kraut, M. J., and Edmondson, J. (1965). *Cancer Res.* **25**, 1876–1881.
Fried, W., Kedo, A., and Barone, J. (1977). *Cancer Res.* **37**, 1205–1209.
Gerchman, L. L., and Ludlum, D. B. (1973). *Biochim. Biophys. Acta* **308**, 310–316.
Gilman, A. (1963). *Am. J. Surg.* **105**, 574–578.
Goldenberg, G. J. (1974). *Cancer Res.* **34**, 2511–2516.
Goldenberg, G. J. (1975). *Cancer Res.* **35**, 1687–1692.
Goldenberg, G. J., Vanstone, C. L., and Bihler, I. (1971). *Science* **172**, 1148–1149.
Goldenberg, G. J., Lee, M., Lam, H.-Y. P., and Begleiter, A. (1977). *Cancer Res.* **37**, 755–760.
Haas, C. D., Stephens, R. L., Hollister, M., and Hoogstraten, B. (1976). *Cancer Treat. Rep.* **60**, 611–614.
Horváth, I. P., and Institóris, L. (1967). *Arzneim.-Forsch.* **17**, 149–155.
Klatt, O., Stehlein, J. S., McBride, C., and Griffin, A. C. (1969). *Cancer Res.* **29**, 286–290.
Kohn, K. W. (1977). *Cancer Res.* **37**, 1450–1454.
Kohn, K. W., and Grimek-Ewig, R. A. (1973). *Cancer Res.* **33**, 1849–1853.

Kramer, B. S., Fenselau, C., and Ludlum, D. (1974). *Biochem. Biophys. Res. Commun.* **56**, 783–788.
Lawley, P. D., and Brookes, P. (1957). *Proc. Chem. Soc., London* p. 290.
Lessner, H. (1968). *Cancer (Philadelphia)* **22**, 451–456.
Loo, T. L., Householder, G., Gerulath, A. H., Saunders, P. H., and Farquahar, D. (1976). *Cancer Treat. Rep.* **60**, 149–152.
Loveless, A. (1969). *Nature (London)* **223**, 206–207.
Luce, J. K., Thurman, W. G., Isaacs, B. L., and Talley, R. W. (1970). *Cancer Chemother. Rep.* **54**, 119–124.
Ludlum, D. B., Kramer, B. S., Wang, J., and Fenselau, C. (1975). *Biochemistry* **14**, 5480–5485.
Reid, B. D., and Walker, I. G. (1969). *Biochim. Biophys. Acta* **179**, 179–185.
Roberts, J. J., Brent, T. P., and Carthorn, A. R. (1971). *Eur. J. Cancer* **7**, 515–524.
Rudden, R. W., and Johnson, J. M. (1968). *Mol. Pharmacol.* **4**, 258–273.
Rutman, R. J., Steele, W. J., and Price, C. C. (1961). *Cancer Res.* **21**, 1134–1140.
Schabel, F. M., Jr., Skipper, H. F., Trader, M. W., and Wilcox, W. S. (1965). *Cancer Chemother. Rep.* **48**, 17–30.
Sebestyén, J., Hidvégi, E. J., and Köteles, G. J. (1972). *Adv. Antimicrob. Antineoplast. Chemother., Proc. Int. Congr. Chemother., 7th, Prague, 1971* **2**, 21–22.
Shealy, Y. F. (1970). *J. Pharm. Sci.* **59**, 1533–1558.
Shealy, Y. F., Struck, R. F., Holum, L. B., and Montgomery, J. A. (1961). *J. Org. Chem.* **26**, 2396–2401.
Skibba, J. L., Beal, D. D., Ramirez, G., and Bryan, G. T. (1970). *Cancer Res.* **30**, 147–150.
Szybalski, W., and Iyer, V. N. (1964). *Fed. Proc., Fed. Am. Soc. Exp. Biol.* **23**, 946–957.
Thomas, C. B., Kohn, K. W., and Bonner, W. M. (1978). *Biochemistry* **17**, 3954–3958.
Tomisek, A. J., Irick, M. B., and Allen, P. W. (1966). *Cancer Res.* **26**, 1466–1472.
Verly, W. G. (1974). *Biochem. Pharmacol.* **23**, 3–8.
Vistica, D. T., Toal, J. N., and Rabinovitz, M. (1977). *Proc. Am. Assoc. Cancer Res.* **18**, 26.
Warwick, G. P. (1963). *Cancer Res.* **23**, 1315–1333.
Weinstein, I. B., Jeffrey, A. M., Jennette, K. W., Blobstein, S. H., Harvey, R. G., Harris, C., Autrup, H., Kasai, H., and Nakanishi, K. (1976). *Science* **193**, 592–595.
Wheeler, G. P. (1962). *Cancer Res.* **22**, 651–688.
Wheeler, G. P., and Alexander, J. A. (1964). *Cancer Res.* **24**, 1338–1346.
Yin, L., Chun, E. H. L., and Rutman, R. J. (1973). *Biochim. Biophys. Acta* **324**, 472–481.

17

MOLECULAR PHARMACOLOGY OF CISPLATIN

Archie W. Prestayko

I. INTRODUCTION

Cisplatin (*cis*-diamminedichloroplatinum II) is one of a group of platinum compounds first shown to have antibiotic activity in 1965 (Rosenberg *et al.*, 1965) and antitumor activity in experimental tumors in 1969 (Rosenberg *et al.*, 1969). Historically, the development of cisplatin is a very interesting series of events and has been reviewed by Rosenberg (1978). In the course of studies on the effects of electrical fields in cell division, Dr. Rosenberg observed that when *Escherichia coli* cells growing in a culture medium were subjected to an electrical current from two platinum electrodes, the cells did not divide but became long, filamentous structures. After ruling out the possibility that the electrical current was responsible for this phenomenon, Dr. Rosenberg identified *cis*-diamminedichloroplatinum, formed from platinum from the electrodes and ammonium and chloride ions in solution, as the agent responsible for the inhibition of *E. coli* cell division.

The *cis*-diamminedichloroplatinum compound was synthesized and tested in experimental animal tumors. It showed antitumor activity in several different

CANCER AND CHEMOTHERAPY, VOL. III

303

animal tumors and cured some of the animals of their tumors. Subsequently, cis-diamminedichloroplatinum was further tested in experimental animal tumors by the National Cancer Institute, which then introduced the drug (now referred to as cisplatin) into human clinical trials in 1972. Since that time, cisplatin has demonstrated antitumor activity as a single agent and in combination chemotherapy in several different human malignancies.

II. CHEMISTRY

Cisplatin is a water-soluble square planar coordination complex containing a central platinum atom surrounded by two chloride atoms and two ammonia molecules as shown in Fig. 1a. This configuration is referred to as the "cis" configuration, indicating that the chloride atoms and ammonia molecules are on the same side of the platinum atom. Figure 1b shows the diamminedichloroplatinum compound with the chloride atoms and ammonia molecules on opposite sides of the platinum atom. This configuration is referred to as the "trans" configuration.

The platinum in the cisplatin compound has a +2 oxidation state. A cisplatin analogue has been synthesized in which platinum has an oxidation state of +4, hence the chemical name of this compound is *cis-* or *trans-*diamminetetrachloroplatinum IV (Fig. 2). In general, the "cis" platinum complexes have demonstrated greater antitumor activity in animal tumors than the corresponding "trans" compounds. An excellent review of the chemistry of cisplatin and analogues has recently been published (Leh and Wolf, 1976).

III. BIOCHEMISTRY AND MECHANISM OF ACTION

A. Bacterial Cell Studies

Subsequent to the demonstration by Rosenberg *et al.* (1965) that cisplatin prevented cell division in *E. coli,* several studies investigated the site of action of cisplatin in the cell (Rosenberg *et al.,* 1967; Howle and Gale, 1970a; Drobnik *et al.,* 1973). These studies and that of Renshaw and Thomson (1967) indicated that the drug or metabolites of the drug were associated with nucleic acids and proteins in the cells and suggested that DNA was the primary target for cisplatin. Renshaw and Thomson (1967) suggested that after cisplatin $[Pt(NH_3)_2Cl_2]$ penetrates the cell wall of *E. coli,* it is metabolized (hydrolyzed?) to intermediates such as $[Pt(NH_3)_2Cl_2]^{2+}$. The monovalent intermediate was shown to inhibit synthesis of DNA, RNA, and protein, whereas the divalent intermediate was highly selective for inhibition of DNA synthesis and was devoid of activity against RNA and protein syntheses.

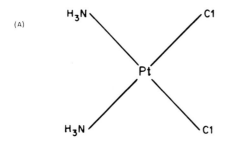

DIAMMINEDICHLOROPLATINUM II (CISPLATIN)
(cis-configuration)

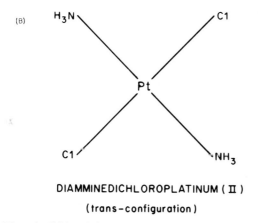

DIAMMINEDICHLOROPLATINUM (II)

(trans-configuration)

Fig. 1. (a) Diamminedichloroplatinum II (cisplatin) (*cis*-configuration). (b) Diamminedichloroplatinum II (*trans*-configuration).

Further evidence suggesting that cisplatin entered bacterial cells and interacted with DNA was provided by Reslova (1971). This study showed that cisplatin could induce lysogenic bacteria; that is, it could cause phage DNA that had been integrated into the bacterial genome to replicate independently and produce phage, which then lysed the bacterial cell. The induction of lysogenic bacteria has been reported to occur as the result of direct interaction of a substance with the bacterial DNA.

B. Animal Cell Studies

In studies carried out in animals bearing tumors, cisplatin caused inhibition of DNA synthesis (Howle and Gale, 1970a; Taylor *et al.*, 1976; Handelsman *et al.*,

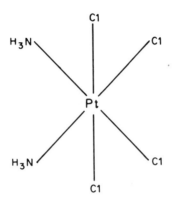

DIAMMINETETRACHLOROPLATINUM IV
(cis-configuration)

Fig. 2.   Diamminetetrachloroplatinum IV (*cis*-configuration).

1974). After a single i.p. injection of cisplatin at 10 mg/kg in mice bearing
Ehrlich ascites tumor cells, followed by *in vitro* incubation of the tumor cells,
there was a marked impairment of incorporation of radioactive labeled precursor
into DNA, RNA, and protein. Subsequently, the rates of incorporation of uridine
and L-leucine returned to control values, and a striking suppression of the rate of
incorporation of thymidine persisted for at least 96 hr. These data were interpreted as indicating a selective inhibitor of DNA synthesis *in vivo*.

The suppression of DNA synthesis in the rat kidney has also been suggested to
proceed via direct interaction of platinum compounds with renal cell nucleic
acid. The change in UV absorption of DNA was measured, and a hyperchromic
change was observed. This change was proposed to be due to a direct interaction
of DDP with bases in DNA (Horacek and Drobnik, 1971).

More direct information showing binding and cross-linking of DNA by cisplatin has recently been demonstrated in mouse leukemia L1210 cells in tissue
culture (Zwelling *et al.*, 1978). Cells were treated with cisplatin and incubated
for various time periods, after which amounts of double-strand DNA resulting
from cross-linking were measured by a DNA alkaline elution technique. The
maximum cross-linking effect of the "cis" cisplatin required about 12 hr of
posttreatment incubation before it was fully developed, whereas the cross-linking
effect of the "trans" isomer of cisplatin was fully developed at the end of 1 hr of
drug exposure.

Electron microscopic and cytologic studies have shown cisplatin to localize in
the nucleus and cause an alteration in nuclear structures. In sarcoma 180 cells in
mice, giant multinucleated cells were observed 4 days after treatment with cisplatin. The nuclei were in communication with each other by thin strands of nuclear

material and were enclosed in a common nuclear membrane. HeLa cells were treated with cisplatin and visualized by electron microscopy and X-ray probe analysis (Khan and Sadler, 1978). Platinum was shown to be localized to the nucleolus and the inner portion of the nuclear membrane. Little platinum was observed in the cytoplasm. Human lymphocytes were treated with cisplatin (Meyne and Lockhart, 1978) and dose dependence was observed for both inhibition of mitotic activity and increased frequency of metaphases with chromosomal aberrations consisting mainly of chromatid breaks. All the studies that showed mammalian cell abnormalities induced by cisplatin suggest that DNA within the nucleus is the primary target for this drug.

C. Molecular Studies

When cisplatin enters the tumor cell (or other tissue cells) in which the chloride concentration is considerably lower, the chloride ions are capable of dissociating, leaving a reactive diammine platinum complex that, probably through reaction with water, can then bind to DNA. Although this binding to DNA may be similar to alkylation, cisplatin probably should not be included in the same group with the classical alkylating agents such as nitrogen mustards for two reasons. First, studies with *E. coli* cells have shown that the filamentous *E. coli* cells revert to normally shaped cells when cisplatin is removed from the medium. In contrast, bacteria are rapidly killed by nitrogen mustardlike compounds. Second, cisplatin has demonstrated antitumor activity in animal tumors that have become resistant to alkylating agents. A discussion of the current knowledge of molecular aspects of cisplatin–DNA interactions follows.

Both *cis*- and *trans*-diamminedichloroplatinum can produce cross-links between two DNA strands. However, since the trans compound is inactive as an antitumor agent, this mechanism would appear to be less important in killing tumor cells. The other mechanism proposed is cross-linking of bases within a DNA strand (intrastrand cross-linking).

Structural measurements on cisplatin and DNA indicate that these molecules are well matched to interact with one another; that is, the distance between the chlorides of cisplatin in the cis position is 3.3 Å and the distance between adjacent bases on the DNA helix (intercalation distance) is 3.4 Å. It seems logical to assume that cisplatin binds to two adjacent bases. However, in the trans configuration, such binding would seem unlikely. The intercalative mode of interaction of cisplatin with DNA has been studied by Lippard (1978) using physicochemical methods and cisplatin was shown to interact with DNA in a manner similar to that of a known intercalative agent, ethidium bromide.

Studies with nucleosides showed that guanosine, adenosine, and cytidine interacted with cisplatin, whereas uridine and thymidine interacted minimally (Mansy and Rosenberg, 1972; Roos *et al.*, 1971). Subsequent studies by Kong and Theophanides (1974) showed that cisplatin formed a bidentate chelate with either the 6-NH_2 and N-7 or the 6-NH_2 and N-1 of adenosine and the 4-NH_2 and N-3 of cytidine. Recent studies have suggested that the N-7 (Kelman *et al.*, 1977) and O-6 (Butour and Macquet, 1978) positions of guanine are likely the initial site(s) of reaction of cisplatin with nucleotides in DNA.

Studies on binding of cisplatin to guanosine were extended to include studies on binding of cisplatin to DNA's with varying guanine/cytosine (G/C) ratios (Stone *et al.*, 1974). The buoyant densities of the DNA–cisplatin complexes were determined and the results showed that the binding of cisplatin to DNA increased as the G/C ratio increased. These results were confirmed by Munchausen and Rahn (1975) with [195]Pt-radiolabeled cisplatin. Using DNA and homopolynucleotides, these investigators showed that cisplatin preferentially binds to guanine residues.

How does the cisplatin–nucleoside interaction result in cessation of cell replication and growth? Butour and Macquet (1978) and Macquet and Butour (1978), using circular dichroism and fluorescence techniques, demonstrated that there are two possible interactions of platinum complexes with DNA. The first is a monofunctional interaction that does not affect the DNA structure. The second is a bifunctional interaction that appears to denature the DNA double helix locally. Figure 3 shows a proposed scheme by which cisplatin interacts and causes local changes in the DNA double helical configuration. Cisplatin reacts with water to form a reactive aquated species that interacts with guanosine in

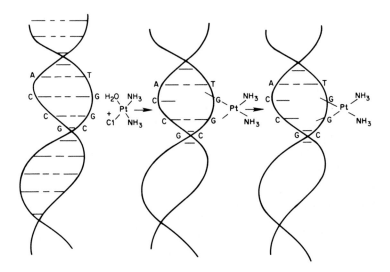

Fig. 3. Proposed scheme for interaction of cisplatin with DNA.

native DNA (A) to form a covalent linkage of cisplatin to DNA (B). As a result of this binding the hydrogen bonds between guanosine and cytidine on opposite DNA strands are broken. The cisplatin molecule then reacts with an adjacent nucleoside (bifunctional binding) to cause further hydrogen bond breakage resulting in local denaturation in the DNA double helix (C). These alterations in the DNA structure probably affect the fidelity of enzymatic DNA replication and RNA transcription, leading to lethal events in the cell. Oher recent studies (Friedman et al., 1978a,b) have implicated cisplatin interactions with various enzymes, including dehydrogenases in events leading to cytotoxicity.

IV. CONCLUSION

Although the precise mechanism of action of cisplatin is not known, the clinical utility of this drug in several human tumors has been confirmed. The proposed mechanism of tumor cell killing by cisplatin appears to be different from that of classical alkylating agents, and cisplatin appears to be synergistic with various alkylating agents and active in tumors that have become resistant to alkylating agents. A proposed mechanism whereby a base substitution mutation is induced in DNA by cisplatin may prove to be a unique mechanism not shared by any other known antitumor drug.

Many cisplatin analogues have shown antitumor activity in experimental tumors, and ongoing studies of the molecular mechanism of action of these agents should establish the mode of action of this unique class of platinum-containing anticancer drugs.

REFERENCES

Butour, J. L., and Macquet, J. P. (1978). *Eur. J. Biochem.* **78,** 455–463.
Drobnik, J., Urbankova, M., and Krekulova, A. (1973). *Mutat. Res.* **17,** 13–20.
Friedman,M. E., Melius, P., Teggins, J. E., and McAuliffe, C. A. (1978a). *Bioinorg. Chem.* **8,** 341–353.
Friedman, M. E., Melius, P., and McAuliffe, C. A. (1978b). *Bioinorg. Chem.* **8,** 355–361.
Handelsman, H., Goldsmith, M. A., Broder, L. E., Carter, S. K., and Slavik, M. (1974). *Cis-Platinum Clin. Brochure* (NSC119875), 6–9.
Horacek, P., and Drobnik, J. (1971). *Biochim. Biophys. Acta* **254,** 341–347.
Howle, J. A., and Gale, G. R. (1970a). *Biochem. Pharmacol.* **19,** 2757–2762.
Howle, J. A., and Gale, G. R. (1970b). *J. Bacteriol.* **103,** 259–260.
Kelman, A. D., Peresie, H. J., and Stone, P. J. (1977). *J. Clin. Hematol. Oncol.* **7,** 440–453.
Khan, A. D., and Sadler, P. J. (1978). *Chem.-Biol. Interact.* **21,** 227–232.
Kong, P. C., and Theophanides, T. (1974). *Inorg. Chem.* **13,** 1167–1170.
Leh, F., and Wolf, W. (1976). *J. Pharm. Sci.* **65,** 315–328.
Lippard, S. J. (1978). *Acc. Chem. Res.* **11,** 211–217.

Macquet, J. P., and Butour, J. L. (1978). *Eur. J. Biochem.* **83,** 375–387.

Mansy, S., and Rosenberg, B. (1972). *Adv. Antimicrob. Antineoplast. Chemother., Proc. Int. Congr. Chemother., 7th, Praque, 1971* **2,** 192–194.

Meyne, J., and Lockhart, L. H. (1978). *Mutat. Res.* **58,** 87–97.

Munchausen, L., and Rahn, R. A. (1975). *Biochim. Biophys. Acta* **414,** 242–255.

Renshaw,E., and Thomson, A. J. (1967). *J. Bacteriol.* **94,** 1915–1918.

Reslova, S. (1971). *Chem.-Biol. Interact. 4,* 66–70.

Roos, I. A. G., Thompson, A. J., and Eagles, J. (1971). *Chem.-Biol. Interact.* **9,** 421–427.

Rosenberg, B. (1978). *Interdiscip. Sci. Rev.* **3**(2), 134–147.

Rosenberg, B., Van Camp, L., and Krigas, T. (1965). *Nature (London)* **205,** 698–699.

Rosenberg, B., Renshaw, E., VanCamp, L., Hartwick, J., and Drobnik, J. (1967). *J. Bacteriol.* **93,** 716–721.

Rosenberg, B., Van Camp, L., Trosko, J., and Mansour, V. H. (1969). *Nature (London)* **222,** 385–386.

Stone, P. J. Kelman, A. D., and Sinex, F. M. (1974). *Nature (London)* **251,** 736.

Taylor, D. M., Tew, D. D., and Jones, J. D. (1976). *Eur. J. Cancer* **12,** 249–254.

Zwelling, L. A., Kohn, K. W., Ross, W. E., Ewig, R. A. G., and Anderson, T. (1978). *Cancer Res.* **38,** 1762–1768.

18

METHOTREXATE: MOLECULAR
PHARMACOLOGY
J. R. Bertino

I. INTRODUCTION

Methotrexate (MTX, 2,4- diamino- N^{10}- methylpteroylglutamic acid) is a widely used drug for the treatment of several human neoplastic diseases, as well as an immunosuppressive agent (Chu and Whitley, 1977; Johns and Bertino, 1973). This folate antagonist supplanted aminopterin (Fig. 1) in the clinic, on the basis of animal studies that indicated that it had a better therapeutic index than aminopterin (Goldin et al., 1955). Dichloro MTX (Fig. 1), on the basis of its success in the treatment of the experimental mouse tumor L1210 (Goldin et al., 1959), also was tested clinically, but in limited trials did not appear to have any superiority over MTX (Frei et al., 1964). During recent years the drug has been tested again utilizing intra-arterial therapy (Cleveland et al., 1969), as well as parenteral administration (Fernbach et al., 1979). Other folate antagonists are also undergoing investigation with the hope that they will have improved selectivity over MTX (Fig. 2). This chapter will cover the chemistry, mechanism of

CANCER AND CHEMOTHERAPY, VOL. III

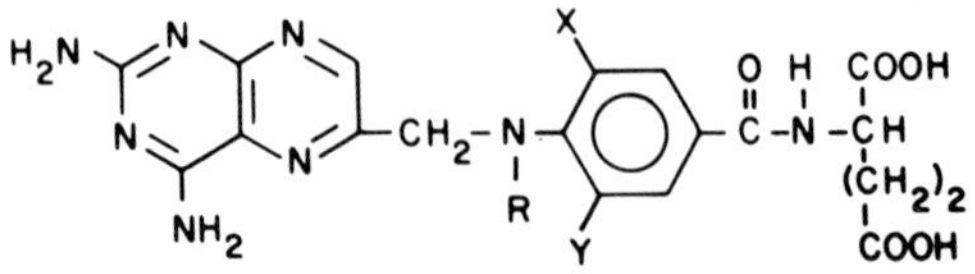

Fig. 1. Structure of classical 2,4-diamino analogues of folic acid.

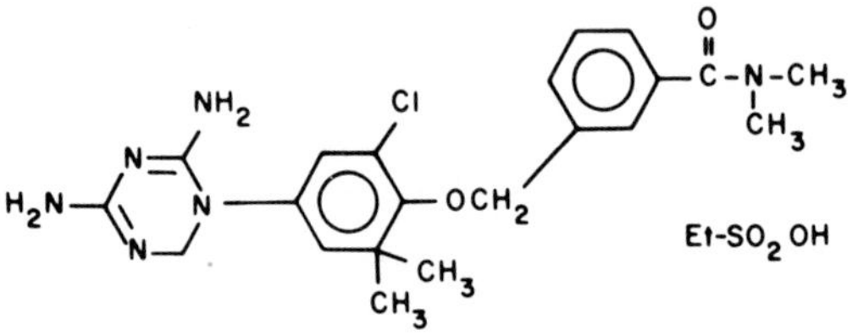

	R	X	Y
AMINOPTERIN	H	H	H
MTX	CH₃	H	H
DICHLOROMTX	CH₃	Cl	Cl

TZT, BAKER'S ANTIFOL, NSC 139105

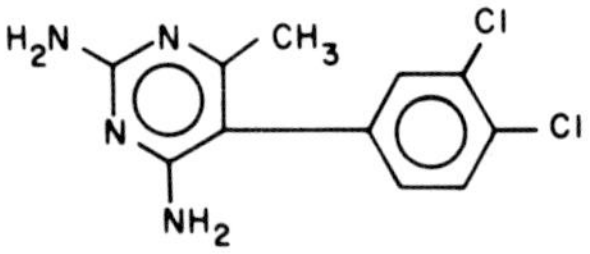

DDMP

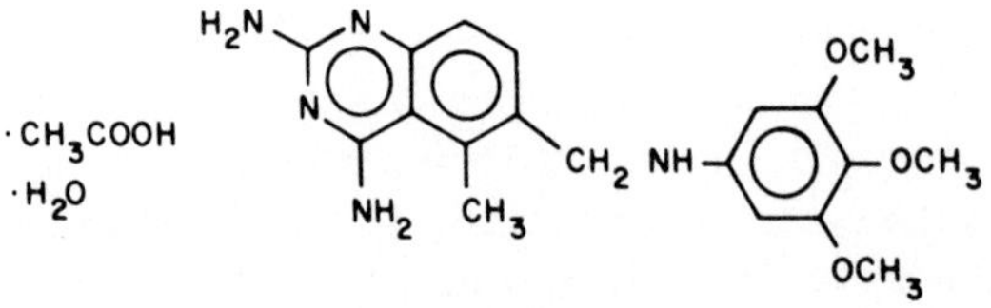

JB-II, NSC 249008

Fig. 2. Structure of "nonclassical" diamino inhibitors of dihydrofolate reductase. TZT, or (Baker's antifol ethanesulfonic acid compound with α[2- chloro- 4- (4,6- diamino- 2,2- dimethyl- *s*-triazine-1(2H)-yl)phenoxyl]-*N, N*-dimethyl-*m*-toluamide (1:1); NSC-139105 is a triazine analogue; DDMP [2,4-diamino, 5-(3′,4′-dichlorophenyl)-6-methylpyrimidine] is a pyrimidine analogue; and JB-11, or TMQ [2,4- diamino- 5- methyl- 6(3,4,5- trimethoxyaniline) methylquinazoline)], is a quinazoline analogue.

action, and effects of MTX and certain other folate antagonists on normal and neoplastic cells. The clinical pharmacology of MTX is discussed elsewhere.

II. CHEMISTRY

MTX is a weak organic acid and its sodium salt is highly soluble in aqueous solution above pH 7.0 (Seegar *et al.*, 1949). Purity may be established by various analytical procedures, including paper or thin-layer chromatography, chromotagraphy on DEAE cellulose, or high-performance liquid chromatography (Watson *et al.*, 1978; Wisnicki *et al.*, 1978). The pure compound is a yellow-orange crystalline material and like folic acid decomposes without melting at about 200°. Concentrations of folate antagonists may be conveniently measured by UV absorption in 0.1 N NaOH (Johns and Bertino, 1973). Lower concentrations in physiologic material (urine, serum, tissues) may be measured after extraction in boiling water and assay by enzyme inhibition (Bertino and Fischer, 1964) or by a competition binding assay (Arons *et al.*, 1975; Kamen *et al.*, 1976; Myers *et al.*, 1975; Raso and Schreiber, 1975). As might be predicted, MTX or its metabolite, 7-OH MTX, is less soluble in acid urine, and this insolubility and precipitation may contribute to the renal toxicity seen with high-dose therapy (Jacobs *et al.*, 1976).

III. MECHANISM OF ACTION AND STRUCTURE–ACTIVITY RELATIONSHIPS

A. Folate Antagonism

The folate coenzymes are involved in several key reactions leading to the synthesis of thymidylate, purines, and the amino acids serine and methionine (Fig. 3). The substitution of a 4-amino group for the 4-hydroxyl Fig. 3 group of folic acid results in a compound (aminopterin) that is a tight binding inhibitor of the enzyme dihydrofolate reductase (DHFR). MTX, as well as dichloro MTX, like aminopterin, are "stoichiometric" inhibitors of this enzyme at pH 6.0 (Bertino *et al.*, 1964; Werkheiser, 1961). This inhibition, although extremely tight, is reversible, and at an alkaline pH, the substrate dihydrofolate can be shown to compete with MTX for binding (Bertino *et al.*, 1964). Although the substitution of a methyl group for a hydrogen on the 10-nitrogen does not decrease binding (MTX), nor does the 3′,5′-dichloro substitution (3′,5′-dichloro MTX), 7-hydroxylation markedly decreases binding of the inhibitor to DHFR (Johns and Loo, 1967). Hydrolysis of the terminal glutamate also markedly decreases binding to the enzyme and has been utilized as a method for MTX inactivation

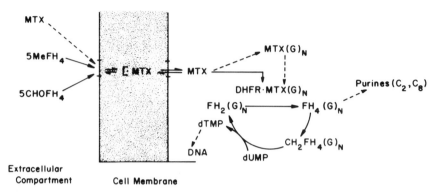

Fig. 3. Mechanism of action of MTX in relation to folate metabolism. Note that inhibition of dihydrofolate reductase (DHFR) by MTX or its polyglutamate (MTX(G_n)) leads to a decrease in formation of tetrahydrofolate (FH_4), and subsequently a decrease in purine and thymidylate (dTMP) biosynthesis. This figure also illustrates the competitive relationship between MTX and 5-methyltetrahydrofolate (5MeFH$_4$) and leucovorin (5-formyltetrahydrofolate, 5CHOFH$_4$) for the membrane transport carrier.

(Abelson *et al.*, 1979; Chabner *et al.*, 1972). In contrast, the addition of gluta-mate side chains to MTX in γ-linkage does not decrease binding of the inhibitor to DHFR. This is of importance, since it is now clear from several studies that MTX is polyglutamated intracellularly (Brown *et al.*, 1974; Jacobs, *et al.*, 1977; Rosenblatt *et al.*, 1978; Whitehead *et al.*, 1975).

In a series of elegant studies, the late B. R. Baker demonstrated that potent inhibition of DHFR could be obtained with compounds that did not resemble folic acid or folate coenzymes (reviewed in Baker, 1967, 1971). These com-pounds maintained the diamino structure, but the binding energy lost by different conformations of the inhibitor was recovered by appropriate hydrophobic sub-stituents (Fig. 2). The value of this approach has been that these molecules can exploit differences in enzyme structure, outside of the active site; these dif-ferences are especially large in the case of bacterial versus mammalian DHFR. Thus potent selective new bacterial agents have emerged from exploitation of this concept by Hitchings, Burchall, and co-workers (Burchall, 1971; Hitchings, 1972, 1975). Several of these "nonclassical" potent inhibitors of mammalian DHFR have been evaluated as antitumor agents, and one of these, Baker's antifol [BAF, TZT (ethanesulfonic acid compound with α[2-chloro-4-(4,6-diamino-2,2-dimethyl-*s*-triazine-1 (2H)-yl)phenoxyl]-*N,N*-dimethyl-*m*-toluamide(1:1); NSC 139105], is now in phase II clinical trials (McCreary *et al.*, 1977; Skeel *et al.*, 1976). It is perhaps ironic that this series of compounds, initially believed to have selectivity on the basis of differences in inhibition of tumor and normal tissue DHFR, enjoyed selectivity in certain experimental tumor systems at least, by virtue of differences in transport (Skeel *et al.*, 1973). As a result of these studies, and a further detailed understanding of the transport process of MTX and folates, there has been renewed enthusiasm for developing more selective folate analogues on this basis (Bertino, 1979). In particular, certain nonclassical quinazoline folate antagonists (Fig. 2) appear to be rapidly accumulated by human neoplastic cells and are under active preclinical investigation (Bertino *et al.*, 1979).

B. Other Sites of Action of MTX

Although it is established that in conventional doses, MTX kills cells primarily via inhibition of DHFR, thus causing thymineless and in some cases, purineless death, the use of high doses of MTX (gm/m^2), as well as the recent finding of polyglutamylation of MTX, has led to a reexamination of this concept in these circumstances. Transport studies have shown that MTX can block uptake of reduced folates into cells, as well as facilitate their efflux (Bertino *et al.*, 1977; Goldman, 1971, 1975). Thus an additional site of action of MTX, especially if MTX is used in a high dose, is to reduce the supply of folates to cells. This relationship is competitive, so that, conversely, high doses of leucovorin (LV, N^{10}-formyltetrahydrofolate) will decrease MTX uptake into cells (Nahas *et al.*, 1972) (Fig. 3). The high extracellular concentrations achieved with high-dose therapy, made safe by leucovorin rescue, hydration, and alkalinization, have also resulted in high intracellular MTX concentrations, although the transport process severely limits the steady-state level of MTX that can be achieved (Goldman, 1975; Sirotnak and Donsbach, 1974; White *et al.*, 1975). It has been postulated that at high intracellular concentrations of MTX (or more properly MTX polyglutamates), inhibition of other folate coenzymes, in particular thymidylate synthetase, may play a role in the antitumor effects of this regimen (Borsa and Whitmore, 1969). Support for this concept derives from studies that show that MTX polyglutamates are more inhibitory to TMP synthetase than MTX (Dolnick and Cheng, 1978). Other folate enzyme systems have not yet been fully examined for MTX polyglutamyl inhibition.

C. Mechanism of Cell Death

When cells are exposed to MTX, depending on the extracellular concentration and the ability of the cells to concentrate the drug, lethal effects may result. Other variables are also important in considering why a cell is or is not killed by MTX. These include the level of the various coenzyme pools within the cell, the level of DHFR and its rate of synthesis, and the availability of performed purines and pyrimidines as well as salvage pathways. Also of great importance is whether or not the cells are in logarithmic growth (Bruce *et al.*, 1966; Hryniuk *et al.*, 1969). Jackson and Harrup (1973) have described a model that attempts to take these factors into consideration to predict MTX effectiveness as a consequence of drug dosage and schedule. A low rate of DNA synthesis and whether cells are in the G_0 or resting state appear to be important factors in determining the natural resistance of certain tumors to the action of MTX, as well as other antimetabolites. Conversely, a population in logarithmic growth with a rapid rate of DNA synthesis, and consequently a short generation time, will be preferentially killed by a short exposure to high levels of MTX (Fig. 4).

As a result of inhibition of TMP synthesis by MTX, cells are unable to synthesize sufficient DNA for subsequent division, and "megaloblast" formation occurs, since in most cells RNA and protein synthesis are not affected to the same degree. At a critical point, cell death ensues, but the exact reason for cell death is not clear. This type of cell death, first described for 5-FU effects in bacteria, has been referred to as "thymineless" death and results in what has also been referred to as unbalanced growth (Cohen, 1971).

In certain cells (e.g., L cell growth in tissue culture), MTX, by virtue of inhibition of RNA and protein syntheses as well as of DNA synthesis, may be a "self-limiting" inhibitor of cell growth, since under these conditions, cell death does not rapidly ensue (McBurney and Whitmore, 1975). Exposure of these cells to a purine in the presence of MTX enhances the rate of cell kill, presumably because this accentuates the unbalanced state. In other cells (L1210), addition of

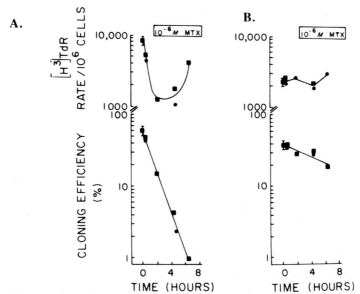

Fig. 4. Effect of short-term exposure of MTX (4.5 hr) on logarithmic versus plateau phase L5278Y cells. Cell survival was measured by the soft agar cloning technique (from Hryniuk *et al.*, 1969). Vertical bars represent standard errors of the geometric means. (A) Log cultures; (B) resting cultures.

purine decreases cell kill by MTX, indicating that MTX can also kill cells by inducing a "purineless" state (Hryniuk et al., 1975). This concept has been extended to in vivo studies, and under the appropriate conditions, the addition of thymidine completely blocks MTX toxicity to normal tissues in both mice (Tattersall et al., 1975) and man (Howell et al., 1977). In mice bearing L1210 leukemia, a tumoricidal effect can be obtained with this combination without toxicity to normal tissues (Semon and Grindey, 1978; Tattersall et al., 1975). Thus far, human tumors have not yet been found that are susceptible to "purineless" death, although this possibility has not been explored adequately. The finding that thymidine protects normal tissues from MTX toxicity has given rise to the use of thymidine as a "rescue" agent following MTX administration, in a similar manner to LV rescue (Ensminger et al., 1976).

Another clinical extension of these findings is that combination chemotherapy with MTX and an inhibitor of either protein or RNA synthesis may result in antagonism of MTX action. An example of this type of antagonism is the concomitant use of MTX and L-asparaginase, an inhibitor of protein synthesis (Capizzi, 1974, 1975; Vadlamudi et al., 1973). However, if asparaginase treatment is delayed 24 hr, this will relieve MTX inhibition at this time, in essence rescuing normal marrow cells, in a similar manner to leucovorin rescue. However, this delayed use of asparaginase after MTX is synergistic for cytotoxicity against neoplastic lymphoblasts that require exogenous asparaginase for cell growth (Capizzi, 1975). This combination has been shown to be highly effective in the treatment of acute lymphoblastic leukemia (Capizzi, 1974).

IV. TRANSPORT OF METHOTREXATE AND RELATED COMPOUNDS

Work from several laboratories has shown that for leukemic cells, MTX is actively transported, with discrete influx and efflux processes (Bender, 1975; Goldman, 1971, 1975; Hakala, 1965; Huennekens et al., 1978; Jackson et al., 1975). MTX utilizes the transport system for reduced folates and in short-term experiments (60 min or less) mouse leukemia cells do not form appreciable amounts of MTX polyglutamates. However, in the case of liver cells, MTX polyglutamates are rapidly formed, and interpretation of transport data becomes more complex (Galivan, 1979). The use of membrane vesicles, prepared for L1210 cells, has recently been reported for MTX transport studies, and these have the advantage that intracellular metabolism is decreased (Yang et al., 1979).

V. MECHANISMS OF RESISTANCE TO FOLATE ANTAGONISTS

Cells become resistant to MTX by one or more of three common mechanisms: increased levels of DHFR, a change in the properties of DHFR so that it binds

MTX less tightly, or decreased uptake of the drug (reviewed in Bertino and Skeel, 1975; Bertino, 1979).

The most common mechanism of acquired resistance observed in experimental mouse tumors has been an increase in the enzyme DHFR (Schrecker *et al.*, 1971). Cell lines have been developed by exposing them to stepwise increases of MTX that contain levels of DHFR 100–300 times higher than the parent sensitive line (Dolnick *et al.*, 1979; Fischer, 1961; Hakala *et al.*, 1961; Nakamura and Littlefield, 1972). This increase of activity of DHFR in the mutant cells has been shown to be due to an increase in the rate at which this enzyme is synthesized, mediated by an increase in mRNA and a corresponding increase in the gene copies that code for DHFR (Alt *et al.*, 1978; Schimke *et al.*, 1977). The amplified gene has been found by *in situ* hydridization techniques to be localized to the No. 2 chromosome of resistant Chinese hamster cells and also the No. 2 chromosome of murine L5178Y cells that have a 300-fold increase in DHFR (Dolnick *et al.*, 1979). Of interest is that this region of the chromosome, which is not present in the parent line, can be easily identified, since it is an area of nonbanding, and it has been referred to as a homogeneous staining region (Biedler *et al.*, 1972). The mechanism of how the DHFR gene is amplified is not known, but is of great interest. Human lines propagated in tissue culture with an increased level of DHFR have also been described (Niethammer and Jackson, 1975), but thus far the mechanism of this increase has not been elucidated. In the clinic a simple *in vitro* biochemical test may be used to detect acquired resistance to MTX, namely, the rate of [^{3}H]deoxyuridine incorporation into DNA in the presence or absence of the inhibitor (Bertino *et al.*, 1975; Bertino, 1979; Hryniuk and Bertino, 1969). In about half the patients thought to be resistant to MTX, a decrease in inhibition of DNA synthesis by MTX (10^{-5}–10^{-7} M) has been noted. In only one such patient has an increase in DHFR activity been found (Bertino, 1979; Hryniuk and Bertino, 1969).

Resistant cell lines with decreased affinity of DHFR for MTX have also been described, thus leading to resistance of this antifol (Flintoff *et al.*, 1976; Gupta, 1977). Jackson *et al.* have measured relatively small decreases in the affinity of DHFR for MTX in several rodent lines and have correlated these differences with natural or intrinsic resistance of these lines to this drug (Jackson and Harrup, 1973). Two leukemic patients demonstrating biochemical resistance to MTX have been shown to have cells containing DHFR with a decreased affinity for DHFR (Bertino and Skeel, 1975).

A third mechanism of resistance to MTX described is decreased uptake of the drug (Fischer, 1960; Hakala, 1965; Hill *et al.*, 1978; Mathe *et al.*, 1978; Sirotnak *et al.*, 1968). In experiments described using the L5178Y line, it was found that the active transport system that results in MTX entry into cells was essentially deleted (Hill *et al.*, 1978). Reduced folates also were not transported actively by this line. However, since folic acid is present in the medium, these cells can thrive in tissue culture. In an L1210 line a double mutant has been described that not only has a 35-fold increase in DHFR but also transports MTX poorly (Lindquist et al., 1978). This line, as might be expected, is highly resistant to MTX. Further characterization and study of these lines could be most rewarding in regard to MTX and reduced folate transport processes.

VI. THE FUTURE FOR FOLATE ANTAGONISTS

Although MTX is a useful drug for the treatment of several human neoplastic diseases, as well as an immunosuppressive agent, it has considerable toxicity in therapeutic doses. Approaches to ameliorating this toxicity and thus to improve the therapeutic index of this drug that is being tested involves the use of various "rescue" agents (i.e., leucovorin, asparaginase, thymidine, carboxypeptidase G_1). This approach has the potential for decreasing toxicity to normal cells and allows the use of large doses of MTX for short periods of time (reviewed in Bertino, 1977). The disadvantages of this technique are the cost of the high doses of MTX administered, the need for careful surveillance of patients, and the relatively short duration of MTX exposure allowable before leucovorin or another rescue agent must be employed; thus tumor cells in G_1 or G_0 may escape from MTX till if they are capable also of utilizing subsequently administered leucovorin.

MTX has been attached to macromolecular carriers to alter its distribution and uptake (Chu and Whitley, 1977; Mathe et al., 1978) and has been encapsulated into erythrocytes (Zimmerman and Pilwat, 1978) and liposomes (Kamen et al., 1976). A very interesting recent publication described the use of liposome encapsulated MTX that could be released at specific sites by local hyperthermia (Weinstein et al., 1979).

Another approach mentioned (vide supra) has been the design of new antifolates that possess greater selectivity for DHFR from neoplastic cells as compared to normal replicating cells. The three-dimensional structure for DHFR from bacterial sources is now known (Mathews et al., 1977, 1978), and it seems likely that in the near future similar information will become available for human enzymes. These advances could allow sophisticated drug design that takes advantage of small differences in normal and neoplastic enzymes, if they exist.

The finding that certain "nonclassical" folate antagonists are accumulated to a greater degree by certain tumor cells than normal tissues has increased interest in this approach. Certain of the 2,4,6-triazine and 2,4-diamino quinazoline inhibitors of DHFR (Fig. 2) are not transported by the active transport system available for MTX, and thus may be accumulated by a much greater degree in neoplastic cells (Bertino, 1979; Skeel et al., 1973). It may therefore be possible to develop this type of agent that not only is a potent inhibitor of DHFR, but is transported selectively by tumor cells as well.

REFERENCES

Abelson, H., Ensminger, W., Rosawsky, A., and Uren, J. (1979). *Chem. Biol. Pteridines, Int. Pteridine Symp., 6th* **4**, 629-633.
Alt, F. W., Kellems, R. E., Bertino, J. R., and Schimke, R. T. (1978). *J. Biol. Chem.* **253**, 1357-1370.
Arons, E., Rothenberg, S., daCosta, M., Fischer, C., and Igbal, M. P. (1975). *Cancer Res.* **35**, 2033-2038.
Baker, B. R. (1967). "Design of Active Site Directed Irreversible Enzyme Inhibitors," pp. 192-263. Wiley, New York.
Baker, B. R. (1971). *Ann. N.Y. Acad. Sci.* **186**, 214-226.
Bender, R. A. (1975). *Cancer Chemother. Rep., Part 3* **6**, 73-82.
Bertino, J. R. (1977). *Semin. Oncol.* **4**, 203.
Bertino, J. R. (1979). *Cancer Res.* **39**, 293-304.
Bertino, J. R., and Fischer, G. A. (1964). *Methods Med. Res.* **10**, 297-309.
Bertino, J. R., and Skeel, R. T. (1975). *In* "Pharmacological Basis of Cancer Chemotherapy" Williams & Wilkins, 681-689 Baltimore, Maryland. U. Texas System Cancer Center, M. D. Anderson Hospital and Tumor Institute, Houston, Texas.
Bertino, J. R., Booth, B. A., Bieber, A. L., Cashmore, A., and Sartorelli, A. C. (1964). *J. Biol. Chem.* **239**, 479-485.
Bertino, J. R., Nixon, P. F., and Nahas, A. (1977). *In* "Folic Acid: Biochemistry and Physiology in Relation to the Human Nutrition Requirements" (Food and Nutrition Board, National Research Council, ed.), pp. 178-187. Natl. Acad. Sci., Washington, DC.
Bertino, J. R., Sawicki, W. L., Moroson, B. A., Cashmore, A. R., and Elslager, E. F. (1979). *Biochem. Pharmacol.* **28**, 1983-1987.
Biedler, J. L., Albrecht, A. M., and Hutchinson, J. D. (1972). *Cancer Res.* **32**, 153-159.
Borsa, J., and Whitmore, G. F. (1969). *Mol. Pharmacol.* **5**, 318-332.
Brown, J. P., Davidson, G. E., Weir, D. G., and Scott, J. M. (1974). *Int. J. Biochem.* **5**, 727.
Bruce, W. R., Meeker, B. E.,and Valeriote, F. A. (1966). *J. Natl. Cancer Inst.* **37**, 233-245.
Burchall, J. J. (1971). *Ann. NY. Acad. Sci.* **186**, 143-152.
Capizzi, R. L. (1974). *Biochem. Pharmacol.* **23**, Suppl. 2, 151.
Capizzi, R. L. (1975). *Cancer Chemother. Rep., Part 3* **6**, 37-41.
Chabner, B. A., Johns, D., and Bertino, J. R. (1972). *Nature (London)* **239**, 395-397.
Chu, B. C., and Whitely, J. M. (1977). *Mol. Pharmacol.* **13**, 80-88.
Cleveland, J. C., Johns, D. G., Farnham, G., and Bertino, J. R. (1969). *Curr. Top. Surg. Res.* **1**, 113.
Cohen, S. S. (1971). *Ann. NY. Acad. Sci.* **186**, 292-301.
Dolnick, B. J., and Cheng, Y.-C. (1978). *J. Biol. Chem.* **253**, 3563-3565.
Dolnick, B. J., Berenson, R. J., Bertino, J. R., Kaufman, R. J., Nunberg, J. H., and Schimke, R. T. (1979). *J. Cell. Biol.* 83:394-402.
Ensminger, W., Frei, E., III, Pitman, S., Wick, M. and Raso, U., *et al.* (1976). *Proc. Am. Assoc. Cancer Res.* **17**, 282.
Fernbach, B., Ohnuma, T., Takahashi, I., Greenspan, E. M., and Holland, J. F. (1979). *Proc. Am. Assoc. Cancer Res.* **20**, 163.
Fischer, G. A. (1960). *Biochem. Pharmacol.* **11**, 1233-1234.

Fischer, G. A. (1961). *Biochem. Pharmacol.* **7,** 75–77.

Flintoff, W. F., Davidson, S. V., and Siminovitch, L. (1976). *Somat. Cell Genet.* **2,** 245.

Frei, E., III, Sparr, C. L., Brindley, C. O., Selawry, O., Holland, J. F., Rall, D. P., Wasserman, L. R., Hoogstraten, B., Shnider, B. I., McIntyre, O. R., Matthews, L. B., and Miller, S. P. (1964). *Clin. Pharmacol. Ther.* **6,** 160–171.

Galivan, J. (1979). *Cancer Res.* **39,** 735–743.

Goldin, A., Venditti, J. M., Humphreys, S. R., et al. (1955). *Cancer Res.* **15,** 742–747.

Goldin, A., Humphreys, S. R., Venditti, J. M., and Mantel, N. (1959). *J. Natl. Cancer Inst.* **22,** 811–823.

Goldman, I. D. (1971). *Ann. NY. Acad. Sci.* **86,** 400–422.

Goldman, I. D. (1975). *Cancer Chemother. Rep., Part 3* **6,** 51–61.

Gupta, R. S. (1977). *Can. J. Biochem.* **55,** 445–452.

Hakala, M. T. (1965). *Biochim. Biophys. Acta* **102,** 198–209.

Hakala, M. T., Zakrewski, S. F., and Nichol, C. A. (1961). *J. Biol. Chem.* **236,** 952–958.

Hill, B. T., Bailey, B. D., and Goldman, I. D. (1978). *Proc. Am. Assoc. Cancer Res.* **19,** 49.

Hitchings, G. H. (1972). *Annu. Rep. Med. Chem.* **7,** 1–5.

Hitchings, G. H. (1975). *In* "Pharmacologic Basis of Cancer Chemotherapy" pp. 25–46. Williams & Wilkins, Baltimore, Maryland.

Howell, S., Ensminger, W., Krishan, A., Parker, I., and Frei, E., III (1977). *Proc. Am. Assoc. Cancer Res.* **18,** 303.

Hryniuk, W. M., and Bertino, J. R. (1969). *J. Clin. Invest.* **48,** 2140–2155.

Hryniuk, W. M., Fischer, G. A., and Bertino, S. R. (1969). *Mol. Pharmacol.* **5,** 557–564.

Hryniuk, W., et al. (1975). *Cancer Res.* **35,** 1427–1432.

Huennekens, F. M., Vitols, K. S.,and Henderson, G. B. (1978). *Adv. Enzymol. Relat. Areas Mol. Biol.* **47,** 313–346.

Jackson, R. C., and Harrup, K. R. (1973). *Arch. Biochem. Biophys.* **158,** 827–841.

Jackson, R. C., Niethammer, D., and Huennekens, F. M. (1975). *Cancer Biochem. Biophys.* *1*:151–155.

Jacobs, S. A., Stoller, R. G., Chabner, B. A., and Johns, D. G. (1976). *J. Clin. Invest.* **57,** 534–538.

Jacobs, S. A., Derr, J. D., and Johns, D. G. (1977). *Mol. Pharmacol.* **26,** 2310–2313.

Johns, D. G., and Bertino, J. R. (1973). *In* "Cancer Medicine" (J. F. Holland and E. Frei, III, eds.), pp. 739–753. Lea & Febiger, Philadelphia, Pennsylvania.

Johns, D. G., and Loo, T. L. (1967). *J. Pharm. Sci.* **56,** 356–359.

Kamen, B. A., Takach, P. L., Vatev, R., and Caston, J. D. (1976). *Anal. Biochem.* **70,** 54–63.

Lindquist, C. A., Moroson, B. A., and Bertino, J. R. (1978). *Proc. Am. Assoc. Cancer Res.* **19,** 165.

McBurney, M. W., and Whitmore, G. F. (1975). *Cancer Res.* **35,** 586–590.

McCreary, R. H., Moertel, C. G., Schutt, A. J., O'Connell, M. J., Hahn, R. G., Reitemeier, R. J., Rubin, J., and Frytak, S. (1977). *Cancer (Philadelphia)* **40,** 9–13.

Mathe, A., Loc, T. B., and Beinard, J. (1978). *C. R. Acad. Sci.* **246,** 1626.

Mathews, D. A., Alden, R. A., Bolin, J. T., Freer, S. T., Hamlin, R., Xuong, N., Kraut, J., Poe, M., Williams, M., and Hoogsteen, K. (1977). *Science* **197,** 452–455.

Mathews, D. A., Alden, R. A., Bolin, J. T., Filman, D. J., Freer, S. T., Hamlin, R., Hol, W. G. J., Kisliuk, R., Pastore, E. J., Plante, L. T., Xuong, N., and Kraut, J. (1978). *J. Biol. Chem.* **253,** 6946–6954.

Myers, C., Lippman, M., Eliott, T., and Chabner, B. (1975). *Proc. Natl. Acad. Sci. U.S.A.* **72,** 3683–3686.

Nahas, A., Nixon, P. F., and Bertino, J. R. (1972). *Cancer Res.* **32,** 1416–1421.

Nakamura, H., and Littlefield, J. U. (1972). *J. Biol. Chem.* **247,** 179–187.

Niethammer, D., and Jackson, R. C. (1975). *Eur. J. Cancer* **11**, 845-854.

Raso, V., and Schreiber, R. (1975). *Cancer Res.* **35**, 1407-1410.

Rosenblatt, D. S., Whitehead, V. M., Dupont, M. M., Vuhich, M.-J., and Vera, N. (1978). *Mol. Pharmacol.* **14**, 210-214.

Schimke, R. T., Alt, F. W., Kellems, R. E., Kaufman, R. J., and Bertino, J. R. (1977). *Cold Spring Harbor Symp. Quant. Biol.* **42**, 649-657.

Schrecker, A. W., Mead, J. A. R., Greensberg, N. H., and Goldin, A. (1971). *Biochem. Pharmacol.* **20**, 716-720.

Seegar, D. R., Cosulich, D. B., Smith, J. M., Jr., and Hultquist, M. E. (1949). *J. Am. Chem. Soc.* **71**, 1753-1759.

Semon, J. H., and Grindey, G. B. (1978). *Cancer Res.* **38**, 2905-2911.

Sirotnak, F. M., and Donsbach, R. C. (1974). *Cancer Res.* **34**, 3332-3340.

Sirotnak, F. M., Kurita, S., and Hutchison, D. J. (1968). *Cancer Res.* **28**, 75-80.

Skeel, R. T., Sawicki, W. L., Cashmore, A. R.,and Bertino, J. R. (1973). *Cancer Res.* **33**, 2972-2976.

Skeel, R. T., Cashmore, A. R., and Bertino, J. R. (1976). *Cancer Res.* **36**, 48-54.

Tattersall, M. H. N., Brown, B., and Frei, E., III (1975). *Nature (London)* **253**, 198-200.

Vadlamudi, S., Krishna, B., Reddy, V. V. S., and Goldin, A. (1973). *Cancer Res.* **33**, 2014-2019.

Watson, E., Cohen, J. L., and Chan, K. K. (1978). *Cancer Treat. Rep.* **62**, 381-387.

Weinstein, J. N., Magin, R. L., Yatvin, M. D., Zaharko, D. S. (1979). *Science* **204**, 188-191.

Werkheiser, W. C. (1961). *J. Biol. Chem.* **236**, 888-893.

White, J. C., Loftfield, S., and Goldman, I. D. (1975). *Mol. Pharmacol.* **11**, 287-297.

Whitehead, V. M., Perrault, M. M., and Stelcner, S. (1975). *Cancer Res.* **35**, 2985-2990.

Wisnicki, J. L., Tong, W. P., and Ludlum, D. B. (1978). *Cancer Treat. Rep.* **62**, 529-532.

Yang, C. H., Peterson, H. F., Sirotnak, F. M., and Chello, P. L. (1979). *J. Biol. Chem.* **254**, 1402-1407.

Zimmerman, U., and Pilwat, G. (1978). *J. Clin. Chem.* **16**, 135.

Part III
Clinical Pharmacology of Selected Neoplastic Agents

19
INTRODUCTION TO CLINICAL PHARMACOLOGY
Steven D. Reich

I. INTRODUCTION

The effects of a drug, both beneficial and adverse, are a function of the pharmacology of the drug, the nature of the disease, and the pathophysiologic state of the patient. These factors are intimately entwined and their interrelationships form the basis for the field of clinical pharmacology, which is the scientific study of drugs in man. Although the principles of clinical pharmacology apply to all drugs, it is especially important to incorporate these principles into clinical practice of cancer chemotherapy. The toxic effects on patients secondary to most cancer chemotherapeutic agents are clinically significant, and can be life threatening, so care and understanding must be used when these drugs are administered.

Although factors that affect the efficacy and toxicity of drugs in man have been considered since ancient times, the scientific discipline of clinical pharmacology is fairly recent and coincides with the explosive increase in new drugs during the past quarter century. Clinical pharmacology encompasses three major areas (Smith and Melmon, 1972). The first of these is the study of the absorption, distribution, metabolism, and elimination of drugs in man. The second involves the study of drug actions as a means of understanding the pathophysiology of diseases of a particular organ system. The third area is the documentation of the

CANCER AND CHEMOTHERAPY, VOL. III

safety and efficacy of drugs in man by appropriate clinical trials. All three of these areas are important to the study of anticancer agents.

The clinical trials necessary to elevate a chemical with antitumor activity to a commercially available drug with beneficial effect on patients with cancer are somewhat different from trials involving a relatively nontoxic drug used for a benign disease. Since most anticancer drugs cause some clinically significant toxicity, phase I trials of these drugs are designed to delineate these toxicities and demonstrate that they are basically predictable and reversible. Anticancer drugs may not be safe, but the risks involved must be significantly less than the adverse reactions that occur if tumor growth is not controlled. Because of the heterogenicity of tumors, phase II trials are designed to determine which patients with specific tumor types will respond favorably to the therapy. Phase III trials are needed to demonstrate that a new drug or therapy has greater benefit than an older therapy. The design and evaluation of clinical trials of anticancer drugs are reviewed elsewhere (Carter, 1979).

The use of anticancer drugs in humans to study the pathophysiology of diseases of organ systems is not often employed. The prime objective of administering chemotherapy to a patient with cancer is control of the tumor. However, an increased understanding of tumor growth and spread, host defenses against cancer, and the host's response to toxic insult has been derived from studies of anticancer drugs administered to humans. No unified approach to this area of clinical pharmacology as it relates to the anticancer drugs has been adopted.

The study of drug disposition in humans provides information necessary for a rational approach to therapeutics. In general, this information is used to design dose regimens of drugs for patient populations and for specific individuals and to correlate aspects of drug disposition with beneficial response and adverse effects. Prediction of efficacy and toxicity can then be made on the basis of measured parameters. When the time course of drug disposition is considered, the term "pharmacokinetics" is used to indicate the field of study. The application of pharmacokinetics to the safe and effective therapeutic management of the individual patient is termed "clinical pharmacokinetics."

II. PHARMACOKINETICS

Pharmacokinetics involves measurement of parameters that are known to have an effect on the pharmacological response of a patient. These measurements include drug plasma concentrations, half-life, clearance, metabolite concentrations, protein binding, and other factors. These parameters are measured in patients under various conditions such as renal or liver dysfunction, limited or extensive disease states, and concomitant administration of other drugs in order to determine the factors that affect response. The measured parameters and the response of patients are integrated by the use of suitable models to interpret the data. Usually, mathematical models are used since the mathematical equations can describe the time course of drug concentrations in the body and can be manipulated to make quantitative predictions of pharmacological effect when changes in the drug, dosage regimen, or the pathophysiologic state of the patient occur.

Although it is true that studies in animals of the interrelationships among host, disease, and drug are inherently easier to perform, the ultimate goal is the therapy of humans, so humans must be the subjects of pharmacological studies (Gold, 1952). Animal experiments can often help establish methodology needed to study drug distribution in humans. Drug metabolism studies in animals can give clues to the metabolism of drug in humans, but they cannot replace human studies because metabolic pathways of humans are often different from those of animals. Animal studies can also give estimates of values not easily obtainable from humans such as blood flow to organs, efficiency of various tissues in extracting a drug, and effects of organ dysfunction on drug disposition and elimination. Toxicology studies in animals can also suggest which organ systems are likely to be damaged by a particular drug.

One of the goals of pharmacokinetic studies is to correlate measurable parameters of drug disposition, metabolism, or elimination with clinical effect. Many drugs show an increasing pharmacological response with an increasing dose and both dose and response can be correlated with plasma concentrations of the drug. Some antitumor drugs, however, do not seem to have a dose–response curve. Sometimes this is related to the mechanism of action of the drug. Cytosine arabinoside, for example, is a cell cycle, phase-specific drug. Cells in the DNA synthetic phase (S) of the cell cycle are most susceptible to the lethal effects of the drug. A dose–response curve can be generated when cells are synchronized in S phase. However, if there is a mixed population of cells, only those in S phase will be killed. Once all cells in S phase have been killed, no further response will be noted as the dose is increased unless other cells are recruited into S phase. The cytokinetics of cells can effect the response of cells to a drug and give the appearance of a lack of relationship between pharmacokinetic parameters and response. This problem must always be kept in mind, since the kinetics of growth of tumors in patients is complex and many antitumor drugs exert their greatest cytotoxic effect on cycling cells. When the interrelationships among mechanism of action, pharmacokinetics, and cytokinetics are known, it is then possible to formulate a model that will describe the kinetics of the system and predict responses to a drug with respect to dose (Lincoln et al., 1976).

III. MATHEMATICAL MODELING

The mathematical model is the basis of pharmacokinetics. A model, simply speaking, is a method of describing or interpreting data. Mathematics is used because it was shown that loss of drugs from the bloodstream could be described by a curve made up of the sum of exponentials (Solomon, 1953). The sophistication of mathematical formulations allows complex systems to be summarized by equations that, when properly interpreted, can add to the understanding of the system.

Numerous observations performed *in vivo* on drug absorption, distribution, and elimination led to the concept that a biological system can be treated as if there were boundaries separating the system into parts, or so-called compartments, and that a drug is transferred to and from compartments in conformance with a set of rules known as first-order kinetics (Dvorchik and Vesell, 1976). It is important to realize that compartmentalized models are not necessary for mathematical modeling (Wagner, 1976), but such models make conceptualization of the system easier for most people.

The term "first-order kinetics" is one that has been borrowed from chemistry. It implies that the rate of a phenomenon such as the decay of a radioactive substance is proportional to the amount of material present. The implication of this relationship is that if there are 100 molecules of an isotope and 50 decay in a time period, during the next period of equivalent time, 25 molecules will decay and not the other 50. In the case where the rate does not depend on concentration, but only on time, as in the case of 50 molecules decaying per unit time, the relationship is called "zero-order kinetics.

When a plot of the numbers of molecules of a radioisotope is made with respect to time on a linear scale, a curve will be generated, as shown in Fig. 1a. The curve will have a steep slope initially but this slope will rapidly decrease. If, however, a logarithmic scale is used to plot the number of molecules with respect to a linear time scale, than a straight line will result, as shown in Fig. 1b. Obtaining a straight line under these conditions is a property of first-order kinetics.

When the concentration of certain drugs is plotted on a logarithmic scale versus a linear time scale, a straight line is obtained, suggesting that the kinetics of the drug approximates the kinetics of a first-order system. This situation can be described by a one-compartment model. Two assumptions must be made in order to use this model. The first assumption is that the drug is administered such that instantaneous and homogeneous distribution to body fluids and tissues occurs. This assumption is not meant to imply that body fluid and tissue levels are uniform in the physiological state. However, this model does assume that the fluid or tissue concentration being measured quantitatively reflects the concentrations of drug in the various body fluids and tissues. The second assumption is that the elimination pathways for the drug are all dependent on the concentration of the drug in the compartment.

The mathematics of a one-compartment model are relatively simple if one is familiar with differential equations. The differential equation of a first-order

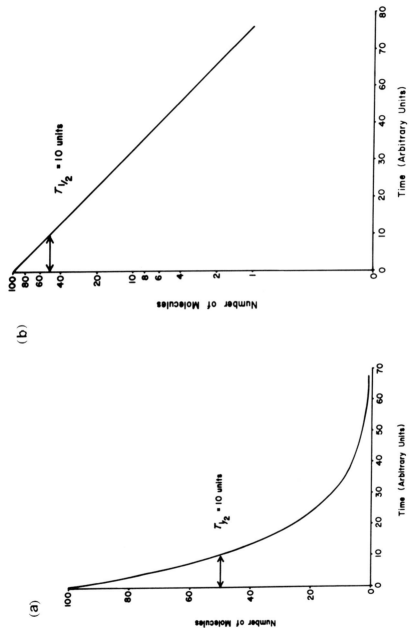

Fig. 1. Time course of the decay of 100 molecules of a radioisotope with a half-life ($T_{\frac{1}{2}}$) of 10 units as an example of first-order kinetics. (a) Linear scale. (b) Semilogarithmic scale.

reaction is $dC/dt = kC$, where C is the concentration of drug, t is time, and k is the first-order or proportionality constant. This equation states that the instantaneous rate of change of concentration dC/dt is directly proportional to the concentration C at time t. The minus sign gives the direction of the change, which in this case is for decreasing concentrations. When the differential equation is integrated, the relationship $C = C_0 \cdot e^{-kt}$ is obtained, where C_0 is the initial concentration at time 0. Logarithms to the base 10 are commonly used, so the expression is sometimes given as $C = C_0 10^{-k't}$ where $k' = k/2.303$. Note that if the logarithm of the equation $C = C_0 \cdot 10^{-k't}$ is taken, the expression log $C = C_0^{-k't}$ is obtained. This expression, when plotted on linear graph paper, will appear as a straight line.

The concentration at the initial time point t_0, i.e., the time when drug was instantaneously delivered to the system, is C_0, which is related to the amount of drug given (A_0), i.e., the dose, by the volume of the compartment, V_d, according to the expression $C_0 = A_0/V_d$. Since the dose is known and the initial concentration of drug is known, or can be found by extrapolating the log concentration versus time curve to the Y intercept at $t = 0$, the volume of the compartment can be readily calculated.

The time it takes to decrease the concentration to one-half is known as the half-life, $t_{\frac{1}{2}}$. A property of a first-order reaction is that no matter what concentration is taken as the reference, one-half that concentration will be present at a time interval equal to $t_{\frac{1}{2}}$. When the concentration is one-half the initial concentration, the equation for drug concentration then becomes

$$0.5C_0 = C_0 e^{-kt\frac{1}{2}} \quad \text{or} \quad e^{-kt\frac{1}{2}} = 0.5$$

When solved for the half-life,

$$t_{\frac{1}{2}} = \frac{\ln 2}{k} = \frac{0.693}{k}$$

Ordinarily, concentrations of drug obtained by sampling plasma at selected times are plotted on semilogarithmic paper with a log to the base 10 scale. The half-life of the drug is determined by inspection, and the Y intercept ($x = T_0$) is determined by extrapolation. The dose of the drug is known. The rate constant of elimination (k) can be calculated from the half-life, and the volume of distribution (V_d) calculated from the dose (A_0) and initial concentration (C_0).

Since data points determined experimentally are subject to various errors of measurement, a straight-line plot is rarely obtained. However, statistical methods such as linear regression analysis of the semilog plot, can give the line that "best fits" the data points (Gibaldi and Perrier, 1975).

Most of the antitumor drugs are given as an intravenous bolus, but some are given by intramuscular or subcutaneous injection and others by the oral route. Occasionally drugs are given as an intravenous infusion, and investigational protocols utilizing continuous administration of a drug over a period of days have been employed. Mathematical models have been derived that incorporate the effects of the route and method of administration. The rate of absorption from muscle, subcutaneous tissues, or the gastrointestinal tract is often proportional to the amount of drug present; that is, it is a first-order process (Koch-Weser, 1974). Absorption from muscle and subcutaneous tissues can usually be considered as complete. Absorption from the gastrointestinal tract may not be complete so another variable must be considered, namely, the fraction of drug absorbed. When absorption is taken into account, the shape of the concentration versus time curve on a linear scale shows an initial concentration of zero, then a rise to a peak concentration, followed by a decrease in concentration. When absorption is rapid, peak concentrations are high and are reached early compared to when absorption is slow. If absorption is not complete, then the peak concentration will be lower, but the time to peak concentration may not be affected. The effects of absorption on the concentration versus time curve are shown in Fig. 2. When the body is considered as a one-compartment model, then a plot of the logarithm of plasma concentration versus time yields a curve with a linear terminal portion. The half-life of decay of this portion of the curve is the same as that obtained by the intravenous administration of drug. The relative magnitudes of the absorption rate constant and the elimination rate constant of a system are important in determining the shape of the curve.

The area under the concentration–time curve (AUC) is an important pharmacokinetic parameter. It is directly proportional to the total amount of drug that reaches the central compartment. AUC is sometimes known as concentration times time (CXT) or drug exposure. For many drugs, response is proportional to CXT and not to peak concentration (Mellett, 1974). When drug absorption is complete, the area under the curve for a first-order process is the same as that for an instantaneous, bolus, intravenous injection. It is important to remember, however, that if a drug is absorbed too slowly, it may not achieve sufficient body levels to produce a desired response or a desired intensity of pharmacological response. The onset of response is also influenced by the rate of absorption (Gibaldi and Perrier, 1975).

The assumption that intramuscular, subcutaneous, and oral absorption is first order aids in pharmacokinetic modeling and in understanding the response of patients to drugs administered by these routes. Experimentally derived data may be hard to fit to such a model (Greenblatt and Koch-Weser, 1976). It has been demonstrated that intramuscular injection may lead to erratic and incomplete absorption (Gibaldi and Perrier, 1975). Drugs given orally can be metabolized to active agents. Measurements of only parent compounds in the blood may give the impression that the amount of drug available to the systematic circulation (bioavailability) is low and give the false impression that activity will be low. Another problem that arises is that absorption may be complete, but because the

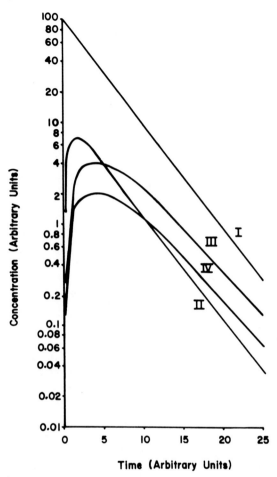

Fig. 2. Effect of route of administration and degree of absorption on plasma concentration curves if a one-compartment model is assumed. (The half-life of the drug is 3 units.) (I) Bolus, intravenous injection. (II) Intramuscular injection (assuming complete absorption by a first-order process with a half-life of 0.5 units). (III) Oral administration (assuming complete absorption by a first-order process with a half-life of 2.5 units). (IV) Oral administration (assuming only half the drug is absorbed by a first-order process with a half-life of 2.5 units).

intestinal venous system drains into the liver, a certain fraction of the dose absorbed may not reach the systematic sampling site because of metabolism within the liver. This process has been termed "first-pass" effect (Gibaldi *et al.*, 1971).

Intravenous infusion of drug into a patient is one of the methods of administration used for methotrexate, cytosine arabinoside, bleomycin, carmustine, cisplatin, and a variety of other drugs. Usually the drug is administered as a certain quantity over a given period of time, which means that the rate of delivery is constant and not concentration dependent as with first-order absorption. A constant infusion of a drug which confers one-compartment characteristics on the body will give concentrations with time that approach a constant level. At that level the rate of infusion equals the rate of elimination from the system. Once the infusion stops, the decay of concentration has the same terminal half-life as a bolus intravenous injection. After an infusion time equal to four times the biological half-life of the drug, the plasma concentration is within 10% of the plateau level. Seven times the drug half-life will bring the plasma concentration to within 1% of the plateau level. Changing the rate of the infusion will change the maximum concentration reached, but will not change the time necessary to reach maximum concentration. Since a drug with a long half-life will require long infusion times in order to reach the plateau level, loading doses are sometimes administered. A bolus intravenous injection is given in order to reach the plateau concentration immediately, and then an infusion is started to maintain that concentration. The loading dose required to attain the steady state can be found by multiplying the concentration at the steady state by the volume of distribution of the drug. The rate of infusion required to maintain the concentration is the loading dose times the elimination rate constant.

The one-compartment model represents the simplest case for pharmacokinetic modeling. Few drugs can be accurately described by this model. Multicompartment models are usually necessary. The body is considered to have a "central" and one or more "peripheral" compartments. The central compartment represents areas of the body where equilibration of drug throughout tissues and fluid is so rapid that the compartment appears homogeneous. The peripheral compartments are areas that take longer for a drug to reach and equilibrate. When a three-compartment model is considered, one peripheral compartment is sometimes called the "shallow" and the other the "deep" peripheral compartment. Deep compartments are considered to be made up of poorly perfused tissues that take a long time to reach equilibrum with the central compartment. Usually drug is administered into the central compartment and drug elimination is from the central compartment. Theoretically, drug may be eliminated from the peripheral compartments as well. Since normally only the central compartment, which includes plasma, is sampled and no direct information on peripheral compartments is obtained, there is usually not enough information to determine which compartment is responsible for drug elimination. Urinary excretion data are not helpful in solving this problem.

Multicompartment models may be quite complex. Some models, often referred to as the Dedrick–Bischoff type, use compartments to represent major organ systems (Bischoff and Dedrick, 1968). Drug transfer among compartments is dependent on blood flow and tissue permeability and affinity for the drug.

Tissue volumes are also necessary. The required parameters are determined in animals and then "scaled up" to human proportions.

The two-compartment model is often employed in discussions of the pharmacokinetics of anticancer drugs. Methotrexate (Huffman *et al.*, 1973), adriamycin (Benjamin *et al.*, 1973), bleomycin (Crooke *et al.*, 1977; Kramer *et al.*, 1978; Prestayko and Crooke, 1978), cisplatin (Patton *et al.*, 1978), and neocarzinostatin (Comis *et al.*, 1979) pharmacokinetics have been described by two-compartment systems, although methotrexate (Reich *et al.*, 1977), adriamycin (Benjamin *et al.*, 1977), and cisplatin (Manaka and Wolf, 1978) require at least three compartments to describe their pharmacokinetics adequately. Drugs that confer the characteristics of a two-compartment model on the body yield a biphasic concentration versus time curve on a semilogarthmic scale as shown in Fig. 3. After an intravenous bolus injection, drug concentration can be represented by the equation

$$C = Ae^{-\alpha t} + Be^{-\beta t}$$

where A, B, α, and β are constants. This equation is the sum of two exponential terms. Each term graphs as a straight line on semilogarithmic graph paper. The two components can be determined by graphic or mathematical techniques (Gibaldi and Perrier, 1975). When this is done the slopes of the two lines are α and β, respectively, and the Y intercepts are A and B, respectively. The initial

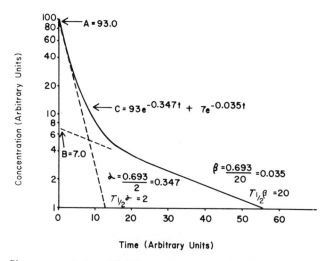

Fig. 3. Plasma concentrations (C) following intravenous administration of a drug that can be described by a two-compartment model. The equation of the curve is given. The graphs of the individual exponential terms are shown. A and B are in concentration units. α and β are in universe time units. Half-life of the distribution phase (α) is 2 units and of the elimination phase (β) is 20 units.

rapid fall in concentration is due to the "alpha" phase, which is the result of distribution of drug into the peripheral compartment. The terminal portion of the curve, the "beta" phase, is due to elimination of the drug from the system once distribution of the drug is complete and equilibrium is reached. The slopes of the curves are related to the half-life of the phases by the expression $t_{\frac{1}{2}}\alpha$ (or β) = 1n $2/\alpha$ (or β) = $0.693/\alpha$ (or β) as is the case with a one-compartment model. The concentrations represented by A and B, when summed, are equal to the concentration at $t = 0$. Since at this time, all the drug is in the central compartment, the apparent volume of the central compartment can be found. Several mathematical methods are available for calculating the apparent volume of the second compartment (Gibaldi and Perrier, 1975; Greenblatt and Koch-Weser, 1975).

Another important parameter is drug clearance, which is a direct index of the elimination of drug from the central compartment (Greenblatt and Koch-Weser, 1975; Dvorchik and Vesell, 1976; Rowland *et al.*, 1973). Clearance is dependent on the elimination constant (k_e). This constant reflects elimination by a variety of methods, including renal elimination, hepatic biotransformation, exhalation by the lungs, and fecal excretion. Clearance of a drug is inversely proportional to its elimination half-life and directly proportional to the total apparent volume of distribution.

Since there is a mathematical relationship among the constants of the concentrations equation of a two-compartment model and the rate constants of drug transfer into and out of compartments, one set of values can be calculated if the other set is known. Usually a curve is graphed and then the half-lives and Y intercepts of the two phases are found. This can be done by curve-stripping techniques where the effects of the elimination phase are subtracted from the concentration curve to find the curve due to distribution alone (Gibaldi and Perrier, 1975). From the half-lives of the α and β phases, the slopes (α and β) of the curves can be calculated. The rate constants for transfer of drug to and from the peripheral compartment and the elimination rate constant can be calculated. Clearance can be calculated using the expression clearance = volume of the central compartment $\times$ elimination rate constant. The units involved for these calculations are those of concentration for A and B and inverse time (time^{-1}) for α, β, and the rate constants. Clearance is expressed as milliliters per minute.

The calculations for one-compartment and two-compartment models for intravenous bolus injection can usually be done with the aid of a simple calculator. However, more complex models require more complex mathematics so programmable calculators and computers are utilized. Several computer programs have been developed to handle basic multicompartment models such as NONLIN (Pedersen, 1977) and CSTRIP (Sedman and Wagner, 1976), complex multicompartment models such as SAAM (Berman and Weiss, 1967), and complex anatomic–physiologic models such as the Dedrick–Bishoff type (Bischoff and Dedrick, 1968). These programs often allow for different methods of drug administration and for simulation of multiple dosing schedules. The ability to simulate multiple dosing schedules can be extremely useful in determining the significance of a drug concentration, since concentrations depend not only on dose and time but also on the previous number of courses of therapy, dosing interval, and whether a loading dose was delivered. Accurate knowledge of drug pharmacokinetics under the conditions of multiple dosing may be clinically helpful for drugs that have "therapeutic windows" where drug concentrations must be kept below a toxic level and above an effective level.

Drug transfer processes are usually considered to be first order with fixed-rate constants. However, some of these processes may be saturable at high concentrations of drug. Under these conditions the rate is not a constant and the term "nonlinear kinetics" is applied (Chau, 1976; Wagner, 1973a). Examples of saturable processes include carrier-mediated transport of a drug across membranes, net secretion of a drug by the kidneys, and enzymes involved in biotransformation. Other mechanisms that could cause nonlinear kinetics include uneven or changing blood flow to an organ system and an inhibitory effect of a metabolic product on an enzyme system. Drugs that classically exhibit nonlinear kinetics include ethanol and phenytoin (Wagner, 1973b). When large doses are given, the half-lives of these drugs are increased. The biotransformation processes are saturated so only a constant amount of drug can be metabolized during a time interval, which means the rate is fixed, or zero order. As the concentration decreases, the mechanisms are no longer saturated and the processes once again become dependent on concentration, or first order. The net effect is to increase the time it takes to eliminate the drug from the body. The mathematics involved in the treatment of nonlinear kinetics is complex and usually requires a computer to solve the various simultaneous differential equations.

An investigation into the pharmacokinetics of some drugs does not account for the pharmacological activity of these drugs. One reason may be that some drugs are metabolized to compounds that also have activity. The pharmacokinetics of the active metabolites must also be considered if accurate predictions of therapeutic response are to be made.

IV. CLINICAL CORRELATIONS OF PHARMACOKINETICS

The pharmacokinetics of a drug can be affected by the actions of other drugs so concomitant therapy must be considered a factor in pharmacokinetic analysis (Chabner and Oliverio, 1975). One drug can displace another from serum albumin, which can raise the concentration of free drug to toxic concentrations. Salicylates, for example, can displace methotrexate from serum proteins (Liegler et al., 1969). One drug can alter the metabolism of another. Microsomal enzyme induction is a classic cause of this alteration. Phenobarbital, for example, is a microsomal enzyme inducer that has been shown to increase the rate of disappearance of adriamycin from the plasma of mice and decrease its antitumor effect (Reich and Bachur, 1976).

Dysfunction of organ systems responsible for the clearance of drug leads to alterations in the clinical pharmacokinetics of drugs. Methotrexate is primarily eliminated by renal excretion and is in itself an agent that can cause renal damage. Administration of methotrexate may cause renal damage, which decreases drug clearance and so increase the plasma concentration of drug. Elevated concentrations can lead to severe myelosuppression, a life-threatening toxicity (Stoller *et al.*, 1977).

The clinical pharmacokinetics of antitumor drugs is further complicated by the fact that chemotherapeutic regimens often consist of several drugs given simultaneously or sequentially. Few of these combinations have been tested to see if the pharmacokinetics of any of the drugs is changed from those when the drugs are given as single agents. Some alterations can be predicted. Cisplatin and methotrexate, for example, are useful agents against tumors of the head and neck region. Cisplatin can be a significant toxin to the kidneys. If renal dysfunction occurs, the pharmacokinetics of methotrexate may be altered from those seen with normal renal function. Methotrexate concentrations may be elevated and drug clearance may be decreased. Some drug interactions may not have been predicted, but in retrospect have a logical basis. The combination of streptozotocin and adriamycin, for example, was tried as a chemotherapeutic regimen for adult sarcomas. Activity of the combination was no different than for adriamycin alone, but the toxicity of the combination was markedly increased (Chang and Wiernik, 1976). Plasma concentrations of adriamycin and metabolites were found to be elevated consistent with liver dysfunction when the drug combination was administered (Chang *et al.*, 1976). It thus appeared that the streptozotocin caused a liver abnormality that decreased the clearance of adriamycin with resultant increased toxicity.

Tumor type and the extent of disease can modify the pharmacokinetics of a drug. Vascular tumors may change blood flow patterns, resulting in a change in the kinetics of a drug from those usually seen. A liver studded with metastatic lesions causing liver dysfunction can markedly affect the kinetics of a drug like adriamycin, which requires liver enzymes for biotransformation and biliary excretion for elimination (Bachur *et al.*, 1977).

The study of pharmacokinetics of antineoplastic drugs leads to a rational approach to chemotherapy. The use of equations and mathematical models allows at least a semiquantitative way of comparing drug therpy (Wagner, 1975). Pharmacokinetic parameters and equations can summarize observed data. The equation of a concentration curve serves as a concise description of the shape of the curve. Pharmacokinetic analysis can increase our understanding of a process involved in the disposition or elimination of a drug from a patient. Studies on the effect of probenecid on methotrexate kinetics, for example, demonstrate that secretory mechanisms are important in eliminating drug from the body by the kidneys (Bourke *et al.*, 1975) and from the cerebrospinal fluid by the choroid plexus (Spector, 1976). Differences in the intensity and duration of biological effect of drug analogues may be explainable by differences in absorption, distribution, metabolism, or elimination. Dichloromethotrexate is an antifol with a shorter half-life and less activity than methotrexate. However, since dichloromethotrexate is excreted primarily by the biliary tract, the drug may find a role in patients with renal failure in whom methotrexate may be contraindicated (Bertino, 1975). Clinical pharmacokinetics can be used to make predictions for patient populations or for individual patients. The effect of changing the route or schedule of drug administration on blood levels can be predicted from an adequate mathematical model. Methotrexate concentrations in blood were predicted by an anatomic–physiologic model when curves were generated by computer to simulate intraperitoneal administration of the drug (Jones *et al.*, 1978). The effect of altered renal function on methotrexate concentrations was predicted by a multicompartment model using nonlinear kinetics to describe renal excretion (Reich *et al.*, 1977). Obtaining a prediction of an appropriate level of methotrexate in a patient with renal dysfunction is clinically helpful. A value above that which was predicted may mean further renal dysfunction and a greater chance of bone marrow toxicity.

One of the major goals of pharmacokinetic research is to relate biological activity quantitatively with pharmacokinetic parameters. Once this is done, the effect of modifying the factors that influence the parameter can be predicted. Because adriamycin, which is a phase-nonspecific compound, has terminal half-life of about 1 day, it could be predicted that a single dose schedule would be as effective as a schedule using daily dosing for 3 days to the same total dose (Benjamin *et al.*, 1974). However, cytosine arabinoside, a phase-specific compound, has a terminal half-life of only 2–3 hr. In order to maintain therapeutic levels, the drug would have to be given frequenctly and an intermittent schedule could be predicted to be suboptimal or even inactive. The drug is currently being given by continuous intravenous infusion to keep concentrations consistantly above the effective level for a period of days, and good clinical results against acute leukemia have been seen (Wiernik, 1978). The area under the concentration versus time curve (AUC) seems to correlate with activity for cell cycle nonspecific agents. Cyclophosphamide, for example, is activated by microsomal enzymes. However, therapeutic activity was shown to be about the same for mice treated with a microsomal enzyme inducer as for control mice. Although metabolism was more rapid in the induced animals, leading to higher peak levels of metabolites with alkylating activity, the AUC of active metabolites and biological activity were about the same for both sets of mice (Hart and Adamson, 1969).

V. DISCUSSION

The pharmacokinetics of antineoplastic drugs such as adriamycin (Chan *et al.*, 1978), methotrexate (Shen and Azarnoff, 1978), 5-fluorouracil (MacMillan *et al.*, 1978), mercaptopurine (Tterlikkis *et al.*, 1977), bleomycin (Crooke *et al.*, 1977; Kramer *et al.*, 1978; Prestayko and Crooke, 1978), cytosine arabinoside (Dedrick *et al.*, 1972), cyclophosphamide (Jao *et al.*, 1972), the nitrosoureas (Oliverio, 1973), and vinca alkaloids (Bender *et al.*, 1977) have been investigated by relatively sophisticated studies. These studies occasionally have led to modifications in treatment programs or served to give a pharmacokinetic rationale to empirically observed phenomenon. The term "enlightened empiricism" has been used to describe the state of the art. Yet attempts have been made to correlate biological activity with such interrelated factors as drug–target interactions, cytokinetics, and pharmacokinetics (Lincoln *et al.*, 1976). We are still a long way from applying pharmacokinetic models routinely to the clinical situation. However, we are beyond the point where pharmacokinetics is simply an esoteric exercise. Clinical pharmacokinetics is a practical discipline that must serve as a tool for the chemotherapist (Greenblatt and Koch-Weser, 1975).

REFERENCES

Bachur, N. R., Riggs, C. E., Jr., Green, M. R., Langone, J. J., Van Vunakis, H., and Levine, L. (1977). *Clin. Pharmacol. Ther.* **21**, 70–77.
Bender, R. A., Castle, M. C., Margileth, D. A., and Oliverio, V. T. (1977). *Clin. Pharmacol. Ther.* **22**, 430–438.
Benjamin, R. S., Riggs, C. E., Jr., and Bachur, N. R. (1973). *Clin. Pharmacol. Ther.* **14**, 592–600.
Benjamin, R. S., Wiernik, P. H., and Bachur, N. R. (1974). *Cancer (Philadelphia)* **33**, 19–27.
Benjamin, R. S., Riggs, C. E., Jr., and Bachur, N. R. (1977). *Cancer Res.* **37**, 1416–1420.
Berman, M., and Weiss, M. F. (1967). "User's Manual for SAAM," Publ. No. 1703. Public Health Serv., (A. C. Sartorelli and D. G. Johns, eds.), Bethesda, Maryland.
Bertino, J. R. (1975). *In* "Handbook of Experimental Pharmacology: Antineoplastic and Immunosuppressive Agents" (A. C. Sartorelli and D. G. Johns, eds.), Vol. 38, Part 2, pp. 468–483. Springer-Verlag, Berlin and New York.
Bischoff, K. B., and Dedrick, R. L. (1968). *J. Pharm. Sci.* **57**, 1346–1351.
Bourke, R. S., Chheda, G., Bremer, A., Watanabe, O., and Tower, D. B. (1975). *Cancer Res.* **35**, 110–115.
Carter, S. K. (1979). *In* "Cancer and Chemotherapy, Introduction to Neoplasia and Antineoplastic Chemotherapy" (S. T. Crooke, A. W. Prestayko, and S. Carter, eds.), Vol. 1, Academic Press, New York.
Chabner, B. A., and Oliverio, V. T. (1975). *In* "Handbook of Experimental Pharmacology: Antineoplastic and Immunosuppressive Agents" (A. C. Sartorelli and D. G. Johns, eds.), Vol. 38, Part 2, pp. 325–342. Springer-Verlag, Berlin and New York.
Chan, K. K., Cohen, J. L., Gross, J. F., Himmelstein, K. J., Bateman, J. R., Lee, Y. T., and Marlis, A. S. (1978). *Cancer Treat. Rep.* **62**, 1161–1171.
Chang, P., and Wiernik, P. H. (1976). *Clin. Pharmacol. Ther.* **20**, 605–610.

Chang, P., Riggs, C. E., Jr., Scheerer, M. T., Wiernik, P. H., and Bachur, N. R. (1976). *Clin. Pharmacol. Ther.* **20**, 611–616.

Chau, N. P. (1976). *J. Pharmacokinet. Biopharm.* **4**, 537–551.

Comis, R. L., Griffin, T. W., Raso, V., and Ginsberg, S. J. (1979). *Cancer Res.* **39**, 757–761.

Crooke, S. T., Comis, R. L., Einhorn, L. H., Strong, J. E., Broughton, A., and Prestayko, A. W. (1977). *Cancer Treat. Rep.* **61**, 1631–1636.

Dedrick, R. L., Forrester, D. D., and Ho, D. H. W. (1972). *Biochem. Pharmacol.* **21**, 1–16.

Dvorchik, B. H., and Vesell, E. S. (1976). *Clin. Chem.* **22**, 868–878.

Gibaldi, M., and Perrier, D. (1975). "Pharmacokinetics." Dekker, New York.

Gibaldi, M., Boyes, R. N., and Feldman, S. (1971). *J. Pharm. Sci.* **60**, 1338–1340.

Gold, H. (1952). *Am. J. Med.* **12**, 619–620.

Greenblatt, D. J., and Koch-Weser, J. (1975). *N. Engl. J. Med.* **293**, 702–705, 964–970.

Greenblatt, D. J., and Koch-Weser, J. (1976). *N. Engl. J. Med.* **295**, 542–546.

Hart, L. G., and Adamson, R. H. (1969). *Arch. Int. Pharmacodyn. Ther.* **180**, 391–401.

Huffman, D. H., Wan, S. H., Azarnoff, D. L., and Hoogstraten, B. (1973). *Clin. Pharmacol. Ther.* **14**, 572–579.

Jao, J. Y., Jusko, W. J., and Cohen, J. L. (1972). *Cancer Res.* **32**, 2761–2704.

Jones, R. B., Myers, C. E., Buarino, A. M., Dedrick, R. L., Hubbard, S. M., and DeVita, V. T. (1978). *Cancer Chemother. Pharmacol.* **1**, 161.

Koch-Weser, J. (1974). *N. Engl. J. Med.* **291**, 233–237, 503–506.

Kramer, W. G., Feldman, S., Broughton, A., Strong, J. E., Hall, S. W., and Holoye, P. Y. (1978). *J. Clin. Pharmacol.* **18**, 346–352.

Liegler, D. G., Henderson, E. S., Hahn, M. A., and Oliverio, V. T. (1969). *Clin. Pharmacol. Ther.* **10**, 849–857.

Lincoln, T., Morrison, P., Aroesty, J., and Carter, G. (1976). *Cancer Treat. Rep.* **60**, 1723–1739.

MacMillan, W. E., Wolberg, W. H., and Welling, P. G. (1978). *Cancer Res.* **38**, 3479–3482.

Manaka, R. C., and Wolf, W. (1978). *Chem.-Biol. Interact.* **22**, 353–358.

Mellett, L. B. (1974). *In* "Handbook of Experimental Pharmacology: Antineoplastic and Immunosuppressive Agents" (A. C. Sartorelli and D. G. Johns, eds.), Vol. 38, Part 2, pp. 330–340. Springer-Verlag, Berlin and New York.

Oliverio, V. T. (1973). *Cancer Chemother. Rep., Part 3* **4**, 13–20.

Patton, T. F., Himmelstein, K. J., Belt, R., Bannister, S. J., Sternson, L. A., and Repta, A. J. (1978). *Cancer Treat. Rep.* **62**, 1359–1362.

Pedersen, P. V. (1977). *J. Pharmacokinet. Biopharm.* **5**, 513–531.

Prestayko, A. W., and Crooke, S. T. (1978). *In* "Bleomycin: Current Status and New Developments." (S. K. Carter, S. T. Crooke, and H. Umezawa, eds.), pp. 117–130. Academic Press, New York.

Reich, S. D., and Bachur, N. R. (1976). *Cancer Res.* **36**, 3803–3806.

Reich, S. D., Bachur, N. R., Goebel, R. H., and Berman, M. (1977). *J. Pharmacokinet. Biopharm.* **5**, 421–433.

Rowland, M., Benet., L. Z., and Graham, G. G. (1973). *J. Pharmacokinet. Biopharm.* **1**, 123–137.

Sedman, A. J., and Wagner, J. G. (1976). *J. Pharm. Sci.* **65**, 1006–1010.

Shen, D. D., and Azarnoff, D. L. (1978). *Clin. Pharmacokinet.* **3**, 1–13.

Smith, W. M., and Melmon, K. L. (1972). *In* "Clinical Pharmacology" (K. L. Melmon and H F. Morrelli, eds.), pp. 3–20. Macmillan, New York.

Solomon, A. K. (1953). *Adv. Biol. Med. Phys.* **3**, 65–97.

Spector, R. (1976). *Cancer Treat. Rep.* **60**, 913–916.

Stoller, R. G., Hande, K. R., Jacobs, S. A., Rosenberg, S. A., and Chabner, B. A. (1977). *N. Engl. J. Med.* **297**, 630–634.

Tterlikkis, L., Ortega, E., Solomon, R., and Day, J. L. (1977). *J. Pharm. Sci.* **66**, 1454–1457.

Wagner, J. G. (1973a). *J. Pharmacokinet. Biopharm.* **1**, 103–121.
Wagner, J. G. (1973b). *J. Pharmacokinet. Biopharm.* **1**, 363–401.
Wagner, J. G. (1975). "Fundamentals of Clinical Pharmacokinetics," pp. 1–51. Drug Intell. Publ., Hamilton, Illinois.
Wagner, J. G. (1976). *Drug Intell. Clin. Pharm.* **10**, 179–180.
Wiernik, P. H. (1978). *Clin. Hematol.* **7**, 259–273.

20

CLINICAL PHARMACOLOGY OF BLEOMYCIN

Stanley T. Crooke

I. INTRODUCTION

The bleomycins are a family of glycopeptide antitumor antibiotics with clinical activity against squamous cell carcinomas of various sites, lymphomas, and testicular carcinomas (Crooke and Bradner, 1976). Until recently relatively little was understood about the clinical pharmacology of bleomycin. This was primarily due to limitations in the assays employed. Initial studies employed a microbiological assay that had limited sensitivity (Fujita, 1971; Ohnuma et al., 1974). Other studies employed bleomycin labeled with radioactive heavy metals, but these were limited by concern that the behavior of bleomycin may be modified by the chelation of metal ions.

More recently, two radioimmunoassays were developed that have greater sensitivity and specificity than the microbiological assay (Broughton and Strong, 1976; Elson et al., 1977). With the development of these assays, the determination of the clinical pharmacological characteristics of bleomycin evolved rapidly, and at present there is significant information relative to its absorption, distribu-

CANCER AND CHEMOTHERAPY, VOL. III

343

tion, and elimination in patients, but essentially no information concerning metabolism or potential metabolites.

II. Newer Clinical Pharmacological Assays for Bleomycin

The first radioimmunoassay developed for bleomycin employs ^{125}I-labeled bleomycin in which the ^{125}I is probably linked via the imidazole moiety (Broughton and Strong, 1976). Preliminary studies demonstrated that the radioimmunoassay did not cross-react with other antitumor agents, or other antibiotics. However, because the antiserum was induced with Blenoxane , the clinically employed material that is a mixture of 13 bleomycin analogues, the specificity of the assay was further characterized. To do this a competitive binding assay was employed in which the unlabeled analogues competed with ^{125}I-labeled Blenoxane for binding sites. Table I shows that different bleomycin analogues interacted to various degrees with the antiserum and that the antiserum is highly selective. Clearly, since neither tallysomycin nor bleomycinic acid cross-reacted, the bleomycinic acid portion of the molecule and a terminal amine structure are essential for interaction with the antiserum. However, the major components in Blenoxane, bleomycin A_2 and B_2, cross-react extensively, and thus the assay specificity is acceptable for clinical pharmacological studies (Strong et al., 1977).

Similar studies employing goat antiserum and ^{125}I-labeled Blenoxane and rabbit antiserum and [57]Co-labeled Blenoxane demonstrated modest differences in

TABLE I

Bleomycin Analogue Immunoreactivity with Rabbit Antisera[a,b]

Bleomycin	Mean concentration (pmole)	SD (pmole)	Cross-reactivity (%)
Sulfate	3.45	±0.11	100
A_2	2.99	±0.22	115.4
B_2	4.63	±0.17	74.5
A_5	29.50	±5.14	11.7
Iso-A_2	13.70	±0.29	25.2
Acid	> 1000.00	—	<1.0
Tallysomycin B	> 1000.00	—	< 1.0
Desamido A_2	8.26	0.51	44.6
B_1	214.2	15.9	1.6

[a] From Broughton et al., 1979.

[b] Indicated quantity of bleomycin analogue was required to produce a 50% inhibition of ^{125}I-labeled bleomycin sulfate bound to antibody. Results are expressed as the mean concentration, in picomols, of the bleomycin analogue determined in five separate analyses.

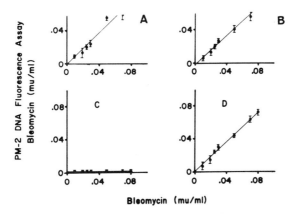

Fig. 1. Bleomycin concentrations in (A) buffer, (B) 5% TCA-treated buffer, (C) serum, and (D) 5% TCA-treated serum, as determined by the PM-2 DNA assay. Varying amounts of bleomycin were added to 1-ml samples of serum, buffer, or TCA-treated serum or buffer; then the bleomycin concentration was determined by the PM-2 DNA assay and the results compared to the amount of bleomycin added. The bars represent the standard deviations about the means.

specificities, but all assays appeared to have specificities acceptable for clinical use (Elson *et al.*, 1979). Furthermore, a radioimmunoassay for tallysomycin was developed that was shown to be non-cross-reactive with the bleomycins, further demonstrating the specificity of the technique (Broughton *et al.*, 1979). That the ^{125}I-labeled and [57]Co-labeled radioimmunoassays gave results comparable to the microbiological assays with the range of sensitivities of the microbiological assay was shown in two studies employing concomitant measurements by all three assays of serum and urine samples of patients receiving Blenoxane (Crooke *et al.*, 1977a,b; Elson *et al.*, 1979).

More recently, another assay has been developed. This assay is designed to be rapid and ultrasensitive and to measure bleomycin activity rather than immunochemical reactivity. It employs covalently closed circular phage PM2 DNA, which is degraded by active bleomycin. The degradation is measured by a decrease in the binding of a fluorescent dye, ethidium bromide. Figure 1 shows a comparison of the results obtained when human serum was assayed for bleomycin with the ^{125}I-RIA and the PM-2 DNA assay. Clearly, the assays gave comparable results (Galvan *et al.*, 1979). This assay may prove particularly useful since it measures "active" bleomycin and is highly sensitive and reproducible.

III. ABSORPTION

With two exceptions, bleomycin is rapidly and extensively absorbed from all sites studied. Although no direct oral pharmacokinetic studies have been reported, bleomycin has been shown to be active after oral administration to mice but to require very high doses (Crooke and Bradner, 1976). It is not absorbed to a significant extent after intravesical administration of doses as great as 120 units (Johnson *et al.,* 1976).

After intramuscular administration to dogs and humans, bleomycin has been shown to be rapidly and extensively absorbed (Prestayko and Crooke, 1978;

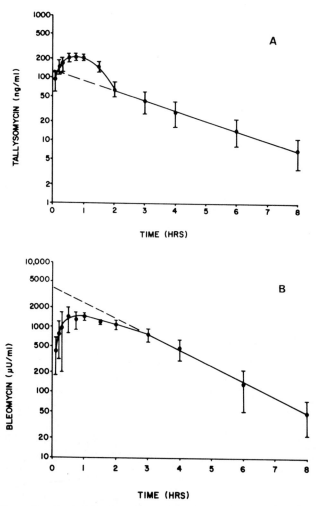

Fig. 2.   Plasma drug levels following intramuscular administration. Samples were collected at the indicated times, and the mean values for four dogs, plus standard deviations, are indicated. (A) Tallysomycin plasma concentrations in dogs administered 3 mg/m² intramuscularly. (B) Bleomycin plasma concentrations in dogs administered 18.5 units/m² intramuscularly.

Crooke *et al.*, 1977a,b; Strong *et al.*, 1979). Figure 2 shows the absorption and elimination from serum of bleomycin administered intramuscularly to dogs. Bleomycin was rapidly absorbed and was shown to be essentially 100% bioavailable in this study. Furthermore, its elimination after intramuscular administration was equivalent to that observed after intravenous administration (Strong *et al.*, 1979). Similar data have been obtained in human beings (Prestayko and Crooke, 1978).

Bleomycin is also rapidly absorbed after intrapleural or intraperitoneal administration. The estimated bioavailability in humans receiving intrapleural or intraperitoneal bleomycin at varying doses was approximately 50% (Alberts *et al.*, 1978). Absorption from subcutaneous sites is probably rapid and extensive, but direct studies have not been reported.

IV. DISTRIBUTION

Studies in mice and rabbits have shown bleomycin to be widely distributed. Tissues tending to accumulate the highest concentrations were skin and spleen, but levels in the kidney, lung, and heart were also high (Fujita, 1971). No significant bleomycin has been found in the brain or cerebrospinal fluid in mice (Fujita, 1971; V. Levin, personal communication). No data are available on the distribution of bleomycin in humans.

V. ELIMINATION

A. Intravenous Bolus Administration

To study the elimination of bleomycin and effects of variations in renal function on the pharmacokinetics of bleomycin after an intravenous bolus, a series of young men with testicular carcinomas was studied. This group of patients was selected because it was felt that they would be relatively homogeneous, and they would be treated with a single regimen, the Einhorn regimen (Table II), and thus potential variability resulting from drug–drug interactions would be reduced.

TABLE II

Treatment Regimen for Metastatic Testicular Cancer

Bleomycin	30 units/week for 12 weeks
Cis-Platinum	20 mg/m^2/day days 1–5 q 3 weeks for 9 weeks
Vinblastine	0.2 mg/kg/day × 2 q 3 weeks

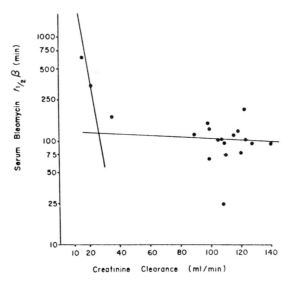

Fig. 3.   Semilogarithmic plot of plasma and serum $t_{\frac{1}{2}}\beta$ of bleomycin versus creatinine clearance from values determined using the radioimmunoassay.

From this and other studies a number of conclusions were derived. First, in all patients and at all levels of renal function studied, a two-compartment model best describes the human pharmacokinetics of bleomycin after an intravenous bolus. Second, the elimination of bleomycin is primarily dependent on renal excretion. Figure 3 shows a semilogarithmic graph of the serum elimination half-life versus the creatinine clearance of the men in this series as determined by the ^{125}I-radioimmunoassay. The elimination half-life was found to be approximately 120 min in patients with creatinine clearances in excess of 25–35 ml/min; the elimination half-life increased exponentially as the creatinine clearance decreased (Crooke *et al.*, 1977a,b).

At creatinine clearances of 50 ml/min or greater, approximately 50% of a dose of bleomycin was found in the urine four hr after dosing, and approximately 70% was recovered within 24 hr. Although bleomycin is not dialyzable, patients in frank renal failure and being treated with chronic hemodialysis had undetectable serum bleomycin concentrations within 48 hr of administration (Crooke *et al.*, 1977a,b). The volume of distribution was approximated 20 liters in all patients regardless of renal function.

B. Prolonged Intravenous Infusion Administration

The serum bleomycin concentrations of four patients who received prolonged intravenous infusions of bleomycin are shown in Fig. 4 (Broughton *et al.*, 1977).

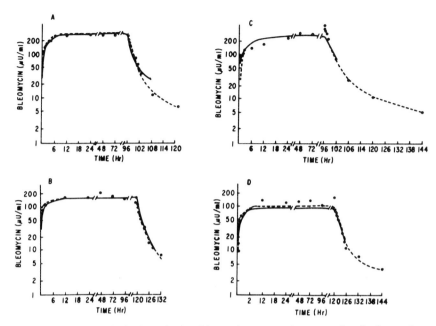

Fig. 4. Semilogarithmic plots of serum bleomycin concentration versus time for four patients receiving 15–30 units per day bleomycin as a continuous 4–5-day intravenous infusion. The experimental data are shown as (●), the curve predicted by the analysis of all the data as (-----), and that predicted by excluding data less than 10 μU/ml as (———). A through D represent patients 1–4, respectively. (From Broughton *et al.*, 1977).

Steady-state concentrations were reached approximately 12 hr after initiation of the infusion and ranged from 0.13 to 0.31 μU/ml. When values less than 10 μU/ml were excluded (the limit of reliability of the assay), the elimination half-life after discontinuation of the infusion was approximately 180 min, and approximately 63% of the administered dose was recovered in the urine. The effects of variations in renal function on the pharmacokinetics of prolonged infusions have not been reported.

C. Intramuscular Administration

As previously discussed, bleomycin is rapidly and extensively absorbed after intramuscular administration. Moreover, the elimination of bleomycin after intramuscular administration is similar to that observed after intravenous administration. The elimination half-life reported was approximately 150 min, and approximately 60% of the administered dose was recovered in the urine within 24 hr after administration (Prestayko and Crooke, 1978). The effects of variations in renal function have not been reported (Crooke, 1979).

VI. CONCLUSIONS

With the development of the radioimmunoassays and the PM-2 DNA fluorescence assay adequate technology now exists for the study of the clinical pharmacology of bleomycin. Clearly, the predominant method of clearance is renal excretion, and the serum elimination half-life is significantly increased in patients with compromised renal function. However, very little is known about the metabolism of bleomycin in human beings with varying renal function, and the impact on the efficacy and toxicity of bleomycin of changes in the clearance rate is not known at present. Future studies should better delineate these characteristics.

REFERENCES

Alberts, D., Chen, H.-S., Liu, R., Chen, J., Mayershorn, M., Perrier, D., Moon, T., Gross, J., Broughton, A., and Salmon, S. (1978). In "The Bleomycins—Current Status and New Developments" (S. K. Carter, H. Umezawa, and S. T. Crooke, eds.), pp. 131–142, Academic Press, New York.

Broughton, A., and Strong, J. E. (1976). Cancer Res. **35**, 1418–1421.

Broughton, A., Strong, J. E., Holoye, P. Y., and Bedrossian, C. (1977). Cancer (Philadelphia) **38**, 2772–2778.

Broughton, A., Strong, J. E., Crooke, S. T., Prestayko, A. W., and Knight, J. (1979). Cancer Treat. Rep. **63**:1829–1832.

Crooke, S. T. (1979). In Cancer Chemotherapy 1979, (H. M. Pinedo, ed) Ann. Cancer Chemother. **1**, pp. 74–93, Excerpta Medica. Amsterdam, 1979.

Crooke, S. T., and Bradner, W. T. (1976). J. Med. (Basel) **7**, 333–428.

Crooke, S. T., Comis, R. L., Einhorn, L. H., Strong, J. E., Broughton, A., and Prestayko, A. W. (1977a). Cancer Treat. Rep. **61**, 1631–1636.

Crooke, S. T., Luft, F. T., Broughton, A., Strong, J. E., Casson, K., and Einhorn, L. (1977b). Cancer (Philadelphia) **39**, 1430–1434.

Elson, H., Oken, M., and Shafer, R. (1977). J. Nucl. Med. **18**, 296–299.

Elson, H., Oken, M. M., Shafer, R. B., Broughton, A., Strong, J. E., Braun, C. T., and Crooke, S. T. (1978). Med. Pediatr. Oncol. **5**,213–218.

Fujita, H. (1971). Jpn. J. Clin. Oncol. **12**, 151–162.

Galvan, L., Strong, J. E., and Crooke, S. T. (1979). Cancer Res. **29**,3948–3951.

Johnson, D. E., Bracken, B., Prestayko, A. W., Brown, T. E., and Crooke, S. T. (1976). J. Am. Med. Assoc. **236**, 1353–1354.

Ohnuma, T., Holland, J. F., Masuda, H., Waligunda, J. A., and Goldberg, G. A. (1974). Cancer (Philadelphia) **33**, 1230–1238.

Prestayko A. W., and Crooke, S. T. (1978). In "The Bleomycins—Current Status and New Developments" (S. K. Carter, H. Umezawa, and S. T. Crooke, eds.), pp. 117–130. Academic Press, New York.

Strong, J. E., Broughton, A., and Crooke, S. T. (1977). Cancer Treat. Rep. **61**, 1509–1512.

Strong, J. E., Schurig, J. E., Issell, B. F., Kramer, W. G., Tavel, A. F., Florczyk, A. P., and Crooke, S. T. (1979). Cancer Treat. Rep. **63**,1821–1827.

21
CLINICAL PHARMACOLOGY OF CISPLATIN
Archie W. Prestayko

I. INTRODUCTION

The overall clinical utility of a drug is determined by its antitumor activity relative to its toxic effects on normal tissues. The therapeutic effectiveness of cisplatin is determined by its metabolism, distribution, and absorption into different tissues, clearance from the blood, and urinary excretion. Various methodologies applied to cisplatin pharmacological studies will be discussed in this chapter and information available on pharmacokinetics of cisplatin in laboratory animals and human cancer patients will be presented. Information on the antitumor activity, toxicity, and mechanism of action will be presented in other chapters in this volume.

II. CISPLATIN PHARMACOKINETICS

A. Laboratory Animals

1. Tissue Distribution

In studies on cisplatin labeled with radioactive platinum, the tumor-to-blood ratio of radioactivity varied from 1:3 to 2:0 in mice bearing sarcoma 180, 4-5

Copyright © 1981 by Academic Press, Inc.

days after injection of the drug (Lange *et al.*, 1972). In rats bearing the Walker 256 carcinosarcoma, the tumor-to-blood ratio was near unity (Wolf and Manaka, 1974). The organ distribution of radioactivity in tumor-bearing animals and control animals was similar. However, the rate of clearance of drug in tumor-bearing animals was significantly higher than that in control animals, suggesting that in tumor animals, the renal clearance mechanism has been altered (Wolf and Manaka, 1974).

In studies with radioactive cisplatin in dogs (Lange *et al.*, 1972; Litterst *et al.*, 1976, 1977; Wolf and Manaka, 1974, 1977) radioactivity was distributed in highest concentrations in kidney, liver, gonads, spleen, and adrenals at 1–2 hr after cisplatin injection but remained significantly elevated only in kidney, liver, ovary, and uterus for up to 6 days after treatment. Only trace amounts of radioactivity were detected in the brain. The tissue/plasma ratio of platinum was 3:1 and 4:1 for kidney and liver, respectively, at 4–6 days after drug administration.

Recently, it has been reported that following injection of [195m]platinum-labeled cisplatin into rats 66% of the radioactivity in the blood at 1 hr was associated with red blood cells. Of the radioactivity in the plasma, approximately 45% was bound to albumin and prealbumin at 1 hr after injection (Manaka and Wolf, 1978). The mechanism whereby cisplatin is released from red cells and from serum proteins and distributed to other cells or eliminated is currently under investigation.

The kidney and liver are the principal targets of localization of platinum compounds (Rosenberg, 1971). Studies on the subcellular distribution of radioactivity indicate that cisplatin is localized mainly in the cytosol as a low molecular weight complex, and to lesser degrees in nuclei, mitochondria, lysosomes, and microsomes (Leh and Wolf, 1976). Renal retention appears to involve irreversible binding of the platinum complex to renal cells.

2. Plasma Clearance and Urinary Excretion

After a single I.V. injection of cisplatin into dogs and rats (Litterst *et al.*, 1976, 1977) the plasma $t_\frac{1}{2}\alpha$ was less than 1 hr and the $t_\frac{1}{2}\beta$ was 4–5 days in dogs and 2 days in rats. Approximately 60–70% of the cisplatin administered was recovered in the urine within 4 hr after dosing as measured by urinary platinum content. Platinum could still be detected in plasma at 10–12 days after dosing.

The plasma $t_\frac{1}{2}\alpha$ of platinum in dogs receiving 12.5 g mannitol or intravenous hydration prior to cisplatin administration was approximately 30 min (Cvitkovic *et al.*, 1977). Blood and urine levels of platinum were not different from levels of platinum in dogs not receiving hydration and diuresis. Although the urine concentration of platinum was different in the three groups of dogs during the first few hours after cisplatin administration, the total amount of platinum excreted in the urine in 48 hr was similar for the three groups of animals, ranging from 76.5 to 100%.

Another study on the effect of diuretics on distribution and excretion of cisplatin in rats (De Simone *et al.*, 1979) has shown that mannitol increased the urinary excretion of cisplatin during the first 24-hr period but did not affect tissue or blood concentrations when compared to animals not receiving mannitol. Biliary excretion of cisplatin was also noted.

B. Humans

1. Distribution

After administration of radioactive [195m]Pt-cisplatin to patients, whole-body scanning was used to determine the organ distribution of radioactive platinum (Lange *et al.*, 1973; Smith and Taylor, 1974). After 3 hr radioactivity was concentrated in the kidneys and in the head regions, but the brain was relatively devoid of radioactivity. After 40 hr organs containing most of the radioactivity were the kidney, liver, and intestine.

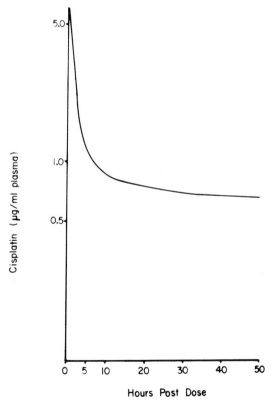

Fig. 1. Plasma concentration of platinum versus time after a rapid intravenous infusion of cisplatin as measured by atomic absorption spectrophotometry.

2. Plasma Clearance

In patients treated with radioactive cisplatin (De Conti *et al.*, 1973; Lange *et al.*, 1973; Smith and Taylor, 1974) levels of radioactivity decayed in a biphasic manner with a $t_{\frac{1}{2}}\alpha$ of 25–49 min and a $t_{\frac{1}{2}}\beta$ of 58–73 hr. During the excretion phase, greater than 90% of the radioactivity in the blood was protein bound. Urinary elimination of the drug was incomplete with only 25–45% of the radioactivity excreted in the first 5 days (De Conti *et al.*, 1973).

Atomic absorption spectrophotometry is currently employed to measure plasma and urine levels of platinum in patients treated with cisplatin. When plasma samples are analyzed for platinum at different times after a cisplatin dose, a typical plasma decay curve for platinum is obtained as shown in Fig. 1. Peak plasma levels of 1–10 μg/ml cisplatin are observed at early times after a therapeutic dose. After about 8 hr, the plasma levels of platinum decrease more slowly over the next several days. Approximately 40–50% of the administered dose can be accounted for in the urine at 5 days after a dose (Fig. 2). After this time the blood and urine levels of platinum are usually below detection and so it is difficult to quantitate accurately the total amount of cisplatin that is eliminated after a dose.

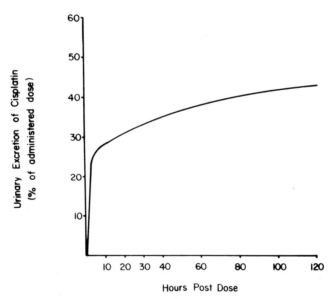

Fig. 2.   Cumulative urinary excretion of platinum versus time after a rapid intravenous infusion of cisplatin as measured by atomic absorption spectrophotometry.

3. Serum Protein Binding

Recently, a method has been described that measures plasma levels of platinum as "free" drug (filterable) and as protein-bound drug (nonfilterable) (Bannister et al., 1977, 1978). Further refinement of this method has made possible the measurement of plasma concentration of parent drug and other species (metabolites or breakdown products) by high-pressure liquid chromatography (Chang et al., 1978). The results of this and another study (Patton et al., 1978) indicated that plasma levels of filterable platinum-containing species after a bolus injection decline in an apparent biphasic mode with a $t_{\frac{1}{2}}\alpha$ of 32–53.5 min. Gormley et al. (1979), using a 1-hr intravenous infusion with saline hydration and mannitol and furosemide diuresis, showed that non-protein-bound platinum was rapidly and biphasically cleared from plasma with a $t_{\frac{1}{2}}\beta$ of 40–45 min and the $t_{\frac{1}{2}}\beta$ of plasma platinum concentration was 67 hr. The plasma $t_{\frac{1}{2}}\beta$ was the same as that obtained from patients who received no hydration or diuretics with cisplatin administration (De Conti et al., 1973). The $t_{\frac{1}{2}}\alpha$ of total plasma platinum observed in earlier studies (De Conti et al., 1973; Lange et al., 1973; Smith and Taylor, 1974) probably represents the plasma clearance of filterable platinum. Within 3 hr after administration of cisplatin, approximately 90% of the platinum in the plasma was protein bound and nonfilterable.

4. Continuous Infusion

The pharmacokinetic data described above were obtained in patients treated with rapid infusion of cisplatin. A recent study was conducted in which patients received a 24-hr continuous infusion of 80 mg/m^2 cisplatin (Jacobs et al., 1978). Peak plasma levels occurred at 24 hr and ranged from 1.03 to 1.90 μg/ml in nine patients with a mean of 1.39 μg/ml. Approximately 14% of the administered dose was excreted during 24 hr compared to a reported 18–30% following rapid infusion of drug. The toxicities of cisplatin were lessened by this long-term infusion without an apparent decrease in effectiveness as compared to other more rapid administration schedules.

5. Plasma Clearance versus Renal Function

Since the major route of excretion of cisplatin is via urine, a decrease in kidney function may change the rate and extent of excretion of cisplatin. Delayed clearance of cisplatin from plasma may cause more severe toxicity of the drug. Currently there are no well-controlled studies in which the relationship of plasma half-life and toxicity to degrees of renal dysfunction has been explored. A report of a patient in acute renal failure with a creatinine clearance <10 ml/min and being maintained by hemodialysis indicated that the $t_{\frac{1}{2}}\beta$ of cisplatin in this patient was approximately 10 days (Prestayko et al., 1979). Further studies are required to define the lowest creatinine clearance above which cisplatin is cleared from plasma at a normal rate.

III. CISPLATIN STABILITY

The reactivity of cisplatin is due to the dissociation of the chloride atoms from cisplatin and formation of charged aquated species (LeRoy 1979). Therefore the stability of cisplatin in solution is dependent on the presence of NaCl in the solution. A recent study by Mariani *et al.* (1980) has investigated the stability of cisplatin in various solutions. Cisplatin is stable for 72 hr at concentrations ranging from 50 to 1000 μg/ml at normal room temperature and light in solutions containing bacteriostatic water, 5% dextrose, and a minimum of 0.225% NaCl. Cisplatin is stable in 5% dextrose in water for only 8 hr.

Reaction with aluminum containing intravenous administration equipment has been reported (Bohart and Ogawa, 1980; Prestayko *et al.*, 1980). Contact of aluminum metal with a cisplatin solution causes platinum to precipitate out of solution lowering the potency of the drug.

IV. CONCLUSION

Since cisplatin is a relatively new antineoplastic drug introduced into cancer chemotherapy regimens, few studies on the clinical pharmacology have been carried out in cancer patients. However, much of the information obtained in animal studies appears to be applicable to the pharmacology of cisplatin in patients.

1. Cisplatin has a long $t_{\frac{1}{2}}\beta$ of 2–3 days that is apparently not affected by administration of hydration and diuretics.
2. Renal mechanisms are primarily involved in the excretion of cisplatin, although some elimination via biliary excretion may occur. Only about 50% of the administered dose of cisplatin can be accounted for in the urine.
3. Hydration and diuretics increase the initial rate of cisplatin excretion but do not appear to increase significantly the total amount of cisplatin excretion after a dose.
4. Cisplatin binds rapidly to serum proteins. Free cisplatin in plasma has a $t_{\frac{1}{2}}\beta$ of 0.5–1.0 hr.

REFERENCES

Bannister, S. J., Sternson, L. A., Repta, A. J., and James, G. W. (1977). *Clin. Chem.* **23,** 2258–2262.
Bannister, S. J., Chang, Y., Sternson, L. A., and Repta, A. J. (1978). *Clin. Chem.* **24,** 877–880.
Bohart, R. D., and Ogawa, G. (1980). *Cancer Treat. Rep.* **63,** 2117–2118.
Chang, Y., Sternson, L. A., and Repta, A. J. (1978). *Anal. Let.* **11,** 449–460.

Cvitkovic, E., Spaulding, J., Bethune, C. P., Martin, J., and Whitmore, W. (1977). *Cancer (Philadelphia)* **39**, 1357-1361.

De Conti, R. C., Toftness, B. R., Lange, R. C., and Creasey, W. (1973). *Cancer Res.* **33**, 1310-1315.

De Simone, P. A., Yancey, R. S., Conpal, J. J., Butts, J. D., and Hoeschele, J. D. (1979). *Cancer Treat. Rep.* **63**, 951-960.

Gormley, P. E., Bull, J. M., LeRoy, A. F., and Cysyk, R. (1979). *Clin. Pharmacol. Ther.* **25**, 351-357.

Jacobs, C., Bertino, J. R., Goffinet, D. R., Fee, W. E., and Goode, R. L. (1978). *Cancer (Philadelphia)* **42**, 2135-2140.

Lange, R. C., Spencer, R. P., and Harder, H. C. (1973). *J. Nucl. Med.* **13**, 328-330.

Lange, R. C., Spencer, R. P., and Harder, H. C. (1973). *J. Nucl. Med.* **13**, 191-195.

Leh, F., and Wolf, W. (1976). *J. Pharm. Sci.* **65**, 315-328.

LeRoy, A. F. (1979). *Cancer Treat. Rep.* **63**, 231-233.

Litterst, C. L., Gram, T. E., Dedrick, R. L., LeRoy, A. F., and Guarino, A. M. (1976). *Cancer Res.* **36**, 2340-2344.

Litterst, C. L., Torress, I. J., and Guarino, A. M. (1977). *J. Clin. Hematol. Oncol.* **7**, 169-179.

Manaka, R. C., and Wolf, W. (1978). *Chem.-Biol. Interact.* **22**, 353-358.

Mariani, E. P., Southard, B. J., Woolever, J. T., Erlich, R. H., and Granatek, A. P. (1980). *In* "Cisplatin: Current Status and New Developments" (A. Prestayko, S. Crooke, and S. Carter, eds.). Academic Press, New York. 305-316.

Patton, T. F., Himmelstein, K. J., Belt, R., Bannister, S. J., Sternson, L. A., and Repta, A. J. (1978). *Cancer Treat. Rep.* **62**, 1359-1362.

Prestayko, A. W., D'Aoust, J. C., Issell, B. F., and Crooke, S. T. (1979). *Cancer Treat. Rev.* **6**, 17-39.

Prestayko, A. W., Cadiz, M., and Crooke, S. T. (1979). *Cancer Treat. Rep.* **63**, 2118-2119.

Rosenberg, B. (1971). *Platinum Met. Rev.* **15**(2), 42-51.

Smith, P. H., and Taylor, D. M. (1974). *J. Nucl. Med.* **15**, 349-351.

Wolf, W., and Manaka, R. C. (1974). "Platinum Coordination Complexes in Cancer Chemotherapy," pp. 124-137. Springer-Verlag, Berlin and New York.

Wolf, W., and Manaka, R. C. (1977). *J. Clin. Hematol. Oncol.* **7**, 79-95.

22
METHOTREXATE: CLINICAL PHARMACOLOGY AND THERAPEUTIC APPLICATION
J. R. Bertino

I. INTRODUCTION

Methotrexate (MTX) continues to be a valuable drug for the treatment of human neoplastic disease. Attempts to increase its efficacy over the years since its introduction into the clinic in 1948 (Farber et $al.$, 1948) have involved evaluation of various dosage schedules, as well as its use in combination with other drugs (Bertino, 1979). Doses have escalated from 1–5 mg/m² per day to very high doses (1–20 gm/m²), followed by leucovorin (LV, N^{10}-formyltetrahydrofolate) "rescue" (Bertino, 1977). The use of MTX in these high doses has led to a reexamination of the clinical pharmacology of this drug in an attempt to prevent serious drug toxicity. This chapter will discuss the clinical

CANCER AND CHEMOTHERAPY, VOL. III

pharmacology and clinical application of MTX, with emphasis on high-dose regimens.*

II. PHARMACOLOGY

A. Mechanism of Action†

The biochemical event that leads to cell death following MTX administration appears to be powerful, and in certain circumstances (pH 6.0), "stoichiometric," inhibition of the enzyme dihydrofolate reductase (DHFR) (Werkheiser 1961; Bertino, 1963; Bertino et al., 1964). Inhibition of this enzyme activity leads to decreased tetrahydrofolate formation, and consequent inhibition of thymidylate and purine biosynthesis (Johns and Bertino, 1974; Chabner and Johns, 1977) (see Fig. 3, Bertino, Chapter 18, this volume). Therefore cells undergoing DNA synthesis during the S phase of the cell cycle are susceptible to MTX, and this drug acts primarily on cells undergoing rapid growth (Bruce et al., 1966; Hryniuk et al., 1969).

In leukemia cells, MTX appears to be transported by an active, carrier-mediated transport system, utilized by the naturally occurring folates, leucovorin (5-formyltetrahydrofolate, LV) and 5-methyltetrahydrofolate (Nahas et al., 1972; Goldman et al., 1968, 1971; Bender, 1975). Folic acid, which is poorly transported, apparently does not use this system (Nahas et al., 1972; Huennekens et al., 1978). MTX, therefore, also acts to compete with reduced folates for transport into cells. MTX also acts to facilitate efflux of reduced folates from cells, thus adding to the relative folate "starvation" caused by impairment of reduced folate transport. Thus MTX not only prevents reduced folate resynthesis by inhibiting DHFR, but also in high concentration inhibits influx of folates and stimulates efflux of reduced folates (Goldman, 1971).

B. Absorption

Methotrexate is a relatively polar, weak dicarboxylic acid (the pK_as of the glutamate carboxyl groups are 4.8 and 5.5) (Seegar et al., 1949; Liegler et al., 1969). In doses of up to 30 mg/m² the absorption is almost complete (Henderson et al., 1965; Huffman et al., 1973). Peak blood levels are reached in 1–2 hr when the patient is in the fasting state. As doses exceed 30 mg/m², proportionally less drug is absorbed (Henderson et al., 1965; Wan et al., 1974), and high-dose regimens are administered via the intravenous route. MTX can also be administered S.C., I.M., or I.P.; peak blood levels are rapidly achieved in 15–30 min.

---

*For other recent reviews, see Bertino (1977), Chabner and Johns (1977), and Bleyer (1978).

† For a more detailed description of the chemistry and mechanism of action of this drug see chapter 18, this volume.

The drug can also be administered intrathecally; in this circumstance the drug slowly leaks out of the cerebrospinal fluid (CSF) and plasma levels are maintained for two to three times longer than would be expected after intravenous administration (Jacobs *et al.*, 1975b). Thus there is more potential for systematic toxicity after intrathecal administration than after a given dose administered parenterally (Jacobs *et al.*, 1975b; Cadman *et al.*, 1976).

C. Plasma Disappearance and Distribution

After intravenous administration, plasma half-life values have been measured, and a triphasic curve has been described (Huffman *et al.*, 1973; Stoller *et al.*, 1975). The initial half-life lasts about 0.75 hr and reflects the distribution phase. Calculations of the volumes of distribution indicate that the drug is distributed initially in the extracellular space and then in total body water (Leme *et al.*, 1975; Henderson *et al.*, 1965). A second phase ($t_{\frac{1}{2}} = 2$–3 hr) can also be identified, which probably reflects the renal clearance of the drug (Isacoff *et al.*, 1976, 1977). A terminal phase can also be measured when plasma levels decrease below 10^{-7} M (24–48 hr after high-dose therapy) (Stoller *et al.*, 1975). This phase has a half-life of 10 hr and may be the result of enterohepatic circulation of the drug. Toxic effects of MTX may be the result of this prolonged third phase, since DNA synthesis in replicating tissues may be inhibited until plasma levels fall below 10^{-8} (Chabner and Young, 1973). Experiments in mice in which this terminal phase is eliminated by carboxypeptidase G_1, an MTX-degrading enzyme, have demonstrated that much of the toxicity of MTX is relieved (Chabner *et al.*, 1972).

Distribution of MTX into the CSF, peritoneal, and pleural cavities occurs slowly. In the presence of pleural or peritoneal effusions, these "third" spaces may act as reservoirs and prolong plasma MTX disappearance with an increase in systemic toxicity (Creavan *et al.*, 1973; Tattersall *et al.*, 1975). When large doses of MTX are used (>500 mg/m^2), high CSF levels are achieved ($>10^{-6}$ M) (Shapiro *et al.*, 1975; Tattersall *et al.*, 1975b). Presumably, these CSF levels are the result of the high plasma levels (10^{-3} M) and reflect a small amount of unchanged drug that penetrates this barrier.

Organ distribution of MTX appears to reflect the presence or absence of specific transport mechanisms, as well as the levels of DHFR present in the cells, and perhaps the amount of conversion to oligoglutamates (Whitehead *et al.*, 1975). The organs that contain the highest levels of MTX and retain it for the longer periods of time are the liver and kidney (Charache *et al.*, 1960; Anderson *et al.*, 1970). A study utilized ^{131}I-labeled aminopterin showed that these organs rapidly took up this folate analogue and retained it for long periods of time (Johns *et al.*, 1968). Until recently it was believed on the basis of displacement of tissue folates into the urine, and characterization of the inhibitor by chromatography and by enzyme inhibition, that the material bound in tissues was unchanged

MTX (Johns *et al.*, 1964). More recently, it has been clearly shown that MTX is present in liver and tumor tissues, at least in part, as oligoglutamates (Whitehead *et al.*, 1975; Jacobs *et al.*, 1975a). Since plasma contains conjugase activity, any oligoglutamates of MTX would be hydrolyzed and the monoglutamate of MTX excreted. The MTX (or oligoglutamates) remaining in these tissues after the plasma level decreases to 10^{-8} M or lower has been shown to be bound primarily or even exclusively to DHFR. In fact, Werkheiser (1961) and Bertino *et al.* (1965) have suggested that liver or blood cells, respectively, can be labeled in this manner, and measurement of the decay of the MTX concentration in these populations can be used to measure the life span of the cells.

Although the rat actively secretes MTX in the bile, biliary excretion is less prominent in humans, and about 1–6% of the drug is estimated to be lost by this route (Creavan *et al.*, 1973). The amount excreted in the bile may be proportional to the dose (Bleyer, 1978).

Approximately 50% of the plasma MTX concentration is weakly bound by plasma proteins, mainly albumin (Liegler *et al.*, 1969; Wan *et al.*, 1974). This binding can be competed for by drugs such as aspirin and sulfa, sulfonamides, and presumably reflects nonspecific binding by the *p*-aminobenzoyl-glutamate part of the molecule (Liegler *et al.*, 1969).

D. Metabolism

When small or conventional doses of MTX are administered to humans, relatively little metabolism of the drug occurs. After most of the drug is excreted in the first 24 hr, a small amount of drug and a metabolite, apparently a pteroate derivative (Johns *et al.*, 1964; Valerino *et al.*, 1972), is excreted in the urine each day for several weeks thereafter, presumably reflecting cell breakdown (Johns *et al.*, 1964). During the terminal phase of the plasma MTX disappearance, some 2,4-diamino-N^{10}-methylpteroic acid can be detected in plasma and the urine (Johns *et al.*, 1964; Y. Wang *et al.*, 1976). This metabolite presumably occurs as a result of metabolism of this drug by bowel bacteria that can hydrolyze the terminal glutamate from MTX (Valerino *et al.*, 1972). Recently, Jacobs *et al.* (1976) have detected an additional metabolite of MTX in the urine and plasma of patients receiving high doses of MTX, namely, 7-OH methotrexate. Large amounts of this metabolite (7–30% of total drug excreted) were found in the urine during the second 12 hr after MTX administration. These investigators postulated that hepatic aldehyde oxidase was responsible for this conversion, and that high MTX levels were necessary to saturate this enzyme in order for the 7-OH compound to be formed. Since the 7-OH compounds is a much less active inhibitor of DHFR, it clearly represents an inactivation of the drug. The role of this metabolite in the toxicity of MTX, especially the renal toxicity, is less clear. Jacobs *et al.*, (1976) have proposed that since this derivative is less soluble than MTX, it could contribute to the nephrotoxicity seen with high-dose therapy.

E. Excretion

MTX excretion is primarily renal, and for all but the smallest doses employed, greater than 90% of the drug is excreted within the first 24 hr after drug administration (Henderson et al., 1965; Pratt et al., 1975; Y. Wang et al., 1976). Two recent studies have indicated that with very large doses (50–200 mg/kg), less than 60% of the MTX could be recovered from the urine at 72 hr (Isacoff et al., 1978; Creaven et al., 1973). At the very low plasma concentrations, MTX may be reabsorbed by the kidney (Huffman et al., 1973), whereas at higher concentrations MTX clearance is greater than insulin clearance, indicating that there is active secretion by tubules as well as filtration (Liegler et al., 1969). A small percentage of an intravenously administered dose (1–2%) is found in the stool as unchanged drug and metabolites; most of the MTX excreted in the bile is reabsorbed. After oral administration, fecal elimination is proportional to dosage; for example, at 30 mg/m², 4–6% was excreted in the feces, and at a dose of 80 mg/m² 28.6% was eliminated by fecal excretion.

F. Drug Interactions

Other drugs may increase or decrease MTX toxicity or therapeutic effects. By displacing MTX from plasma proteins, salicylates and sulfa drugs may increase free MTX levels in plasma, thus making more drug available to tissues and for renal excretion (Liegler et al., 1969; Mandel, 1976). Weak organic acids, such as probenicid and salicylate, may diminish renal tubular transport (Liegler et al., 1969; Bourke et al., 1975). Antibiotics may interfere with the metabolism of the drug by bacterial flora and may decrease reabsorption (Cohen et al., 1976). Other drugs such as vincristine may increase the uptake of this drug by cells (Goldman and Fyfe, 1974), whereas other drugs such as cephalothin and hydrocortisone may decrease its uptake (Bender et al., 1975). In the L1210, but not the P388 mouse, lymphoma allopurinol decreased MTX therapeutic effects, presumably by increasing purines available for the salvage pathway (Grindly and Moran, 1975). It is not clear if allopurinol decreases MTX antitumor effects in patients.

III. CLINICAL APPLICATIONS

A. General Considerations—Guidelines for Use

MTX remains an important drug in the treatment of several human malignancies. MTX is available for both parenteral and oral administration. Use of very high doses (>1.0 gm/m²) is still considered experimental, and 0.5- and 1.0-gm lypholyzed vials for intravenous use without preservatives are only available for protocol studies through the NCI (Catane et al., 1978).

Current regimens in use involve (1) conventional low dosage (p.o. or I.V.) without leucovorin rescue, (2) moderate-dose intermittent regimens with or without LV, (3) high-dose regimens with LV, (4) intrathecal therapy (Table I). The high-dose regimens are administered as a bolus or over 4–6 hr, or by infusion over 20–42 hr (Bertino, 1977; Bleyer, 1978). In poorly perfused tumors or tumors that transport MTX poorly, the bolus approach may result in greater tumor uptake since high extracellular levels are maintained for a few hours; the infusion approach gives a desired blood level that is maintained for the duration of the infusion. Data are not available to choose between these modes of administration; if sufficient MTX is given by bolus to result in a desired 24 or 36 hr blood level, then the advantages of infusion therapy would seem to be minimal. An additional benefit of high-dose regimens is penetration into body cavities, such as the CSF, giving rise to cytocidal concentrations ($> 10^{-7} M$) (Shiparo et al., 1975; Abelson et al., 1979). Guidelines for the use of MTX, based on the experience of this center, as well as others, is given in Tables II and III. Experimental evidence would favor the use of a high MTX dose, e.g., 1–3 g/m^2 as a bolus or 18-hr infusion, to achieve plasma levels of $10^{-6} M$ or greater for 24 hr, then the use of minimal leucovorin rescue (Jacobs and Santicky, 1978). Extremely high doses of MTX (>3.0 g/m^2) may not provide much added benefit, although this point has not been established. Excess LV rescue could protect neoplastic cells from subsequent doses of MTX (Sirotnak et al., 1978; Capizzi et al., 1970; Hryniuk and Bertino, 1969).

MTX effects can also be "rescued" by asparaginase (Capizzi, 1975), thymidine (Tattersall et al., 1975a; Howell et al., 1977), or carboxypeptidase (Chabner et al., 1972; Abelson et al., 1979). The latter two methods are still in the early stages of clinical experimentation, but have some promise. The MTX–asparaginase combination appears to be synergistic in the treatment of human

TABLE I

Dose Schedules of MTX

	Dose	Route	Frequency	LV
I.	Conventional dose			
	a. 15–20 mg/m²	I.V. or p.o.	2 × week	−
	b. 30–50 mg/m²	I.V. or p.o.	Weekly	−
	c. 15 mg/m² × 5 days	I.V. or I.M.	q 2–3 weeks	−
II.	Moderate dose			
	a. 50–150 mg/m²	I.V. push	q 2–3 weeks	−
	b. 240 mg/m²	I.V. infusion (24 hr)	q 4–7 days	+
	c. 0.5–1.0 gm/m²	I.V. infusion (36–42 hr)	q 2–3 weeks	+
III.	High dose			
	a. 1–7.5 gm/m²	I.V. (1–6 hr)	q 1–3 weeks	+

TABLE II

Guidelines for High-Dose MTX Therapy with LV Rescue

1. A normal creatinine clearance should be required before therapy. A normal serum creatinine should be required before each additional course of therapy.
2. Alkalinize the urine before and during the MTX therapy with p.o. sodium bicarbonate (pH 7.0 or higher).
3. Push fluids to 3000 ml/m² day during MTX administration and 24 hr following.
4. Obtain a serum creatinine and plasma or serum MTX 24 hr after starting MTX.
   a. If serum creatinine is more than 50% above pretreatment levels, increase LV to 100 mg q 6 hr and continue until plasma MTX is less than $10^{-8}\ M$.
   b. Adjust LV rescue according to plasma MTX (Table III).

acute lymphatic leukemia as well as for experimental leukemia (Capizzi, 1975). Since asparaginase partly protects patients from MTX toxicity when administered 24 hr later, this technique has allowed relatively large doses of MTX (600–800 mg/m²) to be administered safely at q 9–10 day intervals.

After an intrathecal injection, most patients clear MTX from their CSF within 7 days of injection, and neurotoxicity is rare if drug administration is at 7 or more day intervals (Bleyer, 1978). If MTX is given more frequently, monitoring of spinal fluid levels with appropriate dose modification can reduce the frequency of neurotoxicity (Bleyer et al., 1973a). Guidelines for CSF levels of MTX in patients treated with intrathecal MTX are given in Fig. 1 and may be used to estimate subsequent dose modifications (Bleyer, 1977). Bleyer (1978) has also pointed out that the 12 mg/m² conventional dose (maximum 15 mg total dose) was not adequate to prevent meningeal leukemia in children less than 3 years of age and that body surface measurements do not correlate well with CSF levels of MTX obtained after the 12 mg/m² dose. Table IV indicates the dosage schedule he suggests for intrathecal MTX; note that all patients over the age of 3 receive 12 mg (total) of MTX, irrespective of body surface area.

TABLE III

Leucovorin Rescue Schedules Following High-Dose MTX[a]

Plasma level at 24–30 hrs[b]	LV dose	Duration
$<1.5 \times 10^{-6}\ M$	10–15 mg/m² q 6 h	48 hr
1.5–$5.0 \times 10^{-6}\ M$	30 mg/m² q 6 h	Until plasma level $<5 \times 10^{-8}\ M$
$>5.0 \times 10^{-6}\ M$	60–100 mg/m² q 6 h	Until plasma level $<5 \times 10^{-8}\ M$

[a] Modified from Jacobs and Santicky (1978).

[b] After I.V. bolus or 18-hr infusion therapy (2.5 gm/m²).

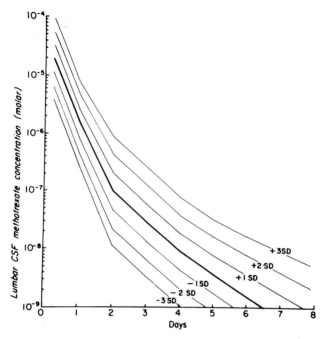

Fig. 1.   Spinal fluid levels after intrathecal MTX administration. Dosage should be adjusted to bring the lumbar CSF MTX concentration between ±1 standard deviation (SD). (After Bleyer, 1977.)

B. Indications

During the past decade the use of high doses of MTX with LV has been evaluated in a variety of human neoplasms. Unfortunately, few comparative trials have been reported comparing results of "conventional" doses of MTX with high-dose leucovorin regimens. The advantages of conventional-dose regimens (see Table I) are relatively low cost and ease of administration. The advantages of high-dose MTX with LV rescue are relatively low toxicity (with

TABLE IV

Guidelines for Intrathecal Therapy

Age (yr)	Total MTX dose (mg)
<1	6
1	8
2	10
≥3	12

TABLE V

Clinical Uses of Methotrexate

A. Diseases in which MTX has established effectiveness
    1. Acute lymphocytic leukemia
    2. Choriocarcinoma
    3. Breast cancer
    4. Oat cell carcinoma
    5. Osteogenic sarcoma
    6. Head and neck cancer
    7. Mycosis fungoides
B. Diseases in which MTX has limited effectiveness
    1. Acute myelocytic leukemia
    2. Burkitt's lymphoma
    3. Diffuse lymphoma
    4. Non-oat cell lung cancer
    5. Soft tissue sarcoma
    6. Gastrointestinal cancer
    7. Melanoma
    8. Ovarian and cervical cancer

---

appropriate monitoring), high levels of drug in the CSF, and, in some circumstances, improved antitumor effects. High-dose regimens with LV can also be incorporated into combination programs with relative safety. MTX plays an essential role in the treatment of several human malignancies (Table V,A). In other tumors MTX does not have major activity as a single agent, but its role in combinations is still under investigation (Table V,B).

C. Toxicity

1. General Considerations

From the previous sections it should be clear that toxicity to normal tissues occurs when cytocidal blood levels are maintained for sufficiently long periods of time. Thus both the plasma concentration of MTX achieved as well as the duration of the respective level are important in predicting toxicity; however, as with other antimetabolites, the toxicity is some *log* function of the extracellular concentration times the duration that this concentration is maintained (Stoller *et al.*, 1975). Thus very large doses of MTX of short duration are well tolerated (Goldie *et al.*, 1972). Moderate doses, if prolonged, may be lethal (Liegler *et al.*, 1969; Chabner and Young, 1973). For example, if plasma concentrations of 10^{-6} M or higher are maintained for greater than 48 hr, irreversible toxicity may occur, presumably because of recruitment of normal marrow and gastrointestinal stem cells into "cycle," thus making them vulnerable to MTX, as S-phase inhibitor. If toxicity is noted, then "rescue" with LV should be maintained until blood levels of MTX decrease to below 10^{-8} M, a level at which DNA synthesis in normal marrow and intestinal mucosa cells resumes (Chabner and Young, 1973). Furthermore, since the relationship between LV and MTX, as regards toxicity, is a competitive one, the higher the blood level of MTX, the higher the LV dose needed for "rescue" (Jacobs and Santicky, 1978; Pinedo et al., 1977). This dose of LV of necessity has been largely empirical, since a practical technique for measuring blood levels of this folate, or its conversion product 5-methyltetrahydrofolate has only just become available (Mehta et al., 1978). These therapeutic recommendations are summarized in Tables II and III.

2. Marrow Toxicity

The limiting toxicities of MTX involve the marrow and the gastrointestinal tract (Hansen et al., 1971). As alluded to earlier, MTX is tolerated well in most dose schedules employed since the stem cell compartment is relatively unaffected by this S-phase inhibitor. As the differentiating compartment is decimated by MTX, however, the stem cell compartment becomes committed, and as a result more vulnerable, if MTX extracellular concentrations are prolonged. It follows that a given dose of MTX would be more toxic in circumstances in which the stem cell compartment of the marrow is already "turned on," i.e., by previous X ray, drug administration, infection, or tumor invasion (Bruce et al., 1966). It follows also that repeated MTX administration in circumstances where the gastrointestinal mucosa and marrow have not completely recovered from the previous administration would be more hazardous. Marrow toxicity may be conveniently measured by the decrease in the granulocyte count, expressed on a logarithmic scale (Bertino and Hryniuk, 1978). Since granulocyte levels reflect events occurring in the marrow 5–7 days earlier, assays of CFU's in marrow would be of greater value, but from the practical sense, the granulocyte count suffices (Bertino and Hryniuk, 1978). Usually a greater than 1.0 log fall of granulocytes to levels below 500 per mm³ carries with it the potential of infection. After a single large dose of MTX (1–5 mg/kg), the nadir is reached in about 10 days, and in 3 weeks from the dose, recovery of the marrow function to normal usually has occurred (Condit et al., 1962; Hansen et al., 1971). Anemia and thrombocytopoenia may also occur after MTX administration, either alone or together with leukopoenia, but these toxicities are usually less in magnitude than the granulocytopoenia (Hansen et al., 1971) and can be more easily handled by appropriate replacement therapy.

3. Gastrointestinal Toxicity

Gastrointestinal toxicity is usually manifested first by oral mucosal lesions, which range from minimal erythema of the buccal mucosa and lower lip to severe ulceration of the oral mucosa and may involve the nasal epithelium (Capizzi et *al.*, 1970). Mucositis may be observed 2–7 days after MTX adminstration and is usually a function of both the drug dose and the duration of the drug administration. It is usually necessary to stop therapy when mucositis occurs and allow for complete healing before the next dose of MTX is administered. Nausea and anorexia, and less commonly, vomiting, may be noted during or after MTX administration, usually with large doses. Diarrhea is also occasionally seen. With toxic doses of MTX, more severe gastrointestinal ulceration and bleeding may be produced.

4. Skin Toxicity

Skin toxicity to MTX occurs in 10–15% of patients and characteristically involves the neck and upper trunk. It can be pruritic and relatively insignificant and unrelated to other signs of systemic MTX toxicity; in other instances it can be related in general to severe MTX toxicity and can progress to severe bullous formation and desquamation (Condit *et al.*, 1962; Jaffe and Traggis, 1975; Lanzkowsky *et al.*, 1976).

5. Hair Loss

Hair loss after MTX administration is uncommon, occurring primarily in older individuals.

6. Renal Toxicity

Renal toxicity is relatively uncommon with conventional doses of MTX, although Condit has described several patients who developed renal failure on conventional doses of this drug (Condit *et al.*, 1969). When this occurs and is not recognized in time, the results are usually disastrous, since the renal failure results in impaired excretion of the drug and consequently prolonged high plasma concentrations. With large doses of the drug renal failure was a major problem leading to several reported deaths (Penta, 1975); if patients are screened carefully using creatinine clearance measurements and are alkalinized and hydrated, this complication may be largely obviated (Pitman *et al.*, 1975; Pitman and Frei, 1976; Isacoff *et al.*, 1977). It would appear therefore that renal toxicity secondary to MTX may be due to either a direct tubular effect, sometimes not a consequence of dose, or, more commonly, secondary to high-dose therapy and precipitation of the drug in the tubules. In both circumstances the renal effects are usually reversible, but unless appropriate action is taken to improve elimination of the drug and to antidote the effects of high concentrations of MTX that result, patients will succumb to the consequences of hematologic and gastrointestinal toxicity. A major problem exists when patients develop renal failure after high-dose MTX. Dialysis, either alone or with charcoal, has not been useful because of the large tissue stores, which then replenish the plasma when dialysis stops (Djerassi *et al.*, 1977); in addition MTX does not dialyze well. (Howell *et al.*,

1978). Carboxypeptidase G_1 has been used with success in lowering MTX levels (Bertino *et al.*, 1974; Howell *et al.*, 1978), but the product of this enzymic inactivation of MTX is 2,4-diamino-N^{10}-methylpteroic acid, even less soluble than MTX in urine. In some circumstances weeks of LV therapy are necessary with close monitoring of blood levels (Bertino, 1977).

7. Hepatic Toxicity

Acute hepatic toxicity is usually not a problem with either conventional or high-dose regimens. When liver function is monitored carefully, transient elevation in SGOT levels is noted, but these usually return to normal. However, patients with impaired liver function should be treated with lower doses of MTX or not at all; enhanced toxicity of this drug may be observed in these circumstances, despite the fact that this drug is excreted primarily unchanged by the kidney and the liver presumably plays only a minor role in drug inactivation. Hepatic fibrosis and cirrhosis have been reported following chronic administration of MTX (Weinstein *et al.*, 1973). Predisposing factors in patients developing this complication have been frequent daily low-dose administration (greater than 12 days/month) (Podurgiel *et al.*, 1973) and in psoriatic patients, associated alcoholism (Roenigk *et al.*, 1971). Intermittent therapy with high doses (80 mg/m² every 2 weeks) did not produce histologic evidence of liver disease, even after 1½ to 2½ years of treatment (McIntosh *et al.*, 1977), nor did weekly treatment using 3–10 mg/m² per week (Mackenzie, 1975).

8. Teratogenic and Mutagenic Effects

MTX is known to be a potent abortifacient, especially if administered during the first trimester of pregnancy (Thiersch, 1962). Thus far there is no evidence that MTX has mutagenic or carcinogenic activity in man (Bailin *et al.*, 1975). Women successfully treated with MTX for choriocarcinoma have not had a high evidence of fetal abnormalities following cessation of therapy nor have they had a higher incidence of secondary malignancies.

9. Neurotoxicity

Neurotoxicity due to MTX can occur both after intrathecal MTX and with systemic administration of large doses (>80 mg/m²).

An acute syndrome has been described following intrathecal administration. This consists of headache, fever, meningismus, and a pleocytosis that may mimic bacterial infection. This syndrome is the most common of the neurologic syndromes associated with intrathecal MTX and appears to be related to high CSF concentration of MTX (Mott *et al.*, 1972; Bleyer *et al.*, 1973b).

A subacute form of CNS toxicity has also been described following intrathecal use; in this circumstance more severe signs of motor dysfunction of the brain are noted: paraplegia, cerebellar dysfunction, cranial nerve palsies and seizures, usually following two or more doses of drug per week (Gagliano and Costanzi, 1976; Weiss *et al.*, 1974). This complication has been correlated with persistently elevated levels of MTX in the CSF (Bleyer, 1977).

In addition to the neurotoxicity reported above after intrathecal MTX, patients receiving high-dose MTX (>50 mg/m^2) parenterally after radiation therapy to the brain (>2000 R) have developed a necrotizing leukoencephalopathy associated with progressive neurologic deterioration (Bresnan *et al.*, 1972; Hendin *et al.*, 1974; Kay *et al.*, 1972; Norrell *et al.*, 1974; Rubenstein *et al.*, 1975; Price and Jamieson, 1975; Shapiro *et al.*, 1973; Smith, 1975; Aur *et al.*, 1976). This may begin insidiously and progress to severe neurologic impairment (dementia, ataxia, seizures, and coma). Bleyer has pointed out that in the 58 cases reported thus far, most of the reported cases were treated with a combination of either systemic or intrathecal MTX (or both) with cranial irradiation (Bleyer, 1977).

10. Miscellaneous Toxicity

Interstitial pneumonitis (Gutin *et al.*, 1976; Sostman *et al.*, 1976; Clarysse *et al.*, 1969) and osteoporosis (Nesbit *et al.*, 1976) have been reported with chronic low-dose administration. Fever (Gottlieb and Serpick, 1970), seizures, recall of radiation of radiation toxicity (Jaffe and Traggis, 1975; Pitman *et al.*, 1975) phototoxicity (Coder *et al.*, 1975), and anaphalactoid reactions (Goldberg *et al.*, 1978) have been reported with high-dose administration. Pleuritic and left upper quadrant pain presumably due to splenic capsule inflammation have also been reported with a moderately high-dose regimen (Hryniuk and Bertino, 1969).

IV. DISCUSSION

This review should serve to illustrate that a large body of information exists on the mechanism of action, pharmacology, and clinical use of MTX. Despite this knowledge, many unanswered questions remain. The value of high-dose MTX as a single agent has not been proved, except possibly for acute lymphocytic leukemia (ALL), diffuse lymphomas, osteogenic sarcoma, and head and neck cancer.

Administration of high-dose MTX in combination with other drugs is now being explored. Use of these regimens either as prophylaxis for meningeal disease (J. O. Wang *et al.*, 1976) or the treatment of CNS disease (Rosen *et al.*, 1977; Abelson *et al.*, 1979) is now also being evaluated. It is probable that the major value of this treatment will be for these purposes.

The limiting factor to successful use of MTX as well as other chemotherapeutic agents is drug resistance, either natural or acquired. Based on data from experimental tumors (Alt *et al.*, 1978) strategies to prevent this resistance that involve combinations of drugs or modalities have been suggested (Bertino,

1979). Possibilities may exist to exploit drug resistance therapeutically (Skipper *et al.*, 1978; Bertino, 1979). The next decade should see the development of more effective drug combinations using MTX as well as the introduction of new folate antagonists with more selectivity into the clinic.

REFERENCES

Abelson, H., Ensminger, W., Rosawsky, A., and Uren, J. (1979). *Chem. Biol. Pteridines, Int. Pteridine Symp.,* **4,** 629–633.

Alt, F. W., Kellems, R. E., Bertino, J. R., and Schimke, R. T. (1978). *J. Biol. Chem.* **253,** 1357–1370.

Anderson, L. L., Collins, G. J., Ojima, Y., and Sullivan, R. D. (1970). *Cancer Res.* **30,** 1344–1348.

Aur, R., Hustu, P., and Simone, J. (1976) *Proc. Am. Assoc. Cancer Res.* **17,** 97.

Bailin, P. L., Tindall, J. P., Roenigk, H. H., and Hogan, M. D. (1975). *J. Am. Med. Assoc.* **232,** 359–362.

Bender, R. A. (1975). *Cancer Chemother. Rep. Part 3* **6,** 73–82.

Bender, R. A., Bleyer, W. A., Frisby, S. A., and Oliverio, V. T. (1975). *Cancer Res.* **35,** 1305–1308.

Bertino, J. R. (1963). *Cancer Res.* **23,** 1286–1306.

Bertino, J. R. (1977). *Semin. Oncol.* **4,** 203–216.

Bertino, J. R. (1979). *Cancer Res.* **39,** 293–304.

Bertino, J. R., and Hryniuk, W. M. (1978). *In* "Clinical Pharmacology: Basic Principles in Therapeutics" (K. L. Melmon and H. F. Morelli, eds.), pp. 802–841. Macmillan, New York.

Bertino, J. R., Booth, B. A., Bieber, A. L., Cashmore, A., and Sartorelli, A. C. (1964). *J. Biol. Chem.* **239,** 479–485.

Bertino, J. R., Johns, D. G., Almquist, P., Hollingsworth, J. N., and Evans, E. A. (1965). *Nature (London)* **206,** 1052–1053.

Bertino, J. R., Skeel, R. T., Makulu, D., McIntosh, S., Uhoch, J., and Chabner, B. (1974). *Clin. Res.* **22,** 483A.

Bleyer, W. A. (1977). *Cancer Treat. Rep.* **61,** 1419–1425.

Bleyer, W. A. (1978). *Cancer (Philadelphia)* **41,** 36–51.

Bleyer, W. A., Chabner, B. A., and Ommaya, A. K. (1973a). *Annu. Meet. Am. Soc. Hematol., 16th* p. 76.

Bleyer, W. A., Drake, J. C., and Chabner, B. A. (1973b). *N. Engl. J. Med.* **289,** 770–773.

Bourke, R. S., Chheda, G., Bremer, A., Watanabe, O., and Tower, D. B. (1975). *Cancer Res.* **35,** 110–116.

Bresnan, M. J., Gilles, F. H., Lorenzo, A. V., Waters, G. V., and Barlow, C. F. (1972). *Trans. Am. Neurol. Assoc.* **97,** 204–206.

Bruce, W. R., Meeker, B. E., and Valeriote, F. A. (1966). *J. Natl. Cancer Inst.* **37,** 233–245.

Cadman, E. C., Lundberg, W. B., and Bertino, J. R. (1976). *Arch. Intern. Med.* **136,** 1321–1322.

Capizzi, R. L. (1975). *Cancer Chemother. Rep., Part 3* **6,** 37–41.

Capizzi, R. L., DeConti, R. C., Marsh, J. C., and Bertino, J. R., (1970). *Cancer Res.* **30,** 1782–1788.

Catane, R., Bono, V. H., Jr., Louie, A. C., and Muggia, F. M. (1978). *Cancer Treat. Rep.* **62,** 178–180.

Chabner, B. A., and Johns, D. G. (1977). *In* "Cancer—A Comprehensive Treatise" (F. Becker, ed.), Vol. 5, pp. 363–377. Plenum, New York.

Chabner, B., and Young, R. (1973). *J. Clin. Invest.* **52,** 1804–1811.

Chabner, B. A., Johns, G., and Bertino, J. R. (1972). *Nature (London)* **239**, 395–397.

Charache, S., Condit, P. T., and Humphries, S. R. (1960). *Cancer (Philadelphia)* **13**, 236–240.

Clarysse, A. M., Cathey, W. J., Cartwright, G. E., and Wintrobe, M. N. (1969). *J. Am. Med. Assoc.* **209**, 1861–1864.

Coder, M., Howely, L. F., and Stone, W. H. (1975). *Oncology* **32**, 275–282.

Cohen, M. H., Creaven, P. J., Fossiede, B. F., Johnston, A. V., and Williams, C. L. (1976). *Cancer (Philadelphia)* **38**, 1556–1559.

Condit, P. T., Schneider, B. I., and Owens, A. H., Jr. (1962). *Cancer Res.* **22**, 706–712.

Condit, P. T., Chanes, R. E., and Joel, W. (1969). *Cancer (Philadelphia)* **23**, 126–131.

Creaven, P. J., Hansen, H. H., Alford, D. A., and Allen, L. M. (1973). *Br. J. Cancer* **28**, 589–591.

Djerassi, I., Ciesielka, W., and Kim, J. S. (1977). *Cancer Treat. Rep.* **61**, 751–752.

Farber, S. L. H., Diamond, R. D., Mercer, R. F., Sylverster, J. R., and Wolff, J. O. (1948). *N. Engl. J. Med.* **238**, 787–793.

Gagliano, R. G., and Costanzi, J. J. (1976). *Cancer (Philadelphia)* **37**, 1663–1668.

Goldberg, N. H., Romolo, J. L., Austin, E. H., Drake, J., and Rosenberg, S. A. (1978). *Cancer (Philadelphia)* **41**, 52–55.

Goldie, J. H., Price, L. A., and Harrap, K. R. (1972). *Eur. J. Cancer* **8**, 409–414.

Goldman, I. D. (1971). *Ann.N.Y. Acad. Sci.* **186**, 400–422.

Goldman, I. D., and Fyfe, M. J. (1974). *Mol. Pharmacol.* **10**, 275–282.

Goldman, I. D., Lichenstein, N. S., and Oliverio, V. T. (1968). *J. Biol. Chem.* **243**, 5007–5017.

Gottlieb, J. A., and Serpick, A. A. (1970). *Cancer Res.* **30**, 2132–2138.

Grindly, G. B., and Moran, R. G. (1975). *Cancer Res.* **35**, 1702–1705.

Gutin, P. H., Wiernik, P. H., Green, M. R., Bleyer, W. A., Bauer, V. L., and Walker, M. D. (1976). *Cancer (Philadelphia)* **38**, 1529–1534.

Hansen, H. H., Selawry, O. S., Holland J. F., and McCall, C. B. (1971). *Br. J. Cancer* **25**, 298–305.

Henderson, E. S., Adamson, R. H., and Oliverio, V. T. (1965). *Cancer Res.* **25**, 1018–1024.

Hendin B., DeVivo, D. C., Torack, R., Lell, M. E., Ragab, A. H., and Vietti, T. J. (1974). *Cancer (Philadelphia)* **33**, 468–482.

Howell, S. B. Ensminger, W., Krishan, A., Parker, I., and Frei, E., III (1977). *Proc. Am. Assoc. Cancer Res.* **18** 303.

Howell, S. B., Blair, H. E., Uren, J., and Frei, E., III (1978). *Eur J. Cancer* **14**, 787–792.

Hryniuk, W. M., and Bertino, J. R. (1969). *J. Clin. Invest.* **48**, 2140–2155.

Hryniuk, W. M., Fischer, G. A., and Bertino, J. R. (1969). *Mol. Pharmacol.* **5**, 557–564.

Huennekens, F. M., Vitols, K. S., and Henderson, G. B. (1978). *Adv. Enzymol. Relat. Areas Mol. Biol.* **47**, 313–346.

Huffman, D. H., Wan, S. H., Azarnoff, D. L., and Hoogstraten, B. (1973). *Clin. Pharmacol. Ther.* **14**, 572–579.

Isacoff, W. H., Townsend, C. M., Eilber, F. R., Forster T., Morton, D. L., and Block, J. B. (1976). *Med. Pediatr. Oncol.* **2**, 319–329.

Isacoff, W. H., Morrison, P. F., Aroesty, J., Willis, K. L., Block, J. B., and Lincoln, T. L. (1977). *Cancer Treat. Rep.* **61**, 1665–1674.

Isacoff, W. H., Eilber, F., Tabbarah, H., Klein, P., Dollinger, M., Lemkin, S., Sheehy, P., Cone, L., Rosenbloom, B., Sieger, L., and Block, J. B. (1978). *Cancer Treat. Rep.* **62**, 1295–1304.

Jacobs, S. A., and Santicky, M. J. (1978). *Cancer Treat. Rep.* **62**, 397–399.

Jacobs, S A., Adamson, R. H., Chabner, B. A., Derr, C. J., and Johns, D. G. (1975a). *Biochem. Biophys. Res. Commun.* **63**, 692–698.

Jacobs, S. A., Bleyer, W. A., Chabner, B. A., and Johns, D. G. (1975b). *Lancet* i, 465–466.

Jacobs, S. A., Stoller, R. G., Chabner, B. A., and Johns, D. G. (1976). *J. Clin. Invest.* **57**, 534–538.

Jaffe, N., and Traggis, D. (1975). *Cancer Chemother. Rep., Part 3* **6**, 31–36.

Johns, D., and Bertino, J. R. (1974). *In* "Cancer Medicine" (J. F. Holland and E. Frei, III, eds.), pp. 739–754. Lea & Febiger, Philadelphia, Pennsylvania.

Johns, D. G., Hollingsworth, J. W., Cashmore, A. R., Plenderleith, I. H., and Bertino, J. R. (1964). *J. Clin. Invest.* **43,** 621–629.

Johns, D. G., Spencer, R. P., Chang, P. K., and Bertino, J. R. (1968). *J. Nucl. Med.* **9,** 530–536.

Kay, H. E. M., Knapton, P. J., O'Sullivan, J. P., Wells, D. G., Harris, R. F., Innes, E. M., Stuart, J., Schwartz, F. C. M., and Thompson, E. N. (1972). *Arch. Dis. Child.* **47,** 344–354.

Lanzkowsky, P., Jayabose, S., Shende, A., and Levy, R. (1976). *Am. J. Dis. Child.* **130,** 675.

Leme, P. R., Creaven, P. J., Allen, L. M., and Berman, M. (1975). *Cancer Chemother. Rep.* **59,** 811–817.

Liegler, D. G., Henderson, E. S., Hahn, M. A., and Oliverio, V. (1969). *Clin. Pharmacol. Ther.* **10,** 849–857.

McIntosh, S., Davidson, D. L., O'Brien, T., and Pearson, H. A. (1977). *J. Pediatr.* **90,** 1019–1021.

Mackenzie, A. H. (1975). *Clin. Pharmacol. Ther.* **17,** 239.

Mandel, M. A. (1976). *Plast. Reconstr. Surg.* **57,** 733–737.

Mehta, B. M., Gisolfi, A. L., Hutchison, D. J., Nirenberg, A., Keliek, M. G., and Rosen, G. (1978). *Cancer Treat. Rep* **62,** 345–350.

Mott, M. G., Stevenson, P., and Wood, C. B. S. (1972). *Lancet* **ii,** 656.

Nahas, A., Nixon, P. F., and Bertino, J. R. (1972). *Cancer Res.* **32,** 1416–1421.

Nesbit, M., Krivit, W., Heyn R., and Sharp, P. (1976). *Cancer (Philadelphia)* **37,** 1048–1057.

Norrell, H., Wilson, C. B., Slagel, D. E., and Clark, D. B. (1974). *Cancer (Philadelphia)* **33,** 923–932.

Penta, J. S. (1975). *Cancer Chemother. Rep., Part 3* **6,** 7–12.

Pindedo, H. M., Zaharko, D. S., Bull, J., and Chabner, B. A. (1977). *Cancer Res.* **37,** 445–450.

Pitman, S. W., and Frei, E., III (1976). *Cancer Treat. Rep.* **61,** 695–701.

Pitman, S. W., Parker, L. M., Tattersall, M. H. N., Jaffe, N., and Frei, E., III (1975). *Cancer Chemother. Rep., Part 3* **6,** 43–49.

Podurgiel, B. J., McGill, D. B., Ludwig, J., Taylor, W. F., and Miller, S. D. (1973). *Mayo Clin. Proc.* **48,** 787–792.

Pratt, C. B., Roberts, D., Shanks, E., and Warmath, c. (1975). *Cancer Chemother. Rep.* **6,** 13–18.

Price, R. A., and Jamieson, P. D. (1975). *Cancer (Philadelphia)* **35,** 306–318.

Roenigk, H. H., Berfeld, W. F., St. Jacques, R., Owens, F. J., and Hawk, W. A. (1971). *Arch. Dermatol.* **103,** 250–261.

Rosen, G., Ghavimi, F., Nirenberg, A., Mosende, C., and Mehta, B. (1977). *Cancer Treat. Rep.* **61,** 681–690.

Rubenstein, L. J., Herman, M. M., Long, T. F., and Wilbur, J. R. (1975). *Cancer (Philadelphia)* **35,** 291–305.

Seegar, D. R., Cosulich, D. B., Smith, J. M., Jr., and Hultquist, M. D. (1949). *J. Am. Chem. Soc.* **71,** 1753–1759.

Shapiro, W. R., Cheriuk, N. L., and Posner, J. B. (1973). *Arch. Neurol. (Chicago)* **28,** 96–102.

Shapiro, W. R., Young, D. F., and Mehta, B. M. (1975). *N. Engl. J. Med.* **293,** 161–166.

Sirotnak, F. M., Moccio, D. M., and Dorick, D. H. (1978). *Cancer Res.* **38,** 345–353.

Skipper, H. E., Schabel, F. M., and Lloyd, H. H. (1978). *Semin. Hematol.* **15,** 207–219.

Smith, B. (1975). *J. Neurol., Neurosurg. Psychiat.* **38,** 810–815.

Sostman, H. D., Matthay, R. A., Putman, C. E., and Smith, G. J. W. (1976). *Medicine (Baltimore)* **55,** 371–388.

Stoller, R. G., Jacobs, S. A., Drake, J. C., Lutz, R. J., and Chabner, B. A. (1975). *Cancer Chemother. Rep., Part 3* **6,** 19–24.

Tattersall, M., Jaffe, N., and Frei, E., III (1975). *Symp. M. D. Anderson Hosp. Tumor Inst., 27th, Houston, Tex. pp. 105–116.*

Tattersall, M. H. N., Brown, B., and Frei, E., III (1975a). *Nature (London)* **253**, 198–200.

Tattersall, M. H. N., Parker, I. M., Pitman, S. W., and Frei, E., III (1975b). *Cancer Chemother. Rep.* **6**, 25–29.

Thiersch, J. B. (1962). *Am. J. Obstet. Gynecol.* **63**, 1298–1304.

Valerino, D. M., Johns, D. G., Zaharko, D. S., and Oliverio, V. T. (1972). *Biochem. Pharmacol.* **21**, 821–831.

Wan, S. H., Huffman, D. H., Azarnoff, D. L., Stephans, R., and Hoogstraten, B. (1974). *Cancer Res.* **34**, 3487–3496.

Wang, J. O., Freeman, A. I., and Sinks, L. F. (1976). *Cancer Res.* **36**, 1441–1444.

Wang, Y., Lantin, E., and Sutow, W. W. (1976). *Clin. Chem.* **22**, 1053–1056.

Weinstein, G., Roenigk, H., Maibach, M., Cosmides, J., Halprin, K., and Millard, M. (1973). *Arch. Dermatol.* **108**, 36–42.

Weiss, H. D., Walker, M. D., and Wiernik, P. H. (1974). *N. Engl. J. Med.* **291**, 127–133.

Werkheiser, W. C. (1961). *J. Biol. Chem.* **236**, 888–893.

Whitehead, V. M., Perrault, M. M., and Stelcner, S. (1975). *Cancer Res.* **35**, 2985–2990.

23

CLINICAL PHARMACOLOGY OF NITROSOUREAS

Steven D. Reich

I. INTRODUCTION

The nitrosoureas are a class of compounds with significant antitumor activity in both animal models and in the clinical situation. A broad spectrum of human malignancies including brain tumors, Hodgkin's disease and other lymphomas, multiple myeloma, malignant melanoma, and gastrointestinal neoplasms appear to respond to therapy with certain nitrosoureas (Wasserman *et al.*, 1975; Schein *et al.*, 1974). Nitrosoureas may have limited value against acute lymphoblastic leukemia (Zubrod, 1967; Schein *et al.*, 1974) and in combination with other agents may be effective against small cell carcinoma of the lung (Hansen *et al.*, 1976).

The nitrosoureas are generally classified as alkylating agents, but because of their chemical structure and activity, they are usually considered separate from the classical alkylating agents. The clinical pharmacology of these drugs is difficult to study because of their high degree of reactivity. However, the disposition and metabolic fate of these compounds is important in terms of understanding their mechanism of action.

The clinically important nitrosoureas in the United States include carmustine (BiCNU) and lomustine (CeeNU), which are commercially available, and semustine, streptozotocin, and chlorozotocin, which are under clinical investigation. Other nitrosoureas, such as a derivative containing a ribofuranosyl group, are being studied in Europe (Mathé and van Putten, 1978).

II. MOLECULAR STRUCTURE

The basic structure of the nitrosoureas is a substituted urea with a nitroso group (NO) on one of the urea nitrogens as shown in Table I. The first of the antitumor nitrosoureas to be used clinically was 1-methyl-1-nitrosourea (Schepartz, 1976). However, this compound was replaced by a more stable drug with better animal antitumor activity. The new compound was 1,3-bis(2-chloroethyl)-N-nitrosourea, (BCNU), which was subsequently given the generic name carmus-

TABLE I

Structures of Clinically Important Nitrosoureas

Structure of nitrosoureas

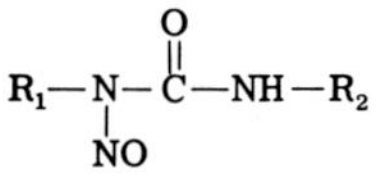

$$R_1 - N - \overset{\overset{\displaystyle O}{\|}}{C} - NH - R_2$$
$$\underset{NO}{|}$$

BCNU

R_1 $ClCH_2CH_2-$
R_2 $-CH_2CH_2Cl$

CCNU

R_1 $ClCH_2CH_2-$

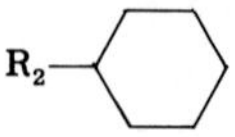

R_2 ⬡

Streptozotocin

R_1 CH_3-

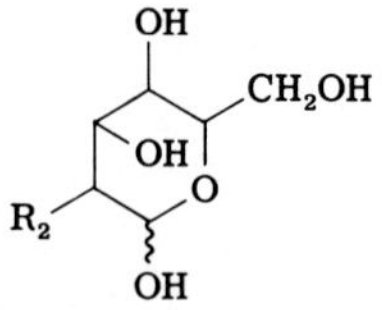

MeCCNU

R_1 $ClCH_2CH_2-$

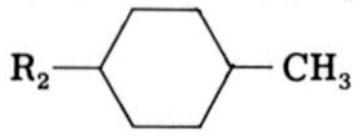

R_2 ⬡ $-CH_3$

Chlorozotocin

R_1 $ClCH_2CH_2-$

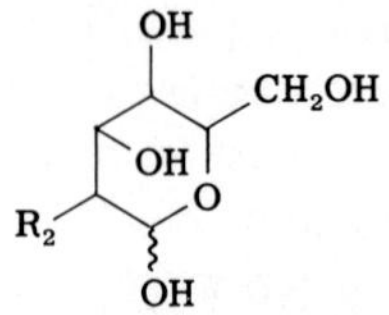

tine. In order to make a more lipid-soluble compound cyclohexyl derivatives were prepared that led to the clinical development of lomustine, 1-(2-chloroethyl)-3-cyclohexyl-1-nitrosourea (CCNU), and of semustine, 1-(2-chloroethyl)-3-(*trans*-4-methylcyclohexyl)-1-nitrosourea (methyl-CCNU). Concurrent with the synthetic work with the nitrosoureas, streptozotocin was isolated from *Streptomyces achromogenes* and characterized as a nitrosourea with a sugar moiety substituted on the 3-nitrogen of methyl nitrosourea (Herr *et al.*, 1967). Chlorozotocin was then synthesized as a chloroethyl derivative of streptozotocin (Johnston *et al.*, 1975a).

The major dose-limiting factor for the administration of BCNU, CCNU, and methyl-CCNU is myelosuppression, which is characteristically delayed. Nadir white blood cell and platelet counts are reached after about 4–6 weeks with 1 or 2 weeks required for recovery. Streptozotocin and chlorozotocin are less myelosuppressive. The mechanism causing this differential in myelosuppression is not known but may involve effects of the sugar moiety.

III. BIOCHEMISTRY AND METABOLISM

Nitrosoureas are capable of alkylation and carbamylation, which means they are able to add alkyl or carbamyl groups to other molecules. Strictly speaking, an alkyl group consists only of carbons and hydrogens linked together by single bonds and a carbamyl group has the following structure: $NH_2(CO)-$. In medical literature, groups with substitutions on the carbon or carbons of an alkyl group and on the nitrogens of a carbamyl group are considered alkyl and carbamyl groups.

The nitrosoureas are chemically unstable in aqueous solutions (Montgomery *et al.*, 1967). BCNU, for example, has a half-life of 305 min in water at 37° and of only 2–3 min in 0.01 N sodium hydroxide solution at 37°. In phosphate-buffered solution at pH 7.2 or in whole blood the half-life is about 1 hour. CCNU is slightly more stable than BCNU in phosphate-buffered solutions at physiologic pH (Panasci *et al.*, 1977b; Montgomery *et al.*, 1967). The nitrosoureas are stable in nonaqueous media at room temperature (Montgomery *et al.*, 1967). Phospholipids, such as phosphatidyl choline, have been shown to maintain the cytotoxicity of CCNU against C-6 glioma cells *in vitro* for longer periods than aqueous media alone (Maker *et al.*, 1978). Phospholipids are present in human plasma and cell membranes, so the interaction of phospholipids with nitrosoureas may affect the cytotoxicity of these drugs in patients.

The aqueous decomposition of the nitrosoureas leads to a variety of reactive chemical species. N-N'-disubstituted nitrosoureas produce an alcohol derived from the groups attached to the nitrosated nitrogen, carbon dioxide, and a symmetric urea, both substituents of which derive from the group attached to the unnitrosated urea nitrogen (Montgomery *et al.*, 1967; Montgomery, 1976). The

N-(2-chloroethyl)-N-nitrosoureas decompose in aqueous solution to yield hydrochloric acid, acetaldehyde, nitrogen, and a primary amine derived from the group attached to the unnitrosated nitrogen (Montgomery, 1976; Montgomery *et al.*, 1975). Possible biologically active moieties resulting from the decomposition of nitrosoureas include carbonium ions and organic isocyanates is shown in Table II (Wheeler, 1975; Colvin *et al.*, 1976; Montgomery, 1976). The specific substituent on the nitrogens of the nitrosoureas determine the mechanism of decomposition of water and the clinical reactivities of the generated entities (Wheeler, 1975).

Metabolism of nitrosoureas has been shown to be mediated by microsomal enzymes (May *et al.*, 1974; Hill *et al.*, 1975; Hilton and Walker, 1975a,b; Johnston *et al.*, 1975b; Reed and May, 1975; Wheeler *et al.*, 1977). BCNU undergoes a denitrosation by microsomal enzymes in the presence of NADPH. Since carbon monoxide only weakly inhibits the reaction, it is probable that cytochrome P-450 is not directly involved in the reaction. CCNU and methyl-CCNU may also be substrates for the denitrosating enzyme, but ring hydroxylation is the more important reaction for these nitrosoureas (Hill *et al.*, 1975). Ring hydroxylation of CCNU and methyl-CCNU occurs rapidly and occurs at a rate faster than that of chemical breakdown (Wheeler *et al.*, 1977). Several isomers have been identified from *in vivo* and *in vitro* experiments with CCNU and the *cis*- and *trans*-4-isomers have been identified in human plasma (Hilton and Walker, 1975a). All the monohydroxy cyclohexyl isomers of CCNU were effective against intracerebrally implanted L1210 leukemia. The half-lives of these isomers were between those of CCNU and chlorozotocin. The 4-isomers had about the same carbamylating activity as parent compound but the 2-isomers were more like chlorozotocin and had low carbamylating activity. The highest alkylating activity was given by the *trans*-2-isomer of CCNU. The biological effects observed following the administration of CCNU and probably methyl-

TABLE II

Possible Biologically Active Moieties Resulting from the Decomposition and Metabolism of BCNU[a]

$$CH_2=CH^+$$
$$ClCH_2CH_2^+$$
$$ClCH_2CH_2OH$$
$$ClCH_2CHO$$
$$ClCH_2CO_2^-$$
$$ClCH_2CH_2N=C=O$$
$$ClCH_2CH_2NH_2$$

[a] From Montgomery (1976).

CCNU are due primarily to the major monohydroxy cyclohexyl metabolites (Wheeler *et al.*, 1977).

IV. CLINICAL PHARMACOLOGY

The rapid degradation and metabolism of the nitrosoureas administered to animals or patients with cancer has made evaluation of the clinical pharmacology of the nitrosoureas difficult. Four major methods have been employed for studying drug concentrations. Radioisotopes of the major nitrosoureas have been synthesized with radioactive atoms in various portions of the molecules (Oliverio, 1973; Mhatre *et al.*, 1978; Adolphe *et al.*, 1975). This allows monitoring the disposition of specific parts of the molecule, but only if a separation technique, such as chromatography, is performed can the disposition of parent drug be determined. Chemical ionization mass spectrometry has been used to quantify BCNU in biological fluids (Weinkam *et al.*, 1978). Chemical methods such as a colorimetric procedure based on decomposition of nitrosoureas to nitrous acid (Loo and Dion, 1965) lack specificity and sensitivity and do not follow parent compound. A biological assay has been developed that measures drug levels by residual antileukemic efficacy in mice (Kline *et al.*, 1968). This method measures antitumor activity but does not give information on the disposition and metabolism of the drug.

Early clinical pharmacological studies on BCNU (DeVita *et al.*, 1967) were done using radiolabeled material with ^{14}C atoms in both chloroethyl groups. Thin-layer chromatography on silica gel G was used to separate parent compound from metabolites. Plasma samples taken as early as 5 min after oral or parenteral administration of BCNU did not contain intact BCNU, although intact drug was found in urine up to one-half hour after drug administration. About two-thirds of the radioactivity was excreted in urine by 96 hr and only less than 1% was recoverable from feces even after oral administration. About 6–10% of drug was exhaled over 24 hr as $^{14}CO_2$. Thirty to forty percent of the isotope could not be accounted for. Plasma half-lives of isotope were 34 hr after oral administration and 67 hr after intravenous administration, which may reflect differences in the distribution of products of degradation and metabolism. Radioactive carbon rapidly entered the cerebrospinal fluid (CSF) of man and equilibrated with plasma radioactivity in about 1 hr. Significant levels of isotope were present after 9 hr.

These early studies demonstrated that BCNU was rapidly degraded or metabolized in man and that portions of the molecule did enter the CSF. However, because both the alkylating and carbamylating portions of the molecule contained radiolabeled chloroethyl groups, no information regarding these reactions was obtained. The presence of radiolabel in the CSF of patients confirmed the finding in animals that the drug rapidly entered the CSF with control of meningeal tumor implants. No information was gained as to why BCNU caused a delayed bone marrow toxicity.

A more recent study (Levin et al., 1977, 1978a) has been performed using selected ion monitoring chemical ionization mass spectroscopy, which gives a sensitive and specific assay for BCNU. This study showed that the rate of chemical decomposition was three times faster in sera than in buffered Ringer's solutions. A heat-labile macromolecule of >25,000 daltons appeared to be responsible for the increase. The lipid content of sera also affected degradation since a meal that produced an elevation of serum triglycerides stabilized BCNU from decomposition in sera. Besides serum concentrations of lipids, body fat was thought to play an important role in BCNU pharmacokinetics and was one of the numerous factors that led to large interpatient variation in BCNU pharmacokinetics. The study confirmed the rapid degradation of BCNU in patients with distribution half-lives on the order of 7 min and terminal half-lives of 4.6 hr. CSF concentrations of BCNU 3 hr after BCNU dosing were about 1 $\mu g/ml$.

The next nitrosourea to enter clinical trials was CCNU. This molecule could be labeled in the chloroethyl, the carbamyl, and the cyclohexyl groups, and so different portions of the molecule could be followed. In animal studies it was found that CCNU had a longer biological half-life than BCNU (Oliverio et al., 1970). CCNU given orally to animals was rapidly degraded and may not have been absorbed as parent compound. The kidneys excreted over 50% oı the metabolites within the first 24 hr. Biliary excretion with reabsorption from the intestinal tract occurred. A significant proportion of the cyclohexyl radioactivity was bound to plasma proteins, but little chloroethyl radioactivity was associated with protein. Levels of radioactivity in the CSF due to the chloroethyl group rapidly exceeded those of plasma and stayed above plasma levels for several hours. Levels of radioactivity in the CSF due to the cyclohexyl group remained below those of plasma. When CCNU was given intravenously, measurable levels of parent compound were obtainable in CSF for about 0.5–1 hr. Plasma CSF and urine levels of radioactivity from CCNU labeled in the chloroethyl or cyclohexyl group after intravenous administration to rhesus monkeys is shown in Fig. 1.

Mice bearing L1210 leukemia cells received CCNU labeled in the cyclohexyl portion and the chloroethyl portion of the molecule. Binding to RNA, DNA, and protein was examined in brain, liver, and tumor tissues and the results are shown in Table III. The alkylating moiety, that is, the chloroethyl group, was found to be bound to RNA, DNA, and protein about equally. The carbamylating moiety was associated to a large degree with the protein of these tissues with little RNA or DNA binding (Cheng et al., 1972).

Pharmacological studies in man using labeled CCNU and methyl-CCNU basically confirmed the animal findings (Sponzo et al., 1973). Both CCNU and methyl-CCNU are rapidly absorbed from the gastrointestinal tract with degrada-

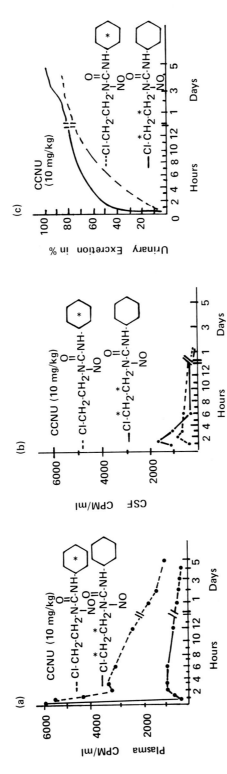

Fig. 1. Levels of radioactivity in rhesus monkeys following a single intravenous injection of 10 mg/kg [ethylene-¹⁴C]CCNU or [cyclohexyl-¹⁴C]CCNU. (Redrawn from Oliverio *et al.*, 1970.) (a) Levels of radioactivity found in plasma. (b) Levels of radioactivity found in CSF. (c) Urinary excretion of radioactivity as a percent of the dose administered.

TABLE III

Binding of Labeled CCNU to Nucleic Acids and Proteins in Tumor-Bearing Mice[a]

Tissue	Radioactivity present (pmoles/mg) in			Radioactivity present (pmoles/mg) in		
	RNA	DNA	Protein	RNA	DNA	Protein
Brain	2.2	–	88.7	17.4		10.4
Liver	0.6	1.1	125.4	18.5	20.6	17.5
Leukemia cells	1.1	9.4	431.6	26.3	26.0	18.5

$$Cl-CH_2-CH_2-N(NO)-\overset{O}{\overset{\|}{C}}-HN-\bigcirc \qquad Cl-CH_2-CH_2-N(NO)-\overset{O}{\overset{\|}{C}}-HN-\bigcirc$$

[a] From Cheng *et al.* (1972).

tion products peaking within 1–6 hr as shown in Fig. 2. Fifty percent of the radioactivity is excreted in urine during the first 24 hr. The entry of degradation products of these drugs into the CSF was prompt and closely paralleled changes in the concurrent plasma levels of radioactivity. No intact drug was found in any body fluid after oral administration.

Individual patients have been studied during surgery for glioma after an oral dose of chloroethyl-^{14}C-labeled CCNU (Walker and Hilton, 1976). In one patient there was prompt absorption with peak radioactivity levels in plasma at 1 hr. At

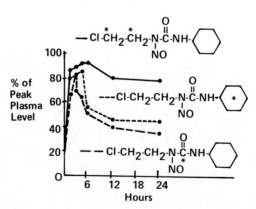

Fig. 2. Average plasma levels of radioactivity after oral CCNU labeled in the cycohexyl, chloroethyl, or carbamyl groups in patients. (Redrawn from Sponzo *et al.*, 1973.)

about 1½ hr both plasma and tumor had comparable concentrations and at 2–2½ hr, concentrations in tumor were greater than those in plasma.

Clinical pharmacological studies of BCNU, CCNU, and methyl-CCNU complemented the studies on the chemistry and mechanism of action of the nitrosoureas. These studies were consistent with rapid degradation and/or metabolism with various disposition of the different reaction products. Drug products, which are active, are able to reach the brain. The carbamylating portion of the molecule binds to plasma proteins and has a half-life consistent with protein metabolism. The radioactivity of the chloroethyl moiety and the carbamyl group appears in expired CO_2, which is consistent with the mechanism of decay determined from the animal experiments.

Animal experiments have delineated two drug–drug interactions involving nitrosoureas, and these interactions may have clinical significance. The effect of phenobarbital pretreatment has been studied in tumor-bearing animals treated with BCNU and CCNU (Muller and Tator, 1978; Levin et al., 1978b). Phenobarbital was studied since it is a microsomal enzyme inducer and nitrosoureas are known to be metabolized by the microsomal enzyme system. The efficacy of the nitrosoureas was significantly decreased in animals pretreated with phenobarbital. However, when phenylethylbiguanide (phenformin) was administered to mice with advanced, subcutaneously implanted, murine L1210 leukemia, an enhancement of the antitumor effect of BCNU was noted (Cohen and Strauss, 1976). The mechanism of this action of phenformin is not known. Since neither of these drug–drug interactions have been studied in patients, the clinical significance of the interactions cannot be assessed.

The clinical pharmacology of streptozotocin has been described (Adolphe et al., 1975). Streptozotocin is nonmyelosuppressive in standard doses, but there were no clues in the distribution, biotransformation, or excretion patterns of the drug as to why the bone marrow is spared. Likewise, pharmacological studies of chlorozotocin in mice were unable to explain why marrow toxicity was decreased compared to the other nitrosoureas. The differential reduction of chlorozotocin toxicity for the normal murine bone marrow could not be explained by the *in vivo* distribution to the marrow since quantitive covalent binding of the chloroethyl group of chlorozotocin was equivalent to that observed for CCNU at an equimolar bone marrow toxic dose (Panasci et al., 1977a). Chlorozotocin will not, however, significantly reduce the DNA synthesis of bone marrow (Schein et al., 1976). At doses of chlorozotocin and BCNU that produce equivalent inhibition of DNA synthesis of L1210 cells *in vivo,* BCNU will suppress bone marrow DNA synthesis to 37% of the control by 24 hr after treatment. These effects could be obtained in an *in vitro* human marrow system as well (Schein et al., 1975).

The clinical pharmacological studies of chlorozotocin complement the animal antitumor data showing this drug has little activity against intracranially implanted L1210 and low concentrations of drug are detected in the brain (Mhatre *et al.*, 1978). This finding is compatible with the drug's relatively high degree of solubility in aqueous solutions.

V. DISCUSSION

In summary, the nitrosoureas represent a group of active antitumor compounds with alkylating activity and some with carbamylating activity. These drugs undergo rapid decomposition and metabolism such that only the first several hours after drug administration are important in terms of the clinical pharmacology of the parent drug The biological half-lives of most metabolites have not been determined. Myelosuppression may be related to the carbamylating activity of the drugs or to the carrier molecule of the nitrosourea, or perhaps to neither of these factors. The reason for the delayed type of myelosuppression after administration of BCNU, CCNU, or methyl-CCNU is also unclear.

Developmental work on the nitrosoureas continues with hundreds of compounds synthesized and several beginning clinical trials (Mathé and van Putten, 1978; Carter and Wasserman, 1976). Perhaps as experience is gained with water-soluble analogues and sugar-modified analogues, structure–activity relationships will become apparent and a nitrosourea with high antitumor activity and minimal toxicity will be designed.

REFERENCES

Adolphe, A. B., Glasofer, E. D., Troetel, W. M., Ziegenfuss, J., Stambaugh, J. E., Weiss, A. J., and Manthei, R. W. (1975). *Cancer Chemother. Rep.* **59**, 547–556.
Carter, S. D., and Wasserman, T. H. (1976). *Cancer Treat. Rep.* **60**, 807–811.
Cheng, C. J., Fukimura, S., Grunberger, D., and Weinstein, I. B. (1972). *Cancer Res.* **32**, 22–27.
Cohen, M. H., and Strauss, B. L. (1976). *Oncology* **33**, 257–259.
Colvin, M., Brundrett, R. B., Cowens, W., Jardine, I., and Ludlum, D. B. (1976). *Biochem. Pharmacol.* **25**, 695–699.
DeVita, V. T., Denham, C., Davidson, J. D., and Oliverio, V. T. (1967). *Clin. Pharmacol. Ther.* **8**, 566–577.
Hansen, H. H., Selawry, O. S., Simon, R., Carr, D. T., Uan Wyk, C. E., Tucker, R. D., and Sealy, R. (1976). *Cancer (Philadelphia)* **38**, 2201–2207.
Herr, R. R., Jahnke, J. K., and Argoudelis, A. D. (1967). *J. Am. Chem. Soc.* **89**, 4808–4809.
Hill, D. L., Kirk, M. C., and Struck, R. F. (1975). *Cancer Res.* **35**, 296–301.
Hilton, J., and Walker, M. D. (1975a). *Proc. Am. Assoc. Cancer Res.* **16**, 103.
Hilton, J., and Walker, M. D. (1975b). *Biochem. Pharmacol.* **24**, 2153–2158.
Johnston, T. P., McCaleb, G. S., and Montgomery, J. A. (1975a). *J. Med. Chem.* **18**, 104–106.
Johnston, T. P., McCaleb, G. S., and Montgomery, J. A. (1975b). *J. Med. Chem.* **18**, 634–637.
Kline, I., Gang, M., Tyrer, D. D., Mantel, N., Venditti, J. M., and Goldin, A. (1968). *Chemotherapy (Basel)* **13**, 28–41.

Levin, V. A., Weinkam, R. J., Hoffman, W., and Wilson, C. B. (1977). *Proc. Am. Assoc. Cancer Res.* **18**, 76.

Levin, V. A., Hoffman, W., and Weinkam, R. J. (1978a). *Cancer Treat. Rep.* **62**, 1305–1312.

Levin, V., Sterans, J., Byrd, A., and Weikam, R. (1978b). *Proc. Int. Congr. Chemother., 10th, Zurich, 1977* **2**, 1164–1165.

Loo, T. L., and Dion, R. L. (1965). *J. Pharm. Sci.* **54**, 809–810.

Maker, H. S., Syed, H. H., and Lehrer, G. M. (1978). *J. Natl. Cancer Inst.* **60**, 1055–1057.

Mathé, G., and van Putten, L. M. (1978). *Cancer Chemother. Pharmacol.* **1**, 5–13.

May, H. E., Boose, R., and Reed, D. J. (1974). *Biochem. Biophys. Res. Commun.* **57**, 426–433.

Mhatre, R. M., Green, D., Panasci, L. C., Fox, P., Woolley, P. V., and Schein, P. S. (1978). *Cancer Treat. Rep.* **62**, 1145–1151.

Montgomery, J. A. (1976). *Cancer Treat. Rep.* **60**, 651–664.

Montgomery, J. A., James, R., McCaleb, G. S., and Johnston, T. P. (1967). *J. Med. Chem.* **10**, 668–674.

Montgomery, J. A., James, R., McCaleb, G. S., Kirk, M. C., and Johnston, T. P. (1975). *J. Med. Chem.* **18**, 568–570.

Muller, P. J., and Tator, C. H. (1978). *J. Can. Sci. Neurol.* p. 349.

Oliverio, V. T. (1973). *Cancer Chemother. Rep., Part 3* **4**, 13–20.

Oliverio, V T., Vietzke, W. M., Williams, M. K., and Adamson, R. H. (1970). *Cancer Res.* **30**, 1330–1337.

Panasci, L. C., Green, D., Nagourney, R., Fox, P., and Schein, P. S. (1977a). *Cancer Res.* **37**, 2615–2618.

Panasci, L. C., Fox, P. A., and Schein, P. S. (1977b). *Cancer Res.* **37**, 3321–3328.

Reed, D. J., and May, H. E. (1975) *Life Sci.* **16**, 1263–1270.

Schein, P. S., O'Connell, J. J., Blom, J., Hubbard, S., Magrath, I. T., Bergevin, P., Wiernik, P. H., Zieglev, J. L., and DeVita, V. T. (1974). *Cancer (Philadelphia)* **34**, 993–1000.

Schein, P. S., Bull, J., McMenamin, M., and Macdonald, J. (1975). *Proc. Am. Assoc. Cancer Res.* **16**, 122.

Schein, P. S., Panasci, L., Woolley, P. V., and Anderson, T. (1976). *Cancer Treat. Rep.* **60**, 801–805.

Schepartz, S. A. (1976). *Cancer Treat. Rep.* **60**, 647–649.

Sponzo, R. W., DeVita, V. T., and Oliverio, V. T. (1973). *Cancer (Philadelphia)* **31**, 1154–1159.

Walker, M. D., and Hilton, J. (1976). *Cancer Treat. Rep.* **60**, 725–728.

Wasserman, T. H., Slavik, M., and Carter, S. K. (1975). *Cancer (Philadelphia)* **36**, 1258–1268.

Weinkam, R. J., Wen, J. H. C., Furst, D. E., and Levin, V. A. (1978). *Clin. Chem.* **24**, 45–49.

Wheeler, G. P. (1975). *In* "Handbook of Experimental Pharmacology: Antineoplastic and Immunosuppressive Agents" (A. C. Sartorelli and D. G. Johns, eds.), Vol. 38, Part 2, pp. 65–84. Springer-Verlag, Berlin and New York.

Wheeler, G. P., Johnston, T. P., Bowdon, B. J., McCaleb, G. S., Hill, D. L., and Montgomery, J. A. (1977) *Biochem. Pharmacol.* **26**, 2331–2336.

Zubrod, C. G. (1967). *Cancer Res.* **27**, Part I, 2557–2560.

INDEX

A

Aclacinomycin A, 126–127, 160, 176
  nucleic acid synthesis inhibition, 238–239
  nucleolar RNA synthesis inhibition, 239–241
  structure–activity relationship, 266
Actinomadura carminata, 159
AD-32, 126, 234
  pharmacokinetics, 119
  pharmacology, molecular, 116, 248–249
AD-41, 234
Adrenalectomy, 192–193
Adriamycin
  activity, animal systems, 256, 258, 261
  activity, clinical
    breast cancer, 121
    gastrointestinal cancer, 125
    genitourinary cancer, 122
    head and neck cancer, 123
    Hodgkin's disease, 120
    leukemia, 120
    lung cancer, 122
    non-Hodgkin's lymphoma, 121
    sarcoma, 122
  chemistry, 112–113
  history, 112, 234–235
  metabolism, 117–118
  pharmacokinetics, 120
    absorption, 117
    distribution, tissue, 117
    plasma clearance, 117
  pharmacology, molecular, 113–116
    nucleic acid synthesis inhibition, 238–239

  toxicity, clinical
    cardiotoxicity, 123–125
    myelosuppression, 123
Adriamycinone, structure, 236
Androgen administration, breast cancer, 194–195
Aklarinone, structure, 236
Alkyl alkane sulfonates, mechanism of alkylation, 292, 293
Alkylating agents, 156–159. *See also* specific types history, 61–63
  mutagenicity, 67
  pharmacology, molecular, 287–301
    cellular resistance, 300–301
    cellular transport, 300
    DNA interaction, 295–299
  toxicity, clinical, 66
Alkylation, 63–65, 288–289
  cellular targets, 295–298
  mitomycin C, 50–52
  nitrosoureas, 39–40
Allopurinol, 17
Alopecia, cyclophosphamide administration, 32
Aminopterin, structure, 313
m-Amsa, 174, 179
  stem cell assay, 216
Anaphylaxis, cisplatinum administration, 149
Anemia
  cisplatinum administration, 149
  methotrexate administration, 368
Anguidine, 165–166, 179
Anthracyclines. *See also* specific types
  activity, clinical, 120–123